Bedside Matters:

The Transformation of Canadian
Nursing, 1900–1990

Kathryn McPherson

UNIVERSITY OF TORONTO PRESS
Toronto   Buffalo   London

Originally published by
© Oxford University Press Canada 1996
© University of Toronto Press Incorporated 2003
Toronto Buffalo London
Printed in Canada

Reprinted 2006

ISBN 0-8020-8679-9 (paper)

Printed on acid-free paper

National Library of Canada Cataloguing in Publication

McPherson, Kathryn M.
Bedside matters : the transformation of Canadian nursing, 1900–1990 /
Kathryn McPherson.

(The Canadian social history series)

Includes bibliographical references and index.
ISBN 0-8020-8679-9
1. Nursing – Canada – History – 20th century.   2. Nurses – Canada –
History – 20th century. I. Title. II. Series.

RT6.A1M36 2003   610.73'0971   C2003-904968-X

University of Toronto Press acknowledges the financial assistance to its publishing program of the Canada Council for the Arts and the Ontario Arts
Council.

University of Toronto Press acknowledges the financial support for its
publishing activities of the Government of Canada through the Book Publishing Industry Development Program (BPIDP)

Contents

List of Tables

Acknowledgements

One of the pleasures of completing a large research project is having the opportunity to formally and publicly thank the people who provided support along the way. While I take full responsibility for all errors and omissions, I also acknowledge the following individuals, collectives, and agencies who facilitated the completion of this manuscript. Research presented here was initiated during my graduate studies at Dalhousie University and Simon Fraser University, where I was privileged to receive supervision from Dr Judith Fingard and Dr Veronica Strong-Boag, respectively. As supervisors they ensured that studying women's history was intellectually challenging and rewarding; they continue to serve as important role models as I make my way through academic life. Greg Kealey, general editor of the Canadian Social History Series, has guided this book through the various phases of revision and publication, generously contributing his time, expertise, and support throughout. Although my formal working relationship with Greg did not begin as soon as initially planned, it was worth the wait. Thanks are also extended to Al Potter for his skilful direction in negotiating through the world of Canadian publishing. Phyllis Wilson and Valerie Ahwee of Oxford University Press kindly expedited the final phases of publication.

I have been fortunate to enjoy ongoing personal and intellectual support from colleagues and friends. Cindy Hahamovitch, Adele Perry, Scott Nelson, and Jay Cassell read drafts of chapters and spent many hours with me hashing over the problems and contradictions of writing social history. Nick Rogers kept reminding me to 'get it done', advice that was sound, if not always graciously received. At a critical point in the publication process, Linda Peake took time away from her own research to copy-edit this manuscript. Meryn Stuart was always willing to listen to ideas, suggest references, and generally keep me connected to developments in nursing and nursing scholarship. And Gina Feldberg has been a faithful ally, providing her careful reading of the manuscript and her critical insights into the history of women and medicine. The academic and scholarly assistance these people contributed were accompanied by large doses of humour and friendship needed to help me juggle teaching, writing, and life in Toronto. Thanks are also due to John Lutz for his thoughtful commentary on research presented in Chapter 5. I have appreciated the intellectual support provided by members of the Margaret Allemang Centre for the History of Nursing and the Toronto Labour Studies Group. Bettina Bradbury, Julie Guard, Craig Heron, Franca Iacovetta, Lynne Marks, Ian Radforth, Robert Storey, Eric Tucker, and Rob Ventresca have been especially generous about sharing their ideas with me. I am grateful to copy-editor Richard Tallman and the anonymous reviewers who, in the final phases of preparing this manuscript, identified useful points of clarification and correction.

I have been fortunate to receive research funding from the following: the Association of Canadian Studies Writing Award, York University Faculty of Arts Research Leave Fellowship, York University Faculty of Arts Research Grant, and the Social Sciences and Humanities Research Council Small Research Grant. That funding allowed me to employ the stellar services of research assistants Virginia McKendry, James Moran, Tracy Shannon, and, most importantly, Lisa Ann Chilton, whose diligence ensured that all the final details were completed. Special thanks are extended to the many archivists across Canada who assisted me, especially the volunteer archivists at nursing association archives for graciously donating their time and knowledge in my search for documentation of nurses' daily lives. I am particularly indebted to the many nurses, both practising and retired, who opened their homes to me, sharing memories and mementoes of the history they have lived. They will not all concur with the conclusions presented here, but I know we share a commitment to recognizing the contributions nurses have made to Canadian society, past and present.

Final thanks belong to my family. Ed Ratz has helped me keep together body and soul, his good cooking and good conversation a constant reminder that nurturing is not the exclusive domain of women. My parents, Margaret and Murray McPherson, have provided unfailing intellectual and emotional support for all my pursuits. Throughout my life they have shared their joy of learning and their commitment to quality education. I hope that I may be as good a parent to my own children, Ella Margaret and Dominik Angus McPherson Ratz. Their arrival (in the last phases of completing this manuscript) has made our lives richer and full of delight. To them I dedicate this book.

1

Gender, Class, and Ethnicity: Reconceptualizing the History of Nursing

In the history of women's work, nursing holds a special place. It is an occupation that embodies the seemingly universal characteristics of feminine healing, caring, and nurturing. The very word 'nurse' evokes the maternal caring we often assume to be central to human existence, and to women's lives. Yet, however long the tradition of women's ministrations to the sick, this archetypally female vocation also has a distinctive history of change. Once the responsibility of informally trained family, friends, servants, or members of religious orders, nursing was transformed in the late nineteenth century from unpaid care to wage labour. In the industrial societies of Europe and North America the occupation came to be the means of subsistence for many women, usually strangers to the patient but formally trained and certified in the curative practices of scientific medicine.

In its modern form, nursing has captured the imagination of a wide range of social commentators. For historians, the transformation of nursing has produced charismatic individuals worthy of scholarly study; individuals such as Florence Nightingale, Edith Cavell, and Sister Kenny have loomed large in international historiography.[1] For the creators and consumers of popular culture, the image of the modern nurse has spawned characters as diverse as Charles Dickens's 'Sarah Gamp' and Ken Kesey's 'Big Nurse', within genres ranging from adolescent literature and Harlequin romance novels to pornography.[2] For artists, nursing has provided powerful feminine imagery as expressed in painting, sculpture, and photography.[3] For 'first wave' feminists, nursing promised a separate sphere in which women could attain financial and personal independence. For contemporary enthusiasts of their family histories, nearly every family can boast of at least one nurse whose adventures inspired oft-repeated tales of humour, drama, and romance.[4]

For women needing and wanting work, nursing has offered relatively decent wages, a non-industrial work environment, public respect, geographic mobility, and, in the modern economy, the option of leaving and rejoining the paid work-force without substantial penalty. It has also been hard work, demanding specific skills, physical strength, emotional resilience, and intellectual acumen. Of course, to say that nursing is, and has been, hard work would come as no surprise to nurses themselves. What is surprising, however, is the infrequency with which historians of nursing have considered the occupation as labour. Historians have examined nursing's educational, legislative, administrative, and organizational pasts, and have explored the vocational calling and professional ethos that inspired the individuals who made their names and careers in the nursing field. Yet few scholars have analysed systematically the fact that for thousands of Canadian women (and some men) in the twentieth century, nursing was in the first instance a means to economic survival. It was work.

One of the reasons for this historiographic trajectory is that much nursing history has been written from within the occupation, by nurses themselves. This is by no means a flaw. Unlike other women's occupations, nursing has been blessed with a tradition of historical writing and with generations of historically conscious and literate women who have struggled to ensure the preservation of primary and secondary source material. This internalist approach has meant that nurse-historians have written for an audience that was well aware of the daily practice of nurses, for whom the actual work was not only self-evident but sometimes shameful.[5] Instead, the activities of the *un*ordinary nurses commanded historical fascination. Dissecting and analysing the work that nurses performed on the job seemed not only unnecessary but unimportant compared to the critical task of celebrating and directing professional achievements and strategies.

This study, then, seeks to re-examine nursing's past by using the tools of social history to probe the everyday lives of 'ordinary' nurses at work. In doing so, this study locates the social history of nursing at the juncture of three related bodies of scholarly literature, those of labour, women's, and medical history. Out of labour history come questions about the labour process, about conditions of work, about attitudes and responses of nurses to their jobs, about the strategies nurses invoked to improve the conditions of their labour, and about how power and resources were allocated and contested at the workplace. At a broader level, labour history provides a framework for considering how working nurses fit within the evolving class structures of twentieth-century Canada. Women's history reminds us that gender played an equally significant role in shaping nurses' lives. Whether focusing on work, sexuality, family, education, or politics, feminist scholarship offers models for understanding the shifting roles and expectations that defined appropriate femininity. This study begins with the premise that nursing was but one employment option from which women had to choose. Thus we must consider working women's shifting occupational options, their changing needs and goals, and the varying social contexts in which they worked. Only then can we understand who became nurses, what they did at the bedside, what features of the job appealed to its members, and why women left nursing. Nursing has remained a largely feminine occupation and female pursuit, but the meaning of sex-segmentation must be explored within specific historical contexts. In pursuing these questions, this study offers a much needed critical analysis of one of the most popular occupational choices for women in this century.

Placing nurses' experiences within the history of medicine is equally important. The medical and political contexts in which nurses worked fundamentally influenced their collective history. Conversely, as the largest patient-care work-force in this century's health-care system, nurses played influential parts in defining that system, but to date few researchers in the field of health-care history have integrated nurses into their narratives. Even the growing influence of the social history of medicine has not substantially increased the historical attention paid to nurses, and, when nurses are considered, they are portrayed as recipients or victims of change, not agents or actors.[6] By focusing on the experiences of nurses, this study explores these links among nursing, scientific medicine, and the political economy of health during a century in which the medical system was undergoing tremendous change. Thus, before proceeding with a discussion of how best to interpret nursing's past, it is first necessary to provide a brief overview of the transformation of nursing and medical care in the modern era.

The Transformation of the Canadian Medical System

Conventional wisdom posits the mid- to late nineteenth century as the formative period when modern medicine was conceived in the Western world. In emerging urban-industrial societies, scientific discoveries such as the germ theory, the reorganization of medical professions, the establishment of state-sponsored public health agencies, and the decline of traditional causes of mortality combined, in differing proportions depending on which author you read, to constitute the modern era of health and health-care services. Within this era, the content and structure of medical care was further revised. In Canada, as elsewhere, the medical system of the 1870–1940 period was significantly different from that of the post-World War II years.

During the 1870–1940 era, patients and their families paid—with cash, with produce, on instalment, or, occasionally, through private insurance plans—for medical and institutional services. If payment could not be arranged, patients had to convince health authorities or private practitioners that charitable attendance was deserved. However reimbursed, most medical care continued to be delivered in patients' homes, although institutions in the years before World War I were attracting increasing numbers of patients from all social classes. Unlike the indigent and incurables who inhabited the pre-modern hospital, the new clientele of the modern hospital expected to be discharged in better, rather than worse, health. Whether in home or hospital, physicians and surgeons promised scientific treatment that included new therapeutics, such as interventionist surgical and obstetrical techniques, while relying on more traditional therapies such as extended periods of rest or the application of fomentations and poultices. Over time, greater numbers of private practitioners sought out hospital facilities to perform the new medical procedures that institutional staffing and equipment permitted.[7] Private and public hospitals for general and specialized care grew in size and number during the last decades of the nineteenth century and the early decades of the twentieth, while parallel developments in mental health led to the establishment of asylums in all provinces to cope with what appeared to be growing numbers of Canadians with mental ailments.[8] The increased popularity of institutional services did not, however, alter the economic structure of the 'fee-for-service' model that characterized the private system, nor did the division of labour change.

Like doctors, most trained or 'graduate' nurses—nurses who had successfully completed a three-year hospital training program—worked for private patients. Engaged for a few days, weeks, or months, the nurse either offered individual care in the patient's home or provided supplementary attendance 'specialing' in private or semi-private hospital rooms. Hired by the patient and under the authority of the doctor, the graduate nurse assisted the medical practitioner with his procedures and, after his departure, stayed on with the patient to carry out the prescribed course of treatment. Not all nurses worked in private care. A very small group of graduates who had acquired extra training could get work with private or government-funded public health organizations or with large companies in industrial nursing.[9] As well, a growing number of positions instructing and supervising the work of student staff were available to graduate nurses in hospitals and in their schools of nursing. By the late 1930s some institutions, particularly small rural hospitals, were hiring graduate nurses to perform direct patient care. Most hospitals, however, relied on the labour of student nurses who apprenticed for three years on the wards in return for formal training and certification. Within this apprenticeship system of staffing and of nursing education, junior, intermediate, and senior student nurses were assigned the numerous tasks involved in patient care and ward maintenance as they advanced up the hierarchy of hospital training. For hospital patients, only the daily encounters with the small staff of male physicians, interns, and orderlies broke the rhythm of female patient care provided by apprenticing students and their graduate supervisors. Thus, in hospital and home care alike, the growing repertoire of therapeutics that constituted patient care was differentiated into medical functions and nursing tasks: the principal division within the health-care work-force was between doctors and nurses, men and women.

In the 1940s, the Canadian health-care system, and nurses' place within it, underwent a fundamental transformation. During and after World War II, public funding for medical institutions increased substantially, as the federal government in particular began considering health a legitimate area for state involvement. Capital grants for hospital construction offered struggling institutions the dollars necessary to expand the size and scope of their community service, which itself increased as new scientific and medical treatments created new patient demands. Recognizing that few patients could afford medical care, insurance companies began to grow, only to be marginalized in 1968 when federal Medicare consolidated health insurance in Canada as a public, rather than private, venture. Even then, doctors and physicians maintained their commitment to private practice. Thus, while access to state-subsidized institutional facilities was critical for doctors, particularly specialists, the Canadian medical profession successfully defended the fee-for-service structure of medical practice, although the 'fee' now came from the state, not from private patients and their families.

By contrast, few nurses supported themselves through private practice in the years after 1942. Rather, most graduate or registered nurses (RNs), whether college, university, or hospital-educated, were paid hourly wages by third-party hospitals, homes, or agencies. Stabilized funding of medical institutions created new demands on and for nursing personnel. The proliferation of highly technological, specialized medical and surgical interventions prompted doctors to relinquish responsibility for certain tasks, such as taking blood pressures and starting intravenous drips. RNs assumed these functions, which in turn intensified the pressure on institutions to guarantee a steady supply of skilled nursing personnel. This demand was met, in part, by the growing numbers of married women who continued to work while also running households and raising families. Labour supply was also secured in other ways. Subsidiary personnel such as ward aides, practical nurses, and nursing assistants were introduced to take responsibility for the many less technological aspects of patient care that RNs had previously performed. As a result, in the contemporary system nurses are but one of many groups of workers in attendance at the bedside and they thus define and defend their position in the work-force relative to practitioners with less formal training, as well as to doctors. Defending interests has meant developing new organizational strategies, foremost among them unions. The older provincial and national professional organizations, which dominated nurses' associational life in the pre-1940 era, continued to oversee licensing and education in the post-war era, while unions have assumed the tasks of improving nurses' working conditions and wages.

Interpreting Nursing's Past

The transformation of the Canadian health-care system, and of nurses' place within it, was not a unique phenomenon. Comparable processes—including the ascent of medical control, the evolution of hospitals from charitable and custodial institutions to socially respectable and therapeutic ones, the growing intervention of the state in health services, and the reformation of skilled nursing—have occurred, with important variations in timing and detail, in most Western nations.[10] Similarities have also emerged in the historical interpretations of nursing's changing face. In the scholarly literature of England, Europe, the United States, Australia, New Zealand, and South Africa, three analytical approaches or frameworks have dominated scholarly writing of nursing history.

The traditional interpretation, which has influenced much of the scholarship generated within nursing itself, addresses the process of professionalization, with particular emphasis on the struggle for professional legitimation and status. Early historians of nursing self-consciously contributed to the professionalizing efforts of their peers by celebrating the noble antecedents of modern nursing.[11] In recent years, authors working within the professionalism paradigm have focused more specifically on twentieth-century efforts to achieve the twin goals of improved educational standards and self-regulation through legislative licensing. Much of this historical writing assessed the contributions of individuals, associations, or events, often identifying key moments when professional status was cemented.[12]

Defining the term 'professional' has inspired substantial scholarly debate. Early theorists emphasized the distinct body of knowledge that delineated professionals from other workers, but more recent scholarship has pointed to the social authority and workplace autonomy that have proved critical determinants of true professional standing.[13] Given this more stringent definition, not all scholars are convinced that professionalization has been a complete or successful process for nursing. Numerous studies have assessed the difficulties nurses faced trying to secure one of the cornerstones of professional status, university education.[14] Recognizing that nursing never achieved completely the self-regulation and workplace autonomy that characterized other professions such as medicine, authors have labelled nursing a 'semi-profession', a 'second-class profession', and a 'dependent profession'.[15] Mary Kinnear's 1995 study, *In Subordination: Professional Women, 1870–1970*, maintained that professionalism remains a useful concept if its gendered dimensions are addressed. Kinnear included nursing as one of the five Manitoba professions she analysed, all of which, she claimed, permitted women 'professional' workplace autonomy, even if female members of those occupations did not enjoy the same privileges or social status as their male peers.[16] Other authors have refined their use of professionalism even further. British scholar Celia Davies acknowledged the theoretical and definitional conundrum that the concept of professionalization has created for historians and concluded that 'as a general concept "professionalization" may confuse more than it clarifies.'[17] Instead, Davies employed the terms 'professional ideology' and 'professionalizing strategy' to signify a particular set of goals and ambitions held by nursing élites. However modified the model, professionalization remains a central preoccupation for many historians and the question of whether nursing has achieved professional status now appears central to any historiographic or introductory essay.[18]

While the debate over professionalism continues, other researchers have turned to a very different paradigm to explain the trajectory of nursing history. This constitutes the second analytic model, that of proletarianization, in which nursing history is conceptualized not as a steady march towards professional stature, but rather as a tale of the inexorable intrusion of capital and industrial modes of production into the realms of service work. The concept of proletarianization is used to describe the conditions of a centralized workplace, rationalization of the work process, the intensification of the pace of work, and the rigid, hierarchical division of labour of 'assembly-line' and factory production, which some authors believed characterized nursing work in the post-World War II era. Within this framework, early twentieth-century nurses were likened to independent producers, sometimes artisans, who, as the twentieth century progressed, were drawn into institutional wage labour.[19] In the process, nursing was 'stripped of its independence from wage labour'.[20] As David Wagner argued:

> In the late 1930s, when hospitals called private duty nurses to accept temporary staff assignments, they threatened resistant nurses with cutting them off the lists of nurses, never again to receive referrals from the hospital or affiliated physicians. Many nurses complained that they were being blackmailed: either become a staff nurse or starve? The process of creating a labor force in nursing was analogous to driving the peasantry off the land in 18th and 19th century England to accept factory work.[21]

The introduction of Marxian categories into nursing history has been extremely important for helping shift research focus away from the minority élite to consider the less vocal majority. This approach has raised questions about authority, power, and control and has introduced dissent and conflict into nursing history.

At the same time that the proletarianization paradigm was being applied to nursing history, other scholars were arguing that a gender, rather than class, analysis best explains the subordination of nurses. In recent years, feminist analyses have begun influencing nursing scholarship, as authors writing from within the occupation, but also from within women's studies, emphasized the continuities of oppression that have characterized nursing history. Authors have concluded that for all the changes nurses have witnessed, the sustained subordination of nurses is best characterized by persisting patriarchy. According to this interpretive framework, in the early twentieth century the male medical establishment exploited the labour and the talents of skilled young women and in the later twentieth century male administrators and legislators, along with doctors, continue to deny nurses the workplace authority or financial remuneration commensurate with nurses' critical role in patient services. This analysis was articulated most vehemently by Ehrenreich and English, whose *Witches, Midwives, and Nurses* analysed nursing in the context of the long-standing 'suppression of female healers by the medical establishment'.[22] While that text received much scholarly criticism, the essence of the argument has resonated through various subsequent publications.[23] Recent Canadian nursing textbooks, such as Baumgart and Larsen's *Canadian Nursing Faces the Future*, now characterize gender as equally important as professionalism in defining nursing work.[24]

Each of these three interpretive frameworks has contributed significantly to our understanding of nursing's past. Professionalism has played a critical role in directing the strategies devised by the organizational élite, as well as in defining working nurses' ethics and the devotion they brought to the bedside. It is also true that the proletarianizing tendencies inherent in hospital employment, such as rationalization of production, exposed nurses to similar forces affecting industrial workers. As well, there is no denying that gender asymmetry has been a persistent influence not only on the structure of the health-care system but also on educational opportunities, job choices, and workplace experiences of the women who become nurses.

Yet these are, to a large extent, competing paradigms that assert mutually exclusive patterns of change and elucidate only part of nursing's complex history. The professionalization paradigm, with its emphasis on the education system and the leadership élite, cannot account for the ongoing subordination of working nurses. The proletarianization framework overstates the autonomy of nurses working within the private health-care market, underestimates the relative privilege of nurses compared to other health-care personnel, and inadequately explains the fragile relationship between nurses and other workers. The emphasis on persisting patriarchy, meanwhile, fails to analyse substantial changes within the occupation, the historical exclusion of non-White women, and ongoing tensions between nursing and feminism. Thus, if each analytic approach contributes something to our understanding of nursing's past, none alone is satisfactory.

Rather than embrace any of these explanatory frameworks entirely, this study argues that nurses occupied a particular position, one simultaneously defined by class and by gender and further complicated by racial/national/ethnic considerations. The mutual, if not always equal, influences of class, gender, and ethnicity need to be considered together in order to explain nurses' position within the health-care system and to understand nurses' strategies to improve that position. Such an approach emphasizes the positions that nurses have occupied in relation to men, to other women, to other workers, and to other ethnic groups. Nurses were simultaneously defined by their subordination to medical men and health service administrators and by their superior status compared to unskilled working women, by their greater opportunities than those of immigrant or non-White Canadians, by their restricted opportunities for work or personal safety compared to working-class men, and by their ambivalent position with respect to patients. These sets of relational positions have not been fixed; the relative influences of class, gender, and ethnic relations have played out in historically specific conditions.

A small number of authors have attempted to map out the particular contours of class, gender, and ethnic relations. Barbara Melosh's 1982 study, 'The Physician's Hand': Work Culture and Conflict in American Nursing, emphasized the divergent approaches to collective action that American nurses embraced and argued that rank-and-file practitioners developed a 'work-culture' distinct from the professional ethos endorsed by nursing's élite. Melosh challenged the current nursing leadership to learn from the past and develop a less exclusive strategy for change that places nurses' interests in line with those of other working-class caregivers, rather than with doctors.[25] Susan Reverby's 1987 publication, Ordered to Care: The Dilemma of American Nursing, 1850–1945, although somewhat more sympathetic to nursing leaders' difficulties in finding an alternate mode of valuing nursing care, concurred with Melosh's general assessment of professionalism's failure to serve nurses' needs. Examining 'the failure of our society to create the conditions under which the desire to care can be valued', Reverby insisted that 'nurses, whatever else can be charged against them, continuously try to meet their obligations to care', but that achieving a basis for political unity, professional or otherwise, was fractured by 'patriarchal constraints from above and differences among women from within'.[26]

For Darlene Clark Hine, author of Black Women in White: Racial Conflict and Cooperation in the Nursing Profession 1890–1950 (1989), differences among American women included significant racial and class barriers that divided élite White leaders from Black practitioners. In particular, Black nurses' continued reliance on private duty work, long after hospital employment became the norm for White nurses, perpetuated 'the deep-seated identification of black women with domestic servitude [which] exacerbated the difficulties black nurses encountered in trying to win acceptance and integration into a status-starved and prestige-hungry profession.'[27] African-American women shared with their European-American sisters gender, which made nursing an appropriate occupational choice, and class, which positioned nurses as a subordinate labour force, but they were fundamentally divided from each other by racial difference and racism.[28]

Shula Marks's 1994 study, *Divided Sisterhood: Race, Class and Gender in the South African Nursing Profession*, builds on Hine's work to analyse the ethnic and class tensions among the British, Afrikaner, and African women who trained as nurses in nineteenth- and twentieth-century South Africa. By considering the political economies of nursing under colonialism, apartheid, and democracy, Marks explores how national, racial, and sexual ideologies intersected to shape who became a nurse and how those women organized politically. Like the American scholars, Marks views professionalism as a strategy with the potential to divide as much as unite.[29]

Canadian scholarship has been less extensive but equally significant. The pioneering work of Judi Coburn provided one of the earliest critiques of professionalism.[30] Although based on limited research, her conclusion that the combined ideologies of professionalism and femininity served to maintain the subordinate position of nursing personnel none the less signalled a promising new direction for Canadian nursing history.[31] The contradictions of professionalism and gender were also raised in Suzann Buckley's 1979 'Ladies or Midwives? Efforts to Reduce Infant and Maternal Mortality', in which the author also challenged nurses' professionalism but for different reasons. Documenting health reformers' unsuccessful attempts in the post-World War I years to decrease maternal mortality by importing British-trained midwives to the poorly serviced Canadian Northwest, Buckley revealed that Canadian nurses, or at least the Canadian Nurses' Association, joined the Canadian Medical Association in resisting the scheme. She asserted that 'despite [nurses'] professed concern for prairie women, other factors, especially professional needs, were more important.'[32] Buckley concluded that nurses' much applauded dedication to service ended when their own professional exclusivity was threatened. While Coburn and Buckley focused on the contradictions of gender and professionalism, Canadian sociologist David Coburn has explored the interplay of professionalism and proletarianization. Arguing that the proletarianization process within Canadian nursing has been retarded by the professionalizing efforts of practitioners and leaders, Coburn characterized proletarianization as an unfinished process, which nurses might successfully resist, but that differences among nurses have created 'formidable obstacles' that threaten to fragment the occupation.[33]

This study will build on these works by focusing on how class, gender, and ethnicity interacted to influence the historical conditions of nursing in Canada. To introduce the relative and changing significance of each of these three sets of social relations, some discussion of how each operated on nursing is first required.

Class, Gender, and Race in Canadian Nursing

One of the most powerful and pervasive features of both historical analysis and popular opinion has been that nurses are, or were, middle class. This is rooted in the long-standing belief that since the nineteenth century, nursing has been an attractive and appropriate occupation for the (redundant) daughters of the bourgeoisie. Martha Vicinus reproduced this claim in her *Independent Women.*[34] Pauline Jardine's 'An Urban Middle-Class Calling: Women and the Emergence of Modern Nursing Education at the Toronto General Hospital 1881–1914' is based on a similar premise.[35] To test these assertions, a number of objective and subjective measures of class could be applied. One would be to identify the occupations of nurses' fathers and/or husbands to determine whether nurses came from middle-class families or married middle-class men. The available evidence pertaining to male heads of households is fragmentary, but the existing documentation indicates that Canadian nurses hailed from a range of family backgrounds—middle class, working class, and agricultural. And, contrary to popular opinion, nurses did not all marry doctors—given that the nursing work-force more than doubled its medical equivalent, this was numerically impossible. Neither did they view nursing as a path of upward mobility through marriage. Nurses who did marry chose husbands with jobs ranging from farmers and manual labourers to white-collar workers and businessmen. Many other nurses did not marry.

Measuring nurses' class by means of the occupation of fathers or husbands is flawed not only for the paucity of empirical data, but also for conceptual reasons. Using male heads of households as an indicator of status implies that class for women is determined in the household, ancillary to production, and not in the sphere of production itself, thereby discounting the experience of class on the job. If we take seriously the Marxian premise that class is defined by one's relationship to the process of production, then measuring status only or entirely in familial terms ignores nurses' workplace experiences. Those theorists who focus on relations of production emphasize two defining elements of class positions: (1) autonomy over or ownership of production and (2) control over the labour process or division of labour.[36] By these objective measures, most nurses do not qualify as middle class or professional because of the dominant position occupied by doctors and health administrators.

In the late nineteenth century the medical profession, seeking to re-establish itself within the medical marketplace, gained legislative authority to define what constituted 'practising medicine'. Since then, control over the distribution of health and medical services has rested with the medical profession, which has ensured that the right to conceptualize and direct patient services—that is, the right to diagnose and prescribe—has remained exclusively a medical prerogative. Occupying the pinnacle of the health-care hierarchy, the medical profession has served as final arbiter in what constitutes legitimate or appropriate medical therapy by using two powerful social forces, science and the law. Scientific experimentation validated the efficacy and assessed the danger of particular medical interventions. The legal system was invoked to prosecute or persecute practitioners, be they within the profession or, more frequently, outside of it, who deviated from scientifically legitimized therapies. Indeed, medical dominance within health care has been so complete that the medical profession is often held up, by academics and aspiring occupational groups alike, as the prototype of successful professionalization.[37]

The ascent of the medical profession was premised, in part, on the creation of a corps of assistants—nurses—who would be both loyal and skilled. Doctors depended on the presence of nurses at the bedside to assist with initial medical treatment, execute subsequent tasks, and monitor patients' progress. If most nurses, labouring at the bedside, were subordinate to the doctor and his directives, they were subordinated precisely because they were skilled. Those skills placed nurses in a privileged position compared to other levels of workers within the health-care hierarchy, over whom nurses sometimes had authority. In the early decades of the century, nurses might have delegated cleaning, cooking, or laundry tasks to domestic workers in the patient's household, whereas institutional nurses might have called on the assistance of the small staffs of orderlies to clean, restrain, or move patients, especially males. In recent decades, hospital nurses have gained the authority to delegate tasks to cleaners, aides, and practical nurses. Throughout, those ancillary personnel have represented competition for nurses and, like skilled workers in industry, nurses have struggled to preserve their jobs in the face of less-skilled, or at least less-trained, and cheaper attendants. In the private market of the early twentieth century, nurses had to distinguish themselves from domestic servants and from informally trained 'nurses', whether neighbours, family members, or practical nurses, who also sought sustenance from health-care work. In the modern era RNs have struggled to maintain their position in the health-care system against threats, explicit or implicit, to replace them with practical nurses and aides. At specific historical moments nurses' alliance with medical practitioners was in part a strategy to preserve an élite, if still subordinate, position at the bedside.

From this perspective, nurses' structural position appears more like that of skilled workers or tradesmen than of professionals, but these similarities have not translated into the subjective conditions of class. Until very recently, nurses rarely demonstrated consistent working-class consciousness as defined by traditional members of the proletariat, such as steelworkers or teamsters. Nurses have been relatively late in organizing, slow to support more broadly based trade union actions and activities, and often hesitant to strike. Within the occupation, a significant number of practitioners remain sceptical or even hostile to unionization.

An important reason for this tangential or marginal relationship to the working class lies in the conditions of service provision. Traditionally, service work has been difficult to organize, but nursing has been especially hard because nurses' relationship to their product is and was a human one. It was much less likely that a worker would feel alienated from a human being who was dependent on her/him than to feel alienated from the product of assembly-line production. However alienated from control over production nurses might have felt, the material and human reality of caring for a dependent human being may have muted or compensated for that alienation. Moreover, at those moments when the human rewards of helping the sick and infirm did not outweigh the frustration and alienation of nurses' position in the production process, using the weapons of working-class resistance, such as the strike, held very different ramifications for nurses than for other workers. Withdrawing labour on the assembly line meant production of goods stopped for a time. Withdrawing labour in the restaurant meant that customers did not get their meals. For nurses, withdrawing labour might mean death or further injury to another human being and, humanity aside, the social and legal ramifications of such action were therefore far greater. Thus, militant action has held very different implications for nurses than for other workers, while the conditions of alienation that provoke militant action have been mitigated by the nature of human service provision.

If the product of nurses' labour is animate, the product is also the consumer. The patient and her/his family constitute another social force in the relations of production that does not exist in industrial production. In the private health-care system of the early twentieth century, patients bought the nurses' service and thus occupied for the duration of the nurses' tenure the position of both consumer and employer. Under health insurance, the state or private company officially paid for nurses' services, but patients and their families still recognized that 'their' tax dollars and government revenues financed health-care work. Thus, whether in the early twentieth-century private system or in the late twentieth-century publicly financed one, patient care has been complicated by consumer demand. Bedside attendants have had to negotiate with family members who often served as patient advocates, invoking personal and family histories in efforts to influence the course of treatment. The social relations of production are thus significantly complicated by the presence of an animate product. For nurses, this has meant that 'class relations' at the bedside have not easily been translated into oppositional positions of managers and workers, doctors and nurses. Family members at times proved a greater source of conflict than doctors, especially if the family members refused to pay the nurse's fee, insisted on hiring non-nurse competition, or lodged a complaint about the nurse's behaviour.

Even if a particular nurse, or group of nurses, did feel alienated from their work, consciousness of that alienation might not take the form of class consciousness. The hierarchical division of labour was as much the product of gender asymmetry as it was of unequal class relations. The uneven relations of production, based on a division of labour and authority, were premised on and reinforced by the hierarchy of gender. Most trained nurses in twentieth-century Canada have been female; however, not just any woman would do. Nursing has been defined by particular feminine paradigms, and nursing educators laboured to ensure that new recruits conformed to these codes of gender-specific behaviour. The dominant feminine paradigm has been a familial one, in which graduate nurses assumed a subordinate wifely position relative to the male doctor and a maternal position relative to the dependent patient. Apprenticing nurses were placed in a filial role, as daughters of the doctor/nurse parental team, apprenticing within the hospital much as domestic servants laboured as daughters of middle-class households. If doctors assumed authority, it was an authority based both on control of ownership of production—as head of the health-care team—and on masculine control over domestic life—as head of the household. At the same time, the personal service tasks demanded in patient care were deemed natural for women to execute. Gender defined and naturalized both the masculine authority of doctors and the social and sexual appropriateness of female nurses.

Bourgeois gentility was endorsed by administrators and nurses alike because gender relations at the bedside were complicated and contradictory. The familial model placed nurses in a figurative (and sometimes literal) heterosexual position *vis-à-vis* doctors. (One suspects that the doctor's sexual respectability depended on the presence of the nurse, who could not only bear witness to the doctor's sexual propriety but could symbolically neutralize the doctor's male sexuality much as the presence of a wife made a man sexually safe, or 'taken'.) But, as genteel women, nurses had to desexualize themselves in order to distance themselves from the only other group of women with intimate knowledge of strangers' bodies—prostitutes. At the same time, nurses lived and worked in the world of an almost exclusively female occupation in which bonds between women were accepted and encouraged. Yet when nurses forged intimate relationships with other women, the norms of compulsory heterosexuality that continued to define nursing's position within the health-care hierarchy served to marginalize or make invisible homoerotic relations. Women and men who pursued careers in nursing negotiated these contradictory demands in different ways at different times, but the example of nursing reveals some of the ways in which 'gender' encompassed more than just sex-typing, but also was informed by sexuality. Nurses' uniforms, seen by many commentators as symbols of oppression and subordination, have for most nurses in this century represented non-sexual femininity that legitimized their place in the work-force, on the streets, and at the bedside.

The politics of class and gender were interwoven in a particular pattern to construct the terrain upon which nurses worked and struggled. Hierarchical relations of production, wherein doctors retained control over conceptualization and organization of medical knowledge and practice, defined nurses in a subordinate position within the modern health-care system. This hierarchy was premised on and reinforced by gender asymmetry. Trained and graduate nurses were introduced into the health-care hierarchy because the sex-segmented work-force ensured that women constituted a cheaper source of labour, but also because feminine respectability would ensure elevated status for modern medical and institutional health services. Significantly, however, the subordinate positions of nurses relative to doctors occurred at the same time that the skilled training of nurses placed them within the élite of women workers. These objective conditions combined to create particular subjective conditions in which nurses interpreted their position as a skilled élite and celebrated their particular definition of femininity as a way both to gain social legitimacy and to distinguish themselves from other women.

The process whereby nurses protected their élite position was not, however, a function of class and gender alone. It was also informed by the social relations of race, ethnicity, and nativity. For most of the twentieth century, nursing in Canada has been the preserve of White and Canadian-born women. As the century progressed the occupation became more ethnically heterogeneous, but the nativist and racist hierarchy remained firmly in place, as newly arrived immigrants and non-White citizens were excluded by virtue of language skills, educational qualifications, or racism. Nursing's racial and cultural exclusivity was not merely the innocent by-product of objective standards or cultural difference; rather, it was promoted by the nursing profession and health-care administrators.

Because nursing relied on an image of feminine respectability to legitimate nurses' presence in the health-care system and their knowledge of the body, respectability was constructed in a racial and national context. Nurses' respectability and definition of gentility were European in origin. White, native-born Canadian women were expected to bring their superior sense of sexual and social behaviour to the bedside, either to act appropriately while caring for their social 'equals' or 'superiors' in private care or to serve as role models for their social 'inferiors', such as immigrants and non-Whites. Visible minorities were not trusted to attend the needs of ailing White Canadians, and until the post-World War II years administrators remained convinced that the very presence of non-White attendants might exacerbate the health problems of White patients. In the eyes of hospital administrators and nursing leaders, Canadian women of non-European heritage could not be relied on to reflect the morality of health at the bedside, to meet the standard of gentility demanded by élite patients, or to negotiate the tricky sexual terrain of patient care. Because vocational calling was embedded in nationalist ideals, 'minority' women were encouraged to pursue nursing only to serve 'their' communities.

Emphasis on the ethnic and racial superiority of nurses reinforced nurses' real or perceived status as an élite among the occupational choices for working women. Although the educational and social criteria for entrance to practice limited access to the occupation for the daughters of unskilled or even semi-skilled workers, nursing never achieved the middle-class composition that some commentators believed. Yet regardless of their class background, the young women who were admitted to training programs were expected to conform to an élite vision of sexual feminine respectability, as defined by European and bourgeois standards, at the same time watching over patients who might be non-English or French-speaking unskilled immigrants. Relations at the bedside of such patients were thus constructed by the labour process, which divided tasks among doctors and nurses, but also by the social relations of ethnicity and gender.   Nursing in Canada may never achieve full professional status, and it has been subordinated by the sexual division of labour and by its relationship to production. But nurses have been privileged by skill, sexual respectability, and racial and ethnic exclusivity. As such, this study argues that within a sex-segmented labour market, nurses were skilled workers positioned at the apex of the occupational hierarchy for women. Neither fully professional nor part of a male-dominated proletariat, the social relations of class, gender, and ethnicity combined to create a distinctive position for nurses.

Five Generations of Trained Nurses

The following chapters explore how these social relations informed the work and lives of the women who trained and worked as graduate nurses in Canada. To capture the specific sets of circumstances that influenced nurses' work, this study proposes that since 1874, when the first training program for nurses was established in Canada, five generations of trained nurses have plied their trade. The first generation, the small cadre of nurses who graduated between 1875 and 1899, pioneered trained nursing in Canada. In the last decades of the nineteenth century they were introduced into hospital wards and then into the community, where they co-existed with and eventually supplanted the untrained domestic caregivers who served as 'nurses' in the pre-modern health-care system. To understand the experiences of the pioneering generation of trained nurses, they must be studied within the context of the nineteenth-century sick room, ward, or institution and in relation to the pre-modern bedside attendants. Such an analysis demands a careful piecing together of the fragmentary documentary evidence pertaining to the health-care services in the diverse regions of nineteenth-century Canada, which constitutes an entire research project beyond the scope of this study. For this reason, although Chapter 2 provides a brief discussion of the first generation of Canadian nurses, the story of nineteenth-century nursing care awaits its own full-length study.

Rather, the story here begins in 1900 with the second generation of Canadian nurses, when the value of trained nursing assistance had been established to the medical profession, to government agencies, and to many sectors of the public. The era of expansion enjoyed by second-generation practitioners contrasted sharply with the crisis conditions confronted by the third generation, trained in hospital apprenticeship programs during the 1920–41 years. After two decades of oversupply and underemployment, World War II sharply inverted the economic and structural basis of work for Canadian nurses. The fourth generation, born into the health-care system of the 1942–67 era, experienced dramatic growth in hospital services and a concomitant demand for more nurses. Federal financing of health insurance, the 1968 program popularly known as Medicare, created the specific context in which the fifth generation of Canadian nurses created new collective vehicles, unions, to defend their interests as workers and as women.

The concept of generation is useful to capture the specific sets of political and economic conditions that have defined nurses' experiences in the health-care system. Beginning with the late nineteenth-century establishment of hospital training schools, the political economy of Canadian health-care conditions substantially changed every 20–5 years, creating a new generation with a unique set of experiences and attitudes. As with biological generations, distinctions between one experiential generation and another are somewhat artificial. Individuals do not always fall neatly into a single category and generations co-exist and overlap. Still, the concept helps to identify chronologically the changes within nursing over the past century and facilitates the analysis of how generations intersected to mediate change. Within the apprenticeship training system, older nurses were responsible not only for teaching students the content of nursing work but also for serving as positive role models of working women. As students graduated from hospital programs, the many nursing organizations served as vehicles through which experienced nurses could initiate new practitioners into the work-force. The occupation's self-conscious élite even sponsored the writing and publication of nursing histories designed to record for future generations the struggles and successes of previous generations. Unlike any other female-dominated occupation, the interaction between generations of nurses—between the experiences of veterans and the expectations of novices—has structured women's initiation into the job of caring and has influenced nurses' understanding of their occupational identity.

The following chapters are organized so as to explore the conditions specific to each generation of nurses and to investigate cross-generational continuities and change. Chapter 2 addresses the second generation of Canadian nurses, trained in the first two decades of this century during an era of hospital expansion and organizational formation. Chapter 3 explores the content of nursing work as it developed over the second and third generations, with specific attention paid to nurses' relationship to science. Chapter 4 focuses on the economic crisis that plagued the third generation of nurses of the inter-war years and considers the ramifications of the demise of private duty and the ascent of hospital-based general duty. Chapter 5 returns to intergenerational issues, examining shifting formulations of femininity as developed for and by nurses between 1920 and 1967. Chapter 6 analyses the structural changes that hospital-based employment wrought upon nursing's fourth generation following World War II and the internal conflicts those structural changes produced. The concluding chapter offers some observations on how the shifting relations of class, gender, and ethnicity have shaped the fifth generation of Canadian nurses in the era of Medicare.

Because this study spans nearly a century and focuses on a nation characterized by diversity, several points of clarification are required. The first pertains to which practitioners qualify as nurses. Over the course of the twentieth century various terms have been used to differentiate informally trained or untrained practitioners from graduates of recognized nursing training programs. In the early twentieth century 'trained' nurses struggled to distinguish themselves not only from untrained competition but also from those women who boasted some training, however limited. The term 'graduate' nurse thus emerged to categorize those practitioners who had successfully completed a three-year apprenticeship. By 1922 nursing organizations in all provinces had achieved legislative definition of the 'registered nurse', a status that still informs nurses' place in the health-care hierarchy. While most graduates of the pre-World War II years chose to gain RN status, not all did. Thus, while the terms 'registered nurses' and 'graduate nurses' are used here interchangeably to establish the parameters of the work-force under study, it is important to note that it was not until the 1940s and 1950s that almost all training school graduates qualified for the legally defined 'registered' status.

The Bachelor of Science in Nursing (B.Sc.N.) title is of little relevance to this study. Acquiring an undergraduate degree as a Bachelor of Science in Nursing has been possible since 1919, when the University of British Columbia initiated Canada's first university degree program in nursing. Until recently, however, university programs were few in number and trained only a small percentage of the nursing work-force. Throughout the twentieth century, RN credentials have remained the mandatory entry to practice, and it has only been in recent years that B.Sc. degrees in nursing have been a prerequisite for specific nursing positions or a meaningful subcategory for defining the nursing work-force. As such, the specific experiences of university-trained nurses do not receive analysis here.

By contrast, distinctions between RNS and registered nursing assistants (RNAS), licensed practical nurses (LPNS), and ward aides are critical. During and after World War II, these subsidiary workers were introduced into Canadian hospitals and assumed many functions previously assigned to apprenticing and graduate nurses. In spite of this commonality of work content, RNAS, LPNS, and other health-care workers have had distinctive histories and traditions, and therefore must be considered separately from RNS. For these reasons the graduate or registered nurse will be the focus of this study, and the experiences of ancillary patient-care personnel will only be considered where relevant to the larger tradition of graduate nurses. So, too, the history of psychiatric nurses, with their distinctive work-force composition and history, is excluded from discussion here.[38] This is not an attempt to privilege the general nurse over other kinds of health-care workers or to create a universal 'nursing history' out of the experiences of one group of workers, however large that group may have been.[39] Rather, this study is structured out of deference for the specific experiences of different groups of nurses and out of recognition of the need for further detailed studies of practitioners such as psychiatric nurses.[40] Public health nurses will be considered more extensively, even though they, too, were a particular subset of the occupation. Public health nurses were required to have post-graduate training, enjoyed significantly more on-the-job autonomy than did other nurses, and, for these reasons, were held up within the occupation as the model of all that nursing could and should be. The number of historical studies on public health nursing, far out of proportion to public health nurses' numerical presence in the work-force, speaks to the symbolic importance that this subset of nursing has represented. Instead of adding to the historical genre that separates public health nursing from other nursing, this study will incorporate that minority experience where relevant. I argue that while public health nurses enjoyed relatively more autonomy and higher wages than did their counterparts in private duty or hospital work, public health nurses shared with other nurses structural constraints and a theoretical basis of work.[41]

A further clarification pertains to the history of nursing in Quebec, which at times fits only partially the model presented here. In that province, Church and State combined to create a system of social services significantly different from that developed elsewhere in Canada. The Quebec Public Charities Act of 1921 rearticulated the historic importance of religious social service work and ensured the Catholic Church's continued dominance as provider of Quebec's institutional health services.[42] In the mid-nineteenth century the number of female orders began to increase, and the number of nuns continued to expand until the 1950s, nearly doubling between 1921 and 1941 alone.[43] Female religious orders provided a pool of skilled administrators for Catholic hospitals, a fact that influenced dramatically the options and experiences of all Quebec nurses. On the one hand, administrative positions were reserved for nuns and thus, relative to their peers elsewhere, laywomen enjoyed limited occupational advancement in Quebec's health-care hierarchy. On the other hand, those nuns who did receive administrative postings in Quebec hospitals were not subordinate to male medical superintendents and thus enjoyed relatively greater authority and autonomy than Protestant or lay nursing administrators.

For all these differences, important similarities between the histories of Quebec nurses and other Canadian nurses do exist. Like hospitals elsewhere, those in Quebec relied on the labours of laywomen apprenticing in their schools of nursing.[44] During the inter-war years, French-speaking nurses did develop a separate organizational forum and publication, but both French- and English-speaking Quebec nurses remained active within their provincial body and the national association.[45] In addition, since World War II, Quebec nurses have unionized to confront workplace issues in a pattern similar to that of other Canadian nurses, and in some instances Quebec nurses preceded or initiated the national trend.[46] Feminist researchers currently investigating the unique circumstances of nursing history in Quebec may conclude that the experiences of Quebecois nurses were so distinctive that their history must be considered separately from that of English-Canadian practitioners.[47] The evidence to date, however, suggests that on many questions the differences do not outweigh the commonalities.

Incorporating Quebec nursing history also serves as a necessary reminder of the significant role played by religious organizations in the development of health services throughout Canada. Catholic, Jewish, Mennonite, Salvation Army, and United Church congregations all engaged in the provision of Canadian hospital and medical services. Like Catholic nuns, the women who occupied administrative and nursing positions within private, religious institutions and organizations sometimes wielded administrative and medical authority that surpassed that of their peers in public, secular hospitals.[48] As well, even at 'lay' hospitals, Christian rituals were made part of student nurses' daily routine.[49] In spite of this, religious influence on social services outside Quebec remains an underdeveloped area of the historical scholarship, in part because of the limited availability of primary documentation. Primary source material from privately administered institutions has less frequently been deposited in public archives and is only now being made available to historians. None the less, segregating Quebec history because of the significance of Catholicism's influence there only serves to marginalize further the religious influences on nursing in the other provinces.

A similar caveat regarding the experiences of minority nurses is also needed. As the following chapters reveal, nursing in twentieth-century Canada has been defined by the ethnic and racial composition of its work-force. It has been an occupation comprised predominantly of women who were White, Canadian-born, English or French-speaking, and of northern European descent. This composition has contributed to nursing's élite status relative to other women's occupations, especially domestic service, but has also shaped the place of minority women in nursing. Further studies of how individuals from ethnic and racial minorities experienced life as student and graduate nurses are needed before we can understand fully the importance of nursing for those individuals and the meaning of 'whiteness' for the occupation. Agnes Calliste's analysis of Caribbean-trained nurses in Canada provides an important model for pursuing these questions.[50] The paucity of nursing-generated primary documentation relating to those minority women who were successful or unsuccessful in their efforts to earn a place in the occupation suggests that researchers will have to consult non-nursing records or conduct extensive oral interviews in order to probe the many influences of ethnic and racial difference on nursing. The analysis of ethnic and racial categorization presented here constitutes only a first step in a much larger scholarly project.

The question of sources has proven a thorny one for historians of nursing everywhere. There are, of course, national sources like the Canadian Nurses' Association records, journals like *Canadian Nurse* (*CN*) and *La Garde-Malade*, as well as published primary sources such as autobiographical accounts. But to study relations at the bedside, sources that document specific workplaces and local health-care economies are required. For this reason, this work combines national and published source material with primary evidence pertaining to three Canadian cities, Halifax, Winnipeg, and Vancouver. As regional centres for the Maritimes, Prairies, and west coast, they were representative of urban health-care systems, in terms of both their substantial medical services and their roles as metropolises for the surrounding rural districts. These particular cities were also selected because of the primary source material available in local archives. The alumnae associations for Halifax's Victoria General Hospital, the Winnipeg General Hospital, and the Vancouver General Hospital were especially active in acquiring and preserving documentation pertaining to their Alma Maters and their local nursing communities and, despite their limited volunteer personnel, in making their archival collections available to outside researchers like myself. School of nursing records, student yearbooks, nursing manuals, student lecture notes and diaries, alumnae minutes and newsletters, nursing association registry lists and minutes, hospital committee reports, and public health nursing documents were available, to varying degrees, in hospital alumnae rooms, associational offices, and the provincial archives of Nova Scotia, Manitoba, and British Columbia. Because sources pertaining to nurses are dispersed among so many institutions and because the Nova Scotia, Manitoba, and British Columbia records were the most easily accessible during the research phases of this project, detailed research into Halifax, Winnipeg, and Vancouver will be presented to substantiate the themes and changes examined in this study, while evidence pertaining to nurses elsewhere will be incorporated when available.

The experiences of 'ordinary' nurses are central to this study, but the names of those women are not. To protect the privacy of individuals whose names appear in 'private' primary sources, such as educational and employment records, pseudonyms have been used. Any similarity between the pseudonym and the original, beyond approximate ethnic background, is coincidental. The names of individuals in the public domain have not been changed. This includes individuals who penned public documents, such as *CN* articles or annual reports, who consented to oral interviews, or who served in official institutional positions, including hospital superintendents, superintendents of nursing, and officers of nursing organizations.

Even with the energies of volunteer archivists, documentation on various features of nurses' work proved hard to locate. Chronic pressure on Canadian hospitals has forced many institutions to destroy old personnel records; constant crises of employment and organizing have forced many nursing associations to focus on nursing's future, not its past; and the more generalized devaluing of women's work has prompted many families to throw out 'mother's old nursing things'. To answer questions about which the documentary evidence was silent I turned, as many social and women's historians have done in recent years, to oral history. My approach to interviewing retired nurses was neither systematic nor representative. While I did try to consult graduates of various classes and institutions, the pressures to interview elderly nurses while their health was good and the reality that not every retired nurse was willing or available to retell her past inevitably skewed my 'sample'.

These limitations aside, the process of consulting retired nurses about their work proved invaluable. Their recollections of daily life on the wards, in homes, and on the streets provided rich descriptions of the work nurses performed and of the human relationships they negotiated. Evocative as these accounts were, the interview material has not merely served to illustrate larger points. Rather, the disjuncture between their own understanding of their history and that of the existing scholarly interpretations led me to re-examine the documentary evidence. Reading it in conjunction with the interview material crystallized the significance of nursing as women's work. Retired nurses, whether living in the eastern, western, or central regions of Canada, were consistent in valuing their patient-care skills and valuing the direct patient care they performed. As the current generation of Canadian nurses confronts further restructuring of health-care work, their foremothers' belief that what happens at the bedside matters stands as both challenge and affirmation.

2

Nursing Classes:
The Second Generation of
Trained Nurses, 1900–1920

In 1901, the superintendent of the Nova Scotia Hospital took advantage of his institution's annual report to applaud the work of its nursing training program. He informed his readers that the school 'has done a great deal towards bettering the condition of our patients and improving their prospects of recovery. The pupils of the school have devoted themselves to their trying and difficult work with a degree of enthusiasm and unselfishness which is deserving of the highest praise and commendation.'[1] The benefits accrued to Nova Scotia's mental health facility were not unique. In the first two decades of the twentieth century, hospital administrators and doctors across the nation came to appreciate the attributes of trained nurses, making the years 1900–20 ones of dramatic change for Canadian nursing. From the small work-force of less than 300 at the turn of the century, the number of student and graduate nurses, almost all women, had surpassed the 20,000 mark by the end of World War I.[2] As the numbers boasting hospital training grew, so, too, did public recognition of the value of trained nursing attendance rise. The heroic efforts of Canadian practitioners in World War I, the 1917 Halifax explosion, and the influenza epidemic of 1917–18 cemented nurses' position as legitimate members of the modern health-care team.

This chapter explores this dynamic second generation of trained nurses, examining the apprenticeship system of hospital staffing and education, the world of graduate nurses, and the organizational structures created in this era. Together, these three elements of nursing life forged a distinctive occupational identity that drew nurses together in spite of the significant differences of rank and experience that separated them. Because the structures of education, work, and collective activity that developed in the the 1900–20 era continued to influence the direction of nursing throughout much of the twentieth century, the second generation of nurses, while meaningful in its own right, is an important point of departure for understanding subsequent historical changes. Before turning our attention to the early twentieth century, however, it is first necessary to consider briefly the nineteenth-century origins of Canada's trained nursing work-force.

From Charwoman to Trained Nurse

The trained nurse stepped onto the Canadian health-care stage in the last decades of the nineteenth century when hospitals joined their American and European counterparts in the radical restructuring of institutional staffing. Hospitals moved to eliminate the old-style nurses, those working-class women who had informally acquired skills, who might be married or widowed, who sometimes lived in the hospital, who provided patients with at least rudimentary bedside care, and who often provided doctors with skilled medical assistance. In their place, hospital administrators introduced student nurses, single women who laboured for two (and later three) years on the wards in exchange for training and certification as 'graduate' nurses. Institutions such as Mack's General and Marine Hospital in St Catharines, Ontario, and the Montreal General recruited 'Nightingale' nurses from London to supervise nursing staffs and to establish hospital training schools. Mack's 1874 opening earned it the title of Canada's first nursing program. Over the next quarter-century, 24 other institutions followed suit, including the Winnipeg General in 1887, Halifax's Victoria General in 1890, Victoria's Royal Jubilee in 1891, and, under the auspices of the Sisters of St Joseph, Toronto's St Michael's Hospital in 1892. The graduates of these programs constituted Canada's first generation of trained nurses.

To twentieth-century observers, trained nurses and the apprentices they supervised appeared an obvious improvement over the working-class domestics who preceded them. In fact, much of what we know about the old-style attendants comes from supporters of the modern nurse who used Dickens's fictional representation of Sarah Gamp—the slovenly, drunken night-watcher presented in *Martin Chuzzlewit*—to signify progress within the occupation.[3] Sir William Osler was one such advocate of change who in 1913 regaled the Johns Hopkins Nurses' Training School alumnae with tales of his student days at the Montreal General. Describing the 'old-time nurses' on staff there in 1868, Osler claimed:

They were generally ward servants who had evolved from the
kitchen or from the backstairs into the wards. . . . Many of them
were of the old type so well described by Dickens, and there are
some of the senior medical men present who remember the
misery that was necessary in connection with that old-fashioned
type nurse.[4]

Much of the 'misery' caused by the old-style nurses was due to drink.
Halifax physician and historian Dr H.L. Scammell echoed Osler's
(and Dickens's) analysis when, in his mid-twentieth-century
manuscript, he described the Victoria General's pre-1877 nursing
staff: 'One of the common causes for the discharge of domestic
servants in Halifax at that time was drunkenness, and not infrequently
these sought and secured employment at the Hospital where they
continued to indulge as often as possible.'[5]

Such unflattering portraits were accurate to a point. Many nineteenth-century nurses were domestics or charwomen who supple-
mented their earnings elsewhere with hospital wages. As members of
working-class communities, they shared cultural values and standards with the indigent or lower working-class patients rather than
with élite doctors and philanthropic administrators. Given working-
class attitudes towards drink, the widespread use of alcohol as a
painkiller, a sedative, and a nutrient, and the horrors of pre-modern
medical treatment witnessed by hospital staff, it was not unusual that
the old-style nurses would indulge in spirits or even appropriate that
prescribed for their patients. But it was also true that untrained
nurses' experience in domestic service often translated into significant skill in attending the sick. Even Osler acknowledged that many
Montreal General nurses, who were 'Dickensian' in looks, were 'in
behaviour, in devotion and in capability equal to the best I have ever
met'. The myth of the pre-modern Sarah Gamp breaks down further
when the nuns who tended patients in Catholic hospitals are factored
in. Those caregivers were often highly skilled, possessed substantial
experience, and enjoyed significant societal respect.[6]

If old-style nurses were a more diverse and skilled group than
twentieth-century observers believed, the difficulties nineteenth-century hospital administrators faced trying to introduce trained nurses
demonstrated that the newly conceived apprenticeship system was
not without problems. In 1875 the Montreal General engaged Maria
Machin, a graduate of the famous English hospital St Thomas's and
friend of Florence Nightingale, to oversee the creation of its nursing
school, but by 1878 conflict over finances between Machin and the

medical board forced Machin's resignation.[7] Further efforts to organize a nursing training program failed until 1890 when Nora Living-
stone, a Canadian-born graduate of the New York Hospital Training
School, permanently established the Montreal General program.
Even after such difficulties were overcome, enrolments in fledgling
programs were small, often numbering as few as three.[8] Thus
throughout the nineteenth century, institutions with and without training schools continued to rely on the labours of ward maids, domestic
servants, matrons, and male attendants to provide patient and ward
care. As late as 1893, the Vancouver Trades and Labor Council complained that while the nursing care during the day at the City Hospital
(later Vancouver General) was excellent, the attendance at night was
insufficient, 'there being but one man to look after 3 wards and that
individual is accustomed to get the worse for liquor and go to sleep'.[9]
In domestic health services, the continued contribution of old-style
nurses was even more pronounced as informally trained nurses
served their local communities, providing home care to the acutely
ill, to accident victims, and to post-partum women.[10] Not until the
close of the century was it apparent that hospital-trained attendants
would dominant the nursing field.

'The Growing Necessities of the Hospital'[11]

By 1900, hospital administrators and medical practitioners throughout North America agreed that the experiment of hospital-trained
nurses had proven a success. In the first two decades of the twentieth
century, institutions across Canada, recognizing the value that nursing
schools had brought to hospitals like Winnipeg General and Halifax's
Victoria General, began establishing their own nursing training programs, hiring members of the first generation of hospital graduates to
oversee the education of the second generation. This expansion of the
apprenticeship system of institutional staffing was part of the larger
process whereby hospitals consolidated their position as respectable,
therapeutically effective sites of medical treatment, while simultaneously coping with increased patient demand. Whether the rising
popularity of hospital care was a function of changes within urban
landscapes, proven confidence in the efficacy of institutional and
medical services, or the machinations of the medical profession bent
on consolidating its élite status has yet to be established by historians
studying the various regions of Canada.[12] Whichever analysis is
emphasized, all agree that the growth in the number of patients and
services was accompanied by the establishment of schools of nursing

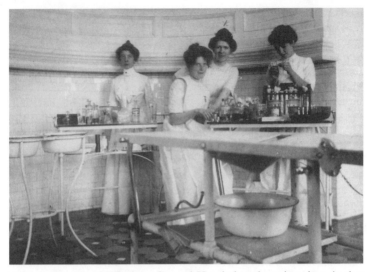

This photograph of Winnipeg General Hospital students is unique in that most images of nurses working in operating theatres were formal poses used to promote the institutional surgical services that hospitals offered. One of the students is Ethel Johns (marked with an X over her head), the Winnipeg General Hospital graduate who went on to become an internationally renowned nursing leader (PAM Winnipeg General Hospital Collection #191).

and a subsequent increase in the number of students admitted. By 1909, 70 hospital schools provided apprenticeship labour to patients, the majority of which required three years of training. By the 1920s, over 200 hospitals relied on the apprenticeship system of staffing.[13]

Young women wishing to pursue a career as trained or graduate nurses began their journey into the ranks by applying to one or more of the available hospital schools, either in their community or, more frequently, in a regional urban centre. If the applicant met the school's requirements of age, education, health, and character, she entered the institution on probationary status. And if, after three months, the 'probie' was deemed suitable, the young apprentice continued on, completing her first year as a 'junior' nurse. A successful first year was marked with the capping ceremony, after which the student continued on to intermediate and then senior nurse status. Apprentices were on duty six and a half days per week and were allowed to take two or three weeks holiday yearly, usually during the summer months when patient demand for hospital services waned. Any days missed due to sickness were noted and had to be made up at the end of year three before graduate status would be conferred. Apprenticing nurses were required to live in hospital residences and conform to the many rules and regulations, whether on or off duty. This apprenticeship system remained the dominant system of staffing Canadian hospitals until the 1940s and persisted as the basis of nursing education until the 1970s.

The apprenticeship system offered Canadian hospitals a number of advantages. The first was volume. Institutions could meet increased patient demand simply by accepting greater numbers of students. At Vancouver General Hospital, for example, the first graduating class, which completed the three-year course in 1901, consisted of three students. By 1920, the graduating class numbered 49, bringing the total number of alumnae for the 1901–20 era to 378.[14] The 25 students and 5 graduate nurses who staffed the wards of Vancouver General in 1905 were responsible for 50 beds. By 1920 the hospital expected 196 student nurses and graduate staff of 45 to service up to 1,200 patients daily.[15] A similar pattern emerged at hospitals elsewhere in the nation. To keep up with demand for patient services, hospitals increased the apprenticeship staff as much as financial and residential resources would permit.

Equally significant was the skill that apprenticing nurses provided. By their intermediate and senior years, students had acquired substantial experience in patient care. Not only were they able to perform most nursing tasks without direct supervision, they could be assigned alone to night-duty shifts and could assume supervisory roles themselves. However unpopular the assignment, senior nurses had a substantial amount of time invested in their training and were unlikely to resign. Hospitals therefore acquired not only skilled but also reliable attendants, who were tied to the hospital for the duration of their training. Student labour also promised a certain flexibility of staffing. Apprentices were expected to rotate through the various wards to gain experience in a range of cases, but the actual amount of time each student spent on each ward could be adjusted as patient load and staffing needs dictated.

Institutions benefited from this skilled and reliable labour at a minimal cost, which helped hospital administrators in their relentless pursuit of fiscal health. Hospital superintendents and volunteer boards of directors struggled to make ends meet on revenues generated from patient fees, government grants, and charitable donations, while facing fixed costs of food, fuel, and supplies. One area in which administrators could economize was salaries and wages. At most institutions, nursing students were granted a monthly stipend of $8, $10, or $12, according to the level of apprenticeship. These financial benefits to institutions were enhanced when hospitals hired out nursing students to perform private-duty service. As the by-laws and regulations of the Victoria General in Halifax explained, 'when they can be spared' pupil nurses could be sent out to different parts of the province to do private nursing. Patient fees were paid directly to the hospital, with no extra wage granted to the nurses on the premise that 'the monthly payments and the instruction afforded in the hospital [are] deemed a full equivalent for the nurses' time'.[16] Annual reports and other hospital publications notified the community of this service. The North Winnipeg Hospital advertised in 1920 that 'the nurses on the staff visit homes; rates maternity cases $10; ordinary visits 50 cents.'[17]

If apprenticing nurses appealed to administrators' sense of economy, they also appealed to medical and lay expectations that servants of the hospital would demonstrate the deference and discipline befitting a subordinate work-force. Deferring to one's superiors was learned early on the job. Probationers entered the hospital at the bottom of the nursing hierarchy, subordinate to juniors, who in turn looked up to intermediates, who deferred to senior students. Seniors were expected to comply with the directives of supervisory graduate nurses, who themselves answered to the superintendent of nursing. Deference extended well beyond merely following orders to include physical demonstrations of differential rank. Nurses were instructed that, when in the presence of more senior nursing staff or any medical practitioners, they were to stand up 'at attention', surrender their place on elevators, and allow superiors to walk ahead.[18] Students remained at each station for a limited amount of time, graduating up and out of the hospital hierarchy over the course of three years.

Hospital administrators insisted that successful apprenticeship programs instruct aspiring nurses to adhere to the rules of the institution and to suppress any desire to challenge or question those rules. In 1901 the superintendent of Halifax's Victoria General reminded his community of the important role 'that peculiar qualification which is known as "tact"' played in good nursing.

> Worst of all are those who are self-opinionated and presumptuous. From all such, any training school may well ask to be delivered. . . . The training which does not ensure that intelligent subordination to the rules, duty and authority which gives the necessary discipline in the wards and effectiveness to the service is not calculated to produce the best results in this important branch of hospital service.[19]

'Intelligent subordination to the rules' applied to all facets of student life. A strict schedule prevailed in the nurses' home. Students had to rise at 6 a.m. and be in their own rooms by 10 p.m., after which no bathing, visiting, or loud noises were permitted. One night per week students were granted late leave until 11:30 and once a month theatre leave extended late leave until midnight. 'Callers' could be received at the home until 9:45 p.m., but students required special permission to entertain patients or ex-patients, and students who had been dismissed from the school were not welcome at any time. Each morning the students had to make their beds and tidy their rooms. Rooms, 'including closets, desks and drawers', had to be 'ready for inspection at all times' and any articles of clothing left lying around the room would be collected and removed by the housekeeping staff. Bathtubs and washrooms had to be cleaned after each use. Moreover, at mealtimes, students were to arrive on time and were not 'allowed to go to the kitchen and give orders to the servants'. Laundry services were provided by the hospital, but only included washing of a specified number of 'plainly made underwear and uniforms' per week. A resident disregarding these rules would 'forfeit the privilege of having her clothes laundered'.[20]

Hospital regulations extended to student behaviour well outside institutional walls. Permission was required to spend the night away from the hospital. Students were allowed to wear their uniforms to the local stores immediately surrounding the hospital, but otherwise were forbidden to wear hospital dress when not on duty. When off duty, students were not allowed on the wards without permission. When on duty they were forbidden to entertain friends. Nurses were also responsible for observing any and all rules posted on the residence bulletin board.

Subordination had both practical and ideological dimensions. The strict rules and regulations that structured daily life at the hospital ensured that the frequently unsupervised students understood the parameters of appropriate action and would police themselves for fear of discipline or fatal error. As well, students were constrained in their behaviour so that they would be rested and ready for working in an environment that was physically taxing and potentially dangerous to their own health. As ideological tools, discipline and subordination helped secure nursing's place within the social category of respectable femininity and thereby accentuated the hospital's position as a respectable environment for middle-class patients to receive treatment. This was especially necessary given the range of class backgrounds of successful applicants to nursing programs. Rural and working-class women had to acquire not only the specific skills of bedside attendance but also 'character' as defined by bourgeois society. As one Nova Scotia nursing educator claimed:

> ... for many of our girls who come to us [hospital training] affords them means of culture they have not had before, particularly those who come from the isolated country districts ... it is very noticeable with many of our pupil nurses that they improve very much in matters of that kind. We notice a change, perhaps in a year.[21]

Character and culture were shaped by religion as well as class. Evelina (Sinclair) Adams recalled her first encounter with Miss Wood, newly appointed superintendent of the Neepawa General Hospital. Before arriving in Manitoba, Wood had worked in a large hospital in Ontario. Adams recalled: 'Our first morning at breakfast, all standing waiting for the lady to be seated, when she looked sternly at me and said "Miss Sinclair you will kindly say Grace." I who had never said a Grace in my life—I have no idea what I said, but the girls assured me it sufficed. Believe me I learned a Grace that evening, which I have never forgotten to this day.'[22] Such formative moments were critical in shaping nurses' perceptions of themselves, as well as their position in the community.

Cementing the ideological position of nurses demanded a fundamental reconfiguration of the social relations of femininity, sexuality, and work. In her analysis of nineteenth-century gender formulations, theorist Mary Poovey has argued that occupations like nursing posed particular contradictions for Victorian societies. Nursing was, in Poovey's terminology, one of the 'border cases' that positioned practitioners between the 'normative (working) man and the normative (nonworking) woman'. Nurses' presence in the work-force and at the bedside had the potential to undermine dichotomized categories of gender and to 'expose the artificiality of the binary logic that governed the Victorian symbolic economy'. According to Poovey, the disruptive potential of nursing was never realized because Florence Nightingale's work and writing ensured that the nurse 'represented a compromise between a series of normative oppositions rather than a destabilizing problem'.[23]

> Not a member of a religious sect, [Nightingale] was able to take up her 'calling' without arousing a religious controversy. Not a 'strong-minded woman' like the would-be lady doctor, she was able to engage in health-care work without antagonizing medical men. Neither a mother nor a professional, she was able to nurture

her wards and to supervise sanitary conditions; she was, in short, able to make the hospital a home and, in so doing, to enhance the reputation of an activity that had been degraded because it was traditionally women's work.[24]

Poovey's analysis of Nightingale's vision for nursing offers a convincing explanation of the successful introduction of nursing training programs in the late nineteenth century, but it infers a closure on the social position of nurses not so easily achieved in most locales. Creating a 'sexless, moralized angel' was a project that challenged nursing administrators and educators throughout the first and second generations of Canadian nurses, and demanded more than just the republication of Nightingale's *Notes on Nursing*.[25]

Throughout the late nineteenth and early twentieth centuries, nursing administrators struggled to resolve the long-standing contradiction between the sexual potential of relations at the bedside and the social respectability demanded by institutions, between genteel femininity and tending the bodies of strangers. Efforts to entice trained nurses to comply with the Victorian ideology of middle-class femininity and sexual respectability, passivity, and ignorance created contradictory conditions for these working women, as events at Halifax's Victoria General Hospital in 1896 revealed. That year, Lady Superintendent Miss Elliot recognized that there were too many male patients needing assistance for the small staff of male 'nurses' to attend. With the support of her medical superintendent, Elliot decided to introduce a 'new rule' mandating that the nursing staff of students be prepared to assume the tasks involved in cleaning and treating male patients' private parts. The female nursing students were appalled and continued to summon male attendants when men on the wards required baths, bedpans, catheters, suppositories, or enemas. As a result, no nurse was actually required to provide such services, but the possibility of direct contact with male genitalia provoked substantial discontent among the nurses, as well as among the patients who found themselves waiting for long periods to receive attention. The situation peaked when one well-to-do male patient complained so vociferously that a commission was struck to investigate the matter.

The commissioners reiterated the hospital's general principle: 'Nursing is a woman's work, for which she is peculiarly fitted', but they conceded that 'there are obviously limitations to her usefulness, imposed both by modesty and her want of physical strength'. They recommended that male nurses should be eliminated altogether and replaced by male orderlies or porters who would perform those duties not suitable for female attendants. In spite of this initial sympathy for the female students' discomfort with the reality of bedside patient care, the commissioners went on to criticize the apprentices for failing to follow orders.

> A young woman entering the profession of nursing ought to make up her mind to the discharge of a great many unpleasant and even repulsive duties for patients, irrespective of sex. If she cannot, then she has no business in the profession, either in a hospital or in private practice. What is wanted is the proper spirit of the profession, and no nurse who possessed that would abuse the privilege of calling for a male nurse in the manner in which many of the nurses appear to have done.

More serious were the flaws Superintendent Elliot displayed. The commission pronounced that while Elliot's motive had been 'the improvement of her department' she had none the less shown herself 'seriously lacking' in tact, gentleness, and carefulness in dealing with the issue. It maintained that 'however desirable the objects aimed at by [Elliot], her attitude toward the nurses, and toward the House Staff and Medical Board, instead of being conciliatory, was rather the reverse.'[26]

This conflict highlighted the central contradiction faced by nurses. The students were applauded for their adherence to feminine sexual distaste over matters of the body, but critiqued for breaking the taboo of female submissiveness and subordination upon which the system of hospital staffing relied. For her part, Elliot was supported in her implementation of the 'new rule' that met the needs of the hospital, but in attempting to teach her students to divorce themselves from their femininity when at work Elliot was condemned for abandoning the feminine persona of tact, gentleness, discretion, and conciliation. Nursing administrators and students were, for different reasons, simultaneously too feminine and not feminine enough. Hospital administrators and doctors alike believed nursing to be women's work and sought to recruit into the hospital schools young women who by virtue of their sex were skilled, subordinate, and inexpensive workers. On the other hand, once on duty, the students had to perform tasks that flew in the face of everything they had learned about feminine sexual respectability.

To resolve this contradiction, administrators of hospital nursing schools implemented codes of dress and behaviour designed to desexualize apprentices and enhance the social status of nursing and hospital care. The strict rules of behaviour on the wards were accompanied by stringent standards of personal and sexual presentation designed to constrain and contain female sexuality. Nursing leaders recognized that the institution itself offered numerous possibilities for male-female social contact. Students were thus forbidden from consorting with male hospital staff, especially orderlies and patients, and were allowed limited opportunity for pursuing relations with doctors. Evidence from early twentieth-century hospitals suggests that, like their late nineteenth-century predecessors, nursing supervisors continued to struggle to mould nurses-in-training into the vision of respectable womanhood necessary for maintaining sterling reputations for both their occupation and institution. Nursing superintendents disciplined students for a range of offences. Apprentices were chastised for any 'objectionable manner' to patients, visitors, and doctors. A common point of conflict emerged when, on being 'corrected' by a superior, students responded in a rude or 'saucy' manner. Gossiping, criticizing the hospital, or simply talking too much also provoked censure. Contraventions of the daily schedule, whether missing morning prayers, arriving late for duty, loitering on the ward after duty, or refusing to stay on duty after hours, resulted in discipline. Other students were chastised for staying out past curfew, especially if caught sneaking back into the residence through a window. Apprentices found flirting, 'posing', or showing 'familiarity' towards male patients, orderlies, or medical staff received stern warnings and were thereafter watched carefully by supervising staff.[27]

Within this moral economy, the uniform played a central symbolic part. In the transition from old-style attendants to the new trained nurses, standardized apparel signified nurses' social position; they were superior to their untrained predecessors but distinct from and subordinate to employers. While each institutional costume included unique details, when first introduced in the late nineteenth century most adopted the basic style of a long blue dress, covered by a white apron and crowned with a cap. Dress and cap were modelled after the habit worn by servants in élite households and, like domestic servants, nurses endured uniform styles that were slightly out of style. Trained nurses were thus expected to dress differently from other working women, but not the same as their patients.[28] Throughout the early twentieth century, the uniform continued to distinguish nurses' social position but also neutralized their sexuality. Playing on class and religious imagery, uniforms signalled both the celibacy that nurses shared with nuns and the sexual repression of Victorian femininity. Like nuns and members of the military, changes in social status were reflected in changes in uniform, representing successful completion of the various stages of their apprenticeship. When it was used

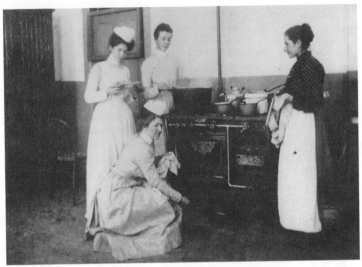

Apprenticing nurses completed a rotation through the 'diet kitchen', where they learned how to cook for and feed infirm patients. Even though hospitals were growing in size and function during the first decades of the twentieth century, many of their features (such as private rooms and the diet kitchen shown here) continued to resemble those in ordinary households (PAM Foote Collection #238).

as a means of discipline, the uniform could hold less positive connotations. Because only graduates could wear the uniform of their school, students who were expelled forfeited not only their training but also the right to identify publicly with graduate nurse status. Expulsion was a relatively rare occurrence. More frequently, apprentices were disciplined by having their caps revoked, a daily reminder that they had transgressed some rule. When one Vancouver General student was caught smoking in her room she lost her cap for six months.[29]

Together, the uniform, the rules, the disciplinary measures, and the celebration of 'character' helped nursing administrators mould apprentices into a labour force that was expandable, skilled, inexpensive, subordinate, and respectable. Nurses' precise position within the hospital hierarchy was shaped by the forces of class and gender. Hospital schools of nursing were designed to provide skilled, subordinate assistants who would carry out the directives of their medical superiors. The largest contingent of patient-care personnel in the early twentieth-century hospital, apprenticing nurses were the 'working class' of institutional services. As skilled workers, however, students did not occupy the lowest rung of the hospital hierarchy. Nurses were subordinate to the male-dominated medical staff—even the highest paid nursing supervisor made half the salary of her medical counterpart—but occupied a position superior to the housekeeping staff.[30] The relationship with orderlies was more complex. While an orderly's salary of $30–$35 per month was far greater than the monthly stipend awarded to student nurses, it was significantly lower than the wages of $50–$75 per month paid to graduate staff nurses. This wage differential symbolized the potential rewards skilled training represented to students who completed their apprenticeship.

Nurses' position within the health-care hierarchy as skilled workers, subordinate to professional doctors but superior to 'untrained' orderlies or domestic servants, was created by a division of labour based not only on class but also on gender. Women's virtual monopoly over nursing work was justified in terms of 'natural' female nurturing, and trained nurses' presence at the bedside was legitimized by their adherence to Victorian codes of femininity. The gendered structure was reinforced by familial and domestic imagery. Modelled on the ideal bourgeois household, hospitals invested male administrators and doctors with tremendous authority. As symbolic wife, the nursing superintendent supported the male head of household by ensuring the smooth functioning of daily patient care. Like daughters, or female servants, apprenticing students were expected to maintain the reputation of the family. Nurses' social position was reflected in the very buildings they inhabited. As architectural historian Annmarie Adams has demonstrated, the many nurses' residences constructed in the early twentieth century were located close to, but distinct from, the hospital itself. Designed to replicate bourgeois homes, these buildings architecturally signified the filial and familial position of female apprentices.[31]

The special treatment accorded the few male nurses served to reinforce female nurses' distinct and lesser position compared to their 'brothers' in the occupation. Victoria General Hospital in Halifax was one of the few general hospitals to train male nurses, perhaps because of the many sailors who used the institution's service. Male applicants to the training school could enter immediately upon acceptance, while successful female applicants had to wait one to two years for a position in the school. Even after 1912, when the Victoria program was extended to three years, male student nurses required only two years to graduate. Until 1916 male staff nurses received higher wages than their female counterparts. When staff nurse William Carpenter broke his leg he received $25 a month compensation, whereas the many female nurses who contracted diseases on the wards received nothing but unpaid time off. Institutions specializing in mental health, such as the Nova Scotia Hospital, relied even more heavily on male nurses and demonstrated even greater concern for maintaining a stable male nursing staff. Men were not exempt from conforming to hospitals' rules of etiquette and deference and, indeed, the frequency with which male students were disciplined for insubordination suggests that most institutional employers appreciated the availability and respectability that female nurses offered. None the less, although nurses of both sexes were positioned as hospitals' skilled work-force, the distinct and relatively privileged position of male nurses stood as testimony to the power of gender asymmetry in the hospital 'family'.[32]

Class and gender also intersected with ethnicity to shape nurses' position. Institutional rules and regulations were designed to inculcate apprentices from a range of class backgrounds in the values and behaviours of middle-class society. The racial homogeneity of the nursing work-force ensured that, as White Canadians, the transformation from rural or working-class woman into the middle-class image of femininity and gentility could be achieved when White students donned the appropriate dress and demeanour. Part of that demeanour was ethnically based. Adhering to institutional standards, indeed, meeting entrance requirements, was a function of language and nativity. Students had to speak English or French and had to acquire the minimum educational standing, prerequisites that eliminated many immigrant women from non-English- or French-speaking nations.[33] On the other hand, if applicants had the necessary language skills, racial privilege, and basic educational requirements, the 'rough edges' of their class background could be smoothed out in the course of their apprenticeship.

The particular configuration of class, gender, and race/ethnicity ensured that the apprenticeship system of staffing served Canadian hospitals well. Whether the apprenticeship system served nurses and nursing well is less clear. Some scholars have characterized the apprenticeship system as fundamentally oppressive and exploitative. Pointing to the long hours of labour demanded of students, the minimal supervision or theoretical instruction they received, and the strict and sometimes arbitrary discipline imposed, authors writing within this framework have claimed that hospitals subordinated educational considerations (and therefore nursing's professional status) to issues of staffing the wards and balancing institutional budgets.[34] Other historians disagree. American scholars Barbara Melosh and Tom Olson in particular have defended the apprenticeship system as a craft-based method of learning that may not have met the professional goals of the occupation's élite but served well the needs of 'rank-and-file' nurses who sought practical skills and valued nursing as work. Historian of medicine Charles Rosenberg has added that apprenticeship training held an economic advantage for women aspiring to become nurses. According to Rosenberg:

> Education and the credentials it legitimated had become both inducement and part payment for a key segment of the hospital's labor force. This was an economic logic too compelling to be ignored. Both hospitals and prospective nurses were capital poor; it was only natural for the two parties to barter: work for diplomas.

Women were willing to barter their labour for training in one of the few skilled occupations that offered formal apprenticeships for women.[35]

Canadian evidence suggests that for all the exploitative features of apprenticeship training, it was no harsher than other forms of female employment and in fact offered women some distinct advantages, as well as some avenues of resistance. Some contemporary observers did criticize nursing training programs. In 1917 a Victoria, BC, citizen wrote to the secretary of the Labour Commission pertaining to the conditions of nurses' labour. Pointing to the 12-hour shifts ('very often this is exceeded by 2 or 3 hours and sometimes in changing duty the Nurse has to work for 24 hours continuously'), the low pay, and the sometimes erratic meal times, the concerned citizen concluded that 'surely this is the worst kind of sweating because to the honour of most of [the students] they do not choose this occupation for money but in order to benefit their fellows'.[36] As the citizen from Victoria recognized, students worked hard and earned every skill they acquired.

At the same time, while hospitals clearly structured nursing education to meet institutional needs and retained the balance of power in relations with nursing students, defining the apprenticeship system as purely exploitative fails to capture the complex relationship between hospitals and aspiring nurses. That apprentices did not necessarily see themselves as powerless or oppressed can be explored in several ways. First, students chose nursing out of a narrow range of occupational options and recognized the potential for community status and financial autonomy that nursing offered. Lacking property, political rights, or substantial options for skilled work, single women viewed nursing training as a realistic and affordable avenue to economic self-sufficiency. Throughout the early twentieth century, domestic service remained the largest and least popular sector of paid work for women, while women in the manufacturing sector were concentrated in sex-specific pockets of industrial production, such as the garment industry, textiles, and food and confectionery processing. Teaching continued to attract large numbers of single women and continued to be plagued by isolation, low wages, and limited possibility of advancement. The most dramatic area of change occurred in the clerical sectors, which grew more than three times faster than the female work-force as a whole in the 1900–21 years. Combined with growth in other tertiary-sector jobs such as telephone operators, white-collar work began to rival blue-collar employment as the preferred sector of employment for many Canadian women.[37]

As one of the white-collar options that involved significant training, credentials, skills, and social status, the popularity of nursing must be understood within this context of women's limited work options. Women inquired about apprenticeship programs in numbers that far outweighed the available positions at local training schools, although it is likely that many submitted applications to more than one training school while others were considering non-nursing options. One page of a 1900–1 register from Halifax's Victoria General lists 30 women who applied to the school. Only seven entered training; the others had 'found another vocation', been accepted elsewhere, withdrew their application, 'failed to report as promised', or simply 'could not be found'.[38] Clearly, many students were shopping around for occupational options and institutional programs, while others did not fulfil entrance requirements.[39]

Canadian administrators thus 'bartered' with working women within an employment context that made nursing a popular option, but not the only option. The presence of so many hospital schools locally and throughout North America gave prospective recruits added bargaining power. Local nursing educators had to compete with schools in other regions of Canada and with American programs that welcomed Canadian recruits enthusiastically. To American and Canadian institutions alike, rural-born women represented the 'sound stock and country childhood' that bred good nurses.[40] Even those who failed to complete one nursing program might face fewer conflicts with their superiors in another school. Nursing administrators were thus obliged to provide sufficient education to their apprentices, to fight for improved accommodation and conditions of work, and to balance discipline with justice; otherwise, they risked tarnishing the reputation of their school and their occupation. For these reasons, superintendents of nursing used hospital annual reports to promote their institutions to prospective students and their parents.

Once enrolled, students expected an education that would prepare them for the rigours of a career in nursing. Educational practices such as 'renting out' students for nursing care in private homes generated income for the hospital and also provided students with experience in private duty, the dominant subsector of graduate nurse employment. Similarly, 12-hour duty, while criticized by some, was one of the usual shifts worked by private-duty nurses and was far shorter than the 24-hour shifts many private-duty nurses worked. Strict residence rules both enhanced the sexual and social reputation of the institution and assured parents that their daughters would be well chaperoned during their apprenticeship. Their distinctive uniform was celebrated by many students and graduates as a valued symbol of hard-earned skills, a symbol that distinguished trained nurses from untrained or informally trained domestic servants, practical nurses, or midwives.

Moreover, administrators had to balance their desire for conformity to nursing procedure and hospital etiquette with the reality that students, especially seniors, represented highly valuable skilled labour. As a result, most dismissals occurred relatively early in students' training, certainly within the first two years and often within the first six months. From then on, as long as they were willing to accept a penalty and appear to repent, apprenticing nurses could bend the formal rules of hospital life quite far without jeopardizing their entire training. Evelina Adams recounted one such instance that occurred during the 1919 Prince of Wales tour. The Prince was scheduled to make a whistle stop at the Neepawa station at 11 p.m. Only one student received late leave per week, but the students were 'determined' to attend the royal visit. After the 10 p.m. curfew, all the nurses except the night nurse on duty left the residence via the fire escape. The next morning the acerbic Superintendent Miss Murray noted 'that it was too bad we had not known about the Prince passing through, or we all might have gone to see him'.[41] Like superintendents in similar situations, Murray was aware of the flagrant and collective disregard for rules, but likely realized that disciplining the entire school would do more harm than good.

Whether nursing administrators excessively disciplined students is central to the debate over relations of exploitation within nursing training programs. Olson's research on Minnesota institutions demonstrated that hospital administrators did not expel students frequently, nor did they impose excessive 'extra time' on students' training

periods. Records from Winnipeg General Hospital confirm his findings. Of the 123 nurses enrolled in the classes of 1903–6, 69 per cent
successfully completed their program, 23 per cent did not graduate,
and the fate of the remaining 8 per cent was not clear from the records.
Among the 28 women who did not complete their apprenticeship, 6
had been dismissed because of some error or conflict, 12 had resigned,
in some cases because of a direct conflict, in other cases for no apparent school-related reason, 4 were forced to resign due to ill health, 3
quit to be married, and another 3 died during training. Of those students who were dismissed or resigned, only one was a senior student,
whose stated reason for leaving, that 'she could not have her afternoon
the day she planned for', likely masked a longer-standing conflict. The
rest of that group were in the first two years of training, with an average length of training completed by non-graduates of one year, three
and one-half months. Winnipeg figures for average length of training
for graduates, 3.03 years, correspond with Olson's findings. Even with
days added on to their training for illness or punishment, most Winnipeg General nurses in this period spent very little time beyond their
three-year commitment. Such data suggest that nursing administrators
were less likely to abuse student nurses, either through unfair dismissal of seniors or through extreme extensions of the length of training, than some historians have proposed.[42]

Precisely because student nurses constituted the predominant hospital work-force, apprentices wielded some power to resist unfair
demands, the final factor to be considered when assessing the degree
of exploitation inherent in the apprenticeship system. Apprentices did
not passively accept dismissal, discipline, or inappropriate educational
practices; rather, they used a range of strategies to defend their position in the work-force, even if those strategies were not always effective. Often, resistance to the system took the form of individual action.
In 1903 the superintendent of Halifax's Victoria General Hospital, Mr
Kenny, reported that: 'About 9 a.m. nurses [Campbell] and [West]
came to me and submitted terms which they would remain on nursing
staff which were that I would guarantee that they should receive satisfactory instruction failing which I should accept a months notice and
furnish them with a recommendation.'[43] Although Kenny's summary
suggested a rather forceful approach, nurses had to use a degree of tact
and diplomacy when directly approaching the superintendent. Mr
Kenny explained to a student who was demanding to return home to
her family 'the demoralizing effect of having a nurse dictate in such a
defiant manner terms of her relations with the Hospital'.[44]

Other students took collective action. Brandon General Hospital pupils appealed to the board of directors when, in 1906, they maintained that Superintendent of Nurses Miss Birtles had gone too far. The incident began when Birtles suspended one nurse, Ruth Winters, for 'insubordination'. The board supported Miss Birtles's discipline and demanded that Winters apologize to her superior. Before long it became clear that Winters had some support, for soon the board was confronted with a letter signed by all 20 students, demanding a reduction in their courseload. Complaining that three years 'is all too short for the amount of work to be covered', they asserted that the recently instituted 'Lectures in Arithmetic, Spelling and Composition' be eliminated. The students insisted that 'these lectures may be advantageous had we the time to spend on them, but we have already received our training along these lines and are now here for a three years training in Hospital work.'[45]

These instances wherein apprentices circumvented the nursing administration to resist unpopular administrative decisions revealed that student nurses were far from powerless and were able, within limits, to resist what they believed to be unfair and unacceptable elements of their training years. These instances of conflict among student and supervisory nurses stand as important indicators that within the hospital hierarchy students had some power, but to conclude that apprentices occupied a position in permanent opposition to nursing administrators is incorrect. However much students objected to the actions of their superiors within the nursing hierarchy, students were equally likely to unite with staff nurses to protest decisions made by upper levels of hospital management. For instance, in August 1902 the Vancouver General matron, Miss Clendenning, attended a meeting of the city's Board of Health, which was investigating the circumstances surrounding a particular patient. At the meeting, the mayor 'was not at all backward in expressing' his negative opinions of Miss Clendenning's assessment. Her nurses were incensed and threatened to resign. Fortunately for the hospital, the assistant matron caught wind of the unrest and 'lost no time in endeavoring to pacify the nurses', but the staff maintained that 'if their matron is subjected to any more insults they will each and every one step down and out'.[46]

Nor was the west coast incident isolated. That same year nurses at Winnipeg General reacted with equal vehemence when four members of the graduate nursing staff were fired. Ethel Johns was one of the student nurses who, believing grounds for dismissal insufficient, submitted a written protest to the board of directors. The board took immediate action, summoning Johns and classmate Isabel Stewart to the board meeting.[47] Johns recalled:

We were sternly asked why we had chosen to break the contract that we had signed when we were accepted as pupil nurses and in which we had solemnly promised to obey the authorities under all circumstances. Did we realize that insubordination could lead to instant dismissal? My heart sank. . . .

Her worst fears did not come to pass. Although the graduate nurses were not reinstated, the students were not disciplined and the 'harsh terms of the contract' were subsequently modified. Later, Johns reflected that although 'the idea of calling a strike had never entered our heads', the threat of one had granted the students some power.

It did not occur to me at the time (although it has since) that the directors may have been a little afraid of us. This must have been the first time that they had encountered an organized protest made on behalf of a traditionally submissive group. . . . The directors knew only too well that if the student working force were to be withdrawn the hospital would be forced to close its doors.[48]

Obviously, she recognized sooner than later the potency of collective action because that same year she again signed a petition. On that occasion, apprenticing nurses supported the staff nurses in protesting the hiring of non-Winnipeg graduates for hospital positions. The nurses reminded the 'sirs' that 'we are told on graduation that our certificates give us an equal standing with nurses from any other Hospital.' Asking for 'a chance of applying for any vacancies that may occur in our own', they pointed out that the previous three staff positions had been awarded to 'strangers, though some of our graduates were willing'.[49]

Such contests for power speak to the interplay of class and gender hierarchies that fostered a complex web of loyalties and relations on the hospital floor. Apprentices could challenge the authority of their nursing superiors by asking hospital boards to intervene with nursing administrators, but this willingness to resist particular policies did not translate into fixed relations of nurse-managers and nurse-workers. Rather, students frequently saw their interests to be in common with those of their superiors, sometimes because of specific economic interests, such as the Winnipeg hospital hiring only 'outside' graduates, and sometimes out of a more general occupational identity that bonded aspiring nurses to their role models on staff. Equally significant was the fact that the finite nature of apprenticeship training diffused permanent antagonisms. Whether they enjoyed their training or resented the discipline, second-generation nurses could endure their three years on the wards knowing that upon graduation they could leave the hospital hierarchy and pursue private-duty work, where practitioners could participate in the relative equality of graduate nurse status.

The World of Graduate Nurses

Successful completion of a three-year apprenticeship granted graduate nurses entry into one of three subsectors of the health-care market: hospital staff positions, private-duty work, and public health service. In the early twentieth century, institutional employment accounted for only one-fifth of all graduates. Those who did seek work on hospital staffs occupied a very different position within the hospital hierarchy than did students. In small, rural hospitals or private hospitals, graduate staffs of one or two nurses performed direct patient care, much as they had in training, but without the extensive hospital hierarchy monitoring their performance.[50] In larger hospitals with training schools, graduate staff performed supervisory duties and only spent time at the bedside when inspecting the work of their subordinates.

Because hospital budgets were tight and most staff nurses were responsible for supervision, not bedside care, graduate staffs remained relatively small in this period. In 1906, the Vancouver General staff consisted of the lady superintendent, the night supervisor, and two head nurses, who together oversaw the daily labours of 34 student nurses. By 1920, hospital expansion to a 1,200-bed facility necessitated a graduate nurse staff of 45 to supervise 196 students.[51] The high ratio of apprentices to staff, and the high volume of patients to be tended, meant that even with the larger supervisory staff, the presence of graduate nurses was often only token. On night duty especially, senior students were placed in charge of wards or floors under the watchful eye of the roaming night supervisor who was responsible for the entire institution. For their part, staff nurses were accountable to the superintendent of nursing, but experienced minimal direct supervision in their daily work.[52]

Rather, staff nurses watched over the performance and behaviour of apprentices, patients, and visitors on their ward or floor. Rules for head nurses emphasized the importance of communication, although the tone and substance of that communication depended on whether the ward housed public or private patients. The former paid little or nothing for the care they received from house medical staff and student nurses. The latter paid the hospital, their own doctor, and, if required or requested, their own special-duty nurse. Not surprisingly, supervisors on private wards were encouraged to use substantially more tact and discretion than were their counterparts on the public wards. For instance, head nurses at Victoria General in Halifax were responsible for ensuring that all student staff understood doctors' orders and for providing a full report of daily or nightly events to the staff nurse coming on duty. On public wards, head nurses monitored the activities of the student or housekeeping staff and disciplined errant nurses, maids, visitors, or patients.[53] On private wards, head nurses had to consult with the paying clientele more frequently and to discipline less often. Consulting was not to become visiting, and private ward staff were warned against allowing visitors to 'deter' them 'where your professional obligations as charge nurses are concerned'. Head nurses had to maintain a high profile for private patients by visiting each patient thrice daily as well as after meals to ensure that residents were satisfied with the quality of bedside care. When specials were on duty, head nurses had to check in on patients without interfering with the private-duty nurse's routine.[54]

In return for their labours, graduate nurses earned a salary, plus board and room. In 1908, female graduate nurses at Vancouver General received $20–$35 per month, male graduate staff $20–$33, and the superintendent of nurses $50.[55] In 1914, salaries ranged from the $125 paid to the lady superintendent to the $50 earned by head nurses on wards.[56] However grandiose this salary would have seemed to the apprenticing student or the domestic worker, it paled by comparison to the salaries paid to the male senior administrative staff.[57] Nursing superintendents earned between one-half and two-thirds the rate paid to hospital superintendents.[58] At Catholic hospitals, nuns served as hospital superintendents and as head nurses, receiving little financial remuneration although perhaps wielding significant authority over male doctors, but lay Catholic nurses received similar rates of pay as their peers in other institutions.[59]

Wage differentials among lay hospital staff revealed the two institutional hierarchies in operation. First, distinct salary levels for graduate nurses reflected the various ranks and statuses among nursing staff. A second, equally significant, differential divided male doctors and administrators from nurses. As was the case between students and their supervisors, conflict on the wards could arise out of either set of hierarchical relationships. A sense of mutual interest and occupational identity sometimes prompted graduates to act in solidarity to protest the actions of male administrators. The Vancouver General staff faced this issue in 1916 when Lady Superintendent Helen

Randal and four staff nurses resigned. The hospital superintendent, Malcolm MacEachern, had ignored Randal's recommended replacement for herself during her leave, a decision that she believed indicated 'she had not the support of the Board nor the Superintendent in carrying out the management of her department'. The board accepted Randal's resignation, but was perplexed by the other four resignations. One of the nurses explained to the board that they supported Randal's protest and did not agree with the 'arrangements made for the carrying on of the work during Miss Randal's leave'.[60] A similar conflict erupted at the St John's General Hospital in 1914 when Medical Superintendent Lawrence Keegan usurped Nursing Superintendent Mary Southcott's authority pertaining to hiring staff nurses. Historian Linda White's analysis of that conflict emphasizes the importance of the nurses' residence in fostering solidarity among staff. In the aftermath of the conflict between Keegan and Southcott over who could appoint ward supervisors, the staff nurses gathered in the residence. Until the wee hours of the morning they planned their protest, indignantly proclaiming that Miss Southcott had been insulted by Keegan and an insult to her was an insult to them all.[61]

Occupational solidarity against injustices perpetrated by male administrators could unite nurses, but on other questions conflict over priorities and protocol divided staff nurses from upper-level nursing management. The 1919 conflict between Mamie Brown and Vancouver General illustrates the different visions held by staff and administrative nurses of how nursing work should be adjudicated. Brown had supervised the case room until she contracted influenza, but when she returned from sick leave she discovered that her job had not been reserved for her and she had been transferred to another part of the hospital. In response to her complaint, Superintendent MacEachern explained that during her absence a certain amount of reorganizing had occurred, that the move 'was nothing against Miss Brown's character', and that, in fact, the nursing superintendent had believed Brown was moving to California for an indefinite length of time. When pushed, however, MacEachern admitted that there had been some concern over Brown's competence, maintaining that 'certain things were going on which would make it appear suspicious in the eyes of the nurses in training' and adding that Miss Brown lacked the teaching credentials necessary for the case room position.[62] Brown insisted that 'after having served for one year and a half in the same department without any suggestion having been made as to her capabilities and without any complaint as to her work' it was unfair 'she should be refused her position upon her return to the hospital'.

Brown's position, and perhaps nerve, was clearly strengthened by the involvement of Dr Carson, a friend of the Brown family. Dr Carson admitted to having served as Brown's informal medical adviser during her recent illness and that he had been the source of the news that Miss Brown might move to California. Carson pointed out that the nursing superintendent could have communicated directly with Miss Brown before assuming the staff nurse would not be returning. One member of the board of directors, Mr Owen, agreed with the plaintiff, stating:

> . . . it appeared to him that an inopportune time had been taken to reorganize the department . . . that it would have been policy to have reinstated Miss Brown and then had the reorganization. He could not see why, after one and a half years of service without any complaint having been made as to Miss Brown's work, that the change should have been made at that particular time. . . .

Owen's remained the dissenting voice, and the decision of the 'officials of the hospital' stood.[63] Nonetheless, the Brown incident revealed the ways in which external male authority could be brought to bear on hospital managers who were concerned about community perceptions of their institution. The conflict also reveals the divergent priorities of staff nurses, for whom nursing was their livelihood and who believed that competence should be measured by performance of bedside care, and nursing administrators, who valued efficiency, educational advancements, and academic credentials.

These conflicts rarely developed into sustained class-based contests of managers versus workers. Not only were staff nurses themselves 'managers' who encountered minimal direct supervision, but when friction between head nurses and senior nursing management did escalate, the many options in private-duty nursing meant that staff nurses simply went elsewhere. In an era when private-duty work was plentiful and when most graduate nurses preferred the autonomy and variety of private health care over the regimentation of institutional work, employment on hospital staffs was relatively easy to acquire. Throughout these early years of hospital growth, administrators constantly complained of difficulties they encountered maintaining adequate graduate nursing staff. In 1910 the Victoria General superintendent reported what by then was a familiar refrain:

> the wards are in the charge of graduate nurses, under the Superintendent of Nurses, and there is generally a graduate in each ward; but as nurses when they graduate desire to go into private practice

or take special courses they cannot be relied on to remain on the staff for more than a short time after their time's completed.[64]

Upon graduation most practitioners sought their fortunes in the private-duty market, providing one-on-one care for individual patients. Calculating the precise proportion of graduates working in private health care is difficult, given nurses' geographic and occupational mobility, but available evidence suggests that between 35 and 45 per cent of graduates were in private-duty work, while 20 to 25 per cent were employed in the hospital and public-health sectors. Approximately 40 per cent of alumnae were married and thus defined as 'inactive' despite the casual labours they might perform in their communities.[65]

For recent graduates especially, private-duty work was a welcome change from the structure of apprenticeship training. To acquire work in private practice, nurses advertised themselves with local nursing employment registries, in the offices of doctors, pharmacists, and morticians, in city directories, in corner stores, and through personal contacts. By 1910, most cities had nursing employment bureaus or 'registries', often operated by local nursing associations and designed to facilitate communication between patients and trained nurses, as well as to ensure fair distribution of work to members. Each practitioner listed a phone number through which she might be reached. Sometimes the number listed was in her own home, but nurses also made arrangements with neighbours and local shopkeepers to serve as informal answering services, taking calls from doctors or patients and notifying nurses that a call had come in.[66] A case might last days, weeks, or months, at the end of which the nurse would seek employment with another client in another home or ward. The duties required of each case would depend on the illness or affliction and on the economic circumstances of the patient's family.

Because the work varied so greatly and because the demand for trained practitioners was relatively high, nurses were selective about which cases they accepted. Winnipeg's registrar asked its members to state their preferred areas of work, including whether they would accept out-of-town cases, so as to expedite the process of assigning registry nurses to the incoming requests. Recognizing that the different branches of nursing ranged in popularity and intensity of labour, nursing associations established wage scales designed to reward nurses who accepted unpopular and difficult assignments. The Brandon Graduate Nurses' Association (BGNA) conformed to the pattern established elsewhere in setting rates of $25 per week for general cases, $28 for maternity, $30 for infectious and mental, and $7 per day for smallpox. Patients were also responsible for transportation costs such as railway tickets and livery.[67]

If nurses received steady work and if they collected their fees, private nursing could provide a degree of financial security. By the end of World War I, nurses working 40 weeks per year could earn potentially up to $1,000 annually, although real earnings averaged between $400 to $750.[68] Women working in industrial production, which like nursing was often seasonal, would be hard pressed to generate that level of income. At Halifax's Moir's Confectionery, female staff earned as much as $23 per week in the rush season and between $10 to $18 weekly the rest of the year. Nor could most white-collar jobs compete with nursing. At Quebec's Banque d'Hochelaga female clerks received a starting wage of $500 per year in 1920. Even taking into account the disparate regional economies, nursing promised the 'living wage' that eluded many working women.[69]

The financial rewards were enhanced by the workplace autonomy that characterized nursing in the private sector. Although private nurses usually worked under a doctor's supervision and instruction, the medical practitioner was only in the work environment a short time. Subsequently, the nurse was alone with the patient, obliged to fulfil the medical directives but able to do so without direct supervision. For example, one Halifax nurse travelled with a doctor to Kentville, Nova Scotia, to perform an appendectomy. She prepared the home and patient for the operation and assisted the doctor during the surgery. The doctor then returned to Halifax, leaving the nurse to provide post-operative care for two weeks. During the time alone with patients, nurses administered whatever medication had been prescribed, changed any dressings, fed the patient if necessary, ensured that patient and linen were kept clean, provided comforts like ice-water, and monitored patient progress, recalling the doctor should the patient's recovery falter.[70]

Not all private care, however, was so isolated. 'Special duty' work, wherein nurses attended private patients in private hospital rooms, required that nurses return to the institutional hierarchy, if only for the duration of the case. Hospital administrators asserted their authority over the specials by insisting that they enter the hospital through the nurses' residence, that they 'register' with the superintendent of nurses at the beginning and end of each case, that they report to the charge nurse before coming on duty each day, and that they 'conform to the rules of the Training School while on duty, and . . . not . . . visit or in any way interfere with patients other than the one they are on duty with.' Within these general guidelines, special nurses were accountable to their patients and their doctors. Specials' position on the periphery of the hospital hierarchy was signified by their dress; they wore the uniform of their Alma Mater rather than that of the host institution.[71]

The relative autonomy of the workplace extended into nurses' private lives. While hospital staff were required to live in institutional residences, private-duty nurses lived alone, with other nurses, or with family members. Of the 261 nurses listed in Toronto's *Might's Directory* for 1910, 80 (or 30 per cent) lived with their families. Many of these were married nurses, who might or might not have been graduates of training programs, or were single women living in the homes of widowed mothers. The remaining 181 women boarded, shared apartments, or took advantage of private residences catering exclusively to nurses. Lillian Smith's home at 9 Pembroke was one such residence that housed 16 nurses, while another seven practitioners co-habited at 7 Ross Ave. Admittedly, private nurses had to pay for accommodation, whereas hospital staff received board and room on top of their wages. But living alone or in a boarding house granted nurses personal freedom impossible under the strict rules of institutional residences. Unfettered by hospital schedules, private-duty nurses took advantage of their freedom to holiday in locations as distant as Bermuda, Florida, and California or to arrange family visits, which sometimes involved returning home to care for relatives.[72]

Occupational flexibility often translated into geographic mobility as well. Nurses were free to take their skills to any part of the continent, and beyond. Within a year of graduation, the Winnipeg General class of 1907 had scattered, with 13 remaining in Winnipeg, 9 working in private-duty or hospital work in western Canada, and 2 pursuing private-duty work in the United States. Maritime women typically travelled south to the 'Boston States', while California attracted many British Columbians.[73] Mobility to the United States was enhanced in the years after 1910 when American states such as New York began to recognize Canadian nursing credentials. This signalled the beginning of formalized 'reciprocity' among Canadian provinces and between Canadian and American nursing organizations. Upon providing proof of their qualifications, graduates of recognized hospital schools could gain 'registered' status in most North American jurisdictions and with it the rights and privileges accorded local graduates, including access to the local nursing registry.[74] A small but significant number of Canadian nurses used their training as passports to travel and work abroad, particularly in the mission fields of China and India where skilled nurses were welcomed.[75]

Counterbalancing these positive features of private duty were the tensions inherent in an unregulated market. To succeed in private duty, nurses had to foster good relations with community members, particularly doctors. In 1918, the Registered Nurses' Association of Nova Scotia (RNANS) registry reported that of 244 calls received, 103 (or 42 per cent) had been from doctors.[76] The Winnipeg registry asked members to list physicians who would provide references for them.[77] Because medical endorsement was essential, the *Canadian Nurse*'s 'Don'ts for Nurses' column reminded readers, 'Don't dilly-dally after you get a call if you want doctors to depend on you.'[78] Registrars fielded calls for nursing services according to whichever member's name was at the top of the list, but the individual physician could still request a specific nurse or recommend one to his patient. This created some tensions for registrars, who had to ignore the registry's roster order to accommodate client preferences. Any hint of criticism prompted registrars to canvass local physicians to ensure that medical confidence in the nursing registries remained strong.[79]

Fostering good relations with superintendents of nursing could also prove critical, especially in smaller centres where nursing administrators arranged for specials to attend private hospital patients. Stories such as that of a nurse who 'suddenly left her patient much to the inconvenience of the Hosp. authorities and the anger of the patient's relatives' and then had the nerve to bill the patient worried registrars that 'instances of this kind are not conducive to improving the status of nursing and such events are unfortunate for all nurses'.[80] Conflict between nurses and their doctors and nursing superintendents jeopardized both the reputation of the registry and the future employment options of the individual nurse.

Relations with patients and their families could be just as complex. While criticisms could stem from inappropriate bedside care, conflict could also arise over questions of etiquette and familial relations. One nursing manual acknowledged:

> the life of a Private Nurse must of necessity be a hard one, and fraught with much discouragement. . . . the days will frequently be long and monotonous, and her own wishes will be frequently put aside. The book that she herself dislikes may be the very one her patient finds interesting and when most tired she may be requested to read it.

The manual insisted that the 'keynote to success' in private duty was discretion: 'even quite trivial remarks made by Nurse, whether wise or otherwise, may be—and often are—detailed again from one member to other of the family.' To prevent getting caught in a web of familial intrigue, nurses were advised:

> When your patient is recovering, you will find that, in course of conversation, there will be remarks made, and questions asked, that had better be left unsaid; but, with practice, you can cultivate quite a vocabulary of your own, for instance, 'Um,' 'Ah,' 'Indeed,' are useful. . . . Need I warn you NEVER, NEVER to discuss the Doctor, relatives, or friends of the Family in a depreciating [*sic*] way.[81]

Avoiding conflict with patients and their families improved nurses' chances for keeping and perhaps prolonging an engagement. This became especially critical once a patient's health improved and reduced nursing care was needed. The Winnipeg General's 'Rules for Special Duty Nurses' included the advice that 'when two nurses have been on duty with a patient and when only one is required the patient keeps which ever one he or she wishes', which suggests the tensions involved in negotiating this key moment in the work cycle of a case.[82]

In many ways, competition among graduate nurses was less troublesome than coping with the many untrained or partially trained practitioners in the community. Throughout the 1900–20 era, non-graduate nurses continued to advertise their services and no clear consensus emerged as to who would claim the category 'nurse' as their own. In 1910 the Halifax registry directly listed 32 'trained nurses', 14 'professional' or 'graduate' nurses, 11 institutional nurses, 5 'male nurses', and 24 undifferentiated 'nurses'. The Winnipeg registry responded to diversity in its work-force by including on its roster women who had completed diverse training programs and who charged varying rates accordingly. Annie McLeod was a graduate nurse who had completed a three-year course at St Michael's Hospital in Toronto and charged $3 per day or $21 per week in 1911 for non-infectious general nursing, or $4 for 'alcohol, drug and mental' cases. Ethel Campbell boasted 10 years of nursing experience, although only one year of formal training at Winnipeg's Misericordia Hospital, and listed rates of $3 per day, $18 per week for general cases and $4 per day or $35 per week for maternity cases. Mrs Perry had attended the City of London Lying-In Hospital's three-month maternity course, which combined with her six years of experience cost prospective patients $2.50 per day or $15–$18 per week. Mrs Hansen demanded lower rates, $2.25 per day or $15 per week, for the benefit of her 13 years of experience, but no formal training, in maternity nursing.[83]

As long as demand for private nursing continued to grow, the presence of these less-qualified practitioners could be accommodated by nursing registries. The Halifax registry, originally maintained at nurse Eveline Pemberton's private hospital 'Restholme', received only nine calls in its first month of operation in June 1910. By 1911 the registrar was facing an insufficient number of graduate nurses to meet patient demand and on several occasions sent uncertified nurses 'as substitutes'. The shortage persisted, only to be exacerbated by the outbreak of World War I. The 1917 Halifax explosion added to the demand and the 1918–19 influenza epidemic extended the emergency conditions of wartime. Elsewhere in Canada, the war and epidemic also required increased nursing attention. Twenty per cent of Winnipeg General Hospital graduates were engaged in military or Red Cross nursing by 1916 and the proportion pursuing private work had diminished to 19 per cent. As a result, Canadians living in 'frontier' conditions of rural western provinces often found they could not 'get a nurse for love nor money'.[84] Such conditions prompted a staff nurse at the Canora, Saskatchewan, hospital in 1920 to write a colleague in Halifax, inquiring 'How is nursing in Halifax? We find we cannot get nurses to come here for Contagious cases. There were six on the Registry in Regina last week "on call" and not one would come here.'[85] In these circumstances, the presence of unlicensed nurses did not present a direct challenge and, at times, allowed registries to foster community goodwill by supplying some form of bedside attendance, even if not by a graduate nurse. Only in the 1920s would the market reverse and employment become scarce.

Within the early twentieth-century political economy of private care, the presence of untrained or partially trained practitioners shaped the conditions of labour that graduate nurses experienced in other, more subtle, ways. For instance, graduate nurses' ability to limit their work to the sick room often depended on the availability of other domestics. In some cases, the presence of domestic servants could lighten a nurse's load. In other cases, the absence of such personnel meant that nurses were obliged to perform whatever domestic tasks were necessary to keep the household running. Nurses' unwillingness to assume domestic chores outside the sick room might prompt a patient to replace her with a less-trained, but more versatile, employee. As well, nurses' abilities to control the hours of labour and pay were directly related to the labour market in domestic service. Mrs George Cran, a trained maternity nurse and advocate of English women's immigration to western Canada, acknowledged in 1916 that in isolated communities nurses could not be 'certain' about receiving their fee:

. . . under stress of fear and love any one can pardon a man for
promising any fee to have his wife tended, and understand too that
with fear allayed and a new expense safely launched on a slender
purse that however willing he might delay payment and perhaps
need a nurse again before the first obligation was discharged. . . .[86]

In the winter of 1918–19, as the influenza epidemic raged, RNANS registrar Sibella Barrington confronted not only 265 requests for nurses
but also numerous complaints from registry members that they had
not been paid. Barrington was not forthcoming about her tactics, but
'was instrumental in arranging for the collection of nearly $150 for
nurses who otherwise would not have received their just remuneration from the public.'[87]

Controlling the hours of labour also confounded the second generation of trained nurses. Over the course of the 1900s and 1910s, 24-
hour attendance was supplanted by 12-hour duty as the dominant
shift. Registries stipulated that members called to 24-hour cases were
owed at least six hours of sleep and two hours during the day for 'out-
door recreation'.[88] Asserting standard hours was a delicate matter,
more so when the patient was acutely ill or when the doctor prescribed extended care and expected the nurse to accommodate the
patient's needs. Graduate nurses could, collectively, insist on adhering to the set 12- or 24-hour schedule, but did so knowing that medical men might recruit untrained competition to replace them. When
Dr Harry Watson provided Winnipeg's registrar with a letter of recommendation for Mrs Dunlop in 1919, his statement that she 'has
done considerable nursing for me & although not qualified I consider
her very valuable in every respect' revealed that such practitioners
remained popular with members of the medical profession.[89]

Within the early twentieth-century health-care hierarchy, private-
duty nurses shared with their counterparts on hospital staffs a specific
location. Required by law to defer to medical decisions and directives, nurses were subordinate to doctors, but boasted formal skills
and certification compared to informally trained female caregivers in
the community. Unlike institutional nurses, however, practitioners in
private duty plied their trade independent of direct supervision by
other nurses. Released from the hierarchy of hospital training and
work, nurses found that the perils inherent in the unregulated private
health-care market were more than compensated for by the autonomy,
variety, mobility, and equality they enjoyed.

Nurses working in the third subsector, public health, experienced
slightly different conditions of labour than did either hospital or

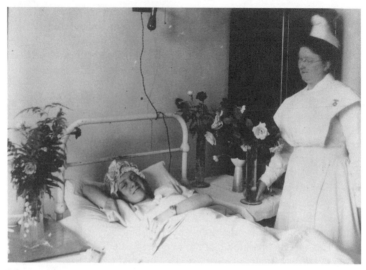

Most graduate nurses worked in the private-duty market, providing one-on-one bedside care either in patients' homes or as 'specials' in private hospital rooms. This is a patient and her special-duty nurse at the Winnipeg General Hospital (PAM Foote Collection #137).

private nurses. Throughout Canada, initial efforts to manage public health through sanitation, inspection, and collection of data had, by the first decades of the twentieth century, given way to more interventionist programs designed to bring the benefits of medical science into working-class homes and neighbourhoods. In this crusade for the people's health, nurses played a special role. To public and private health agencies alike, nurses constituted relatively inexpensive, skilled personnel who could provide domestic and community attendance and education on behalf of or in advance of the more expensive labour of doctors.

The medical profession was not always supportive of public health nursing programs. The oft-told story of medical opposition in 1897 to the establishment of the Victorian Order of Nurses (VON) testified to doctors' concern over competition from nurses, but by the early 1900s much of this kind of opposition had dissolved and medical officers agreed that nurses were logical and loyal allies in the emerging public health movement. VON branches were initiated in most urban centres, usually under the direction of middle-class volunteer women but with occasional input from male administrators.[90] Some Canadian cities also supported charitable nursing agencies such as Winnipeg's Margaret Scott Nursing Mission. Founded in 1904 at 99 George St, the Mission nurses continued the work of Mrs Margaret Scott, who, since 1898, had been providing food, clothing, and moral support to destitute families in the city's North End. In Montreal, religious orders such as the Soeurs de l'Espérance joined Les Gouttes de lait and Assistance maternelle in providing subsidized public health services to needy citizens.[91] In Halifax, the Massachusetts-Halifax Health Commission (MHHC), organized in the years after the Halifax explosion, constituted one of the most innovative and comprehensive public health programs, modelled on the American settlement house system.[92] These privately administered agencies augmented, and sometimes received funding from, state-run public health programs. Municipal and provincial school nurse programs as well as government-sponsored visiting nurse services were concentrated initially in urban centres, but during and after World War I they extended into underserviced rural regions.[93]

For graduate nurses, opportunities in public health work offered several advantages. Like private duty, public health involved a great variety of cases and nurses often travelled significant distances between patients. Nurses ran prenatal and postnatal home nursing classes, well-baby clinics, clean milk depots, and instructional booths at local fairs. They provided obstetrical assistance to local doctors, postnatal attendance for individual mothers, and bedside nursing for chronic and acute patients. Throughout their day, public health nurses enjoyed even greater autonomy from immediate medical supervision than their peers in the hospital or private sectors. Rather than follow up the instructions of physicians, public health nurses decided when a doctor should be consulted. Celebrating the independence of thought and action inherent in public health work, Ethel Johns proclaimed, with her usual rhetorical flourish:

> You are not tied to routine duties like your sisters in the hospitals, you are not harassed with 1001 petty interruptions; you have time to think and read and plan, and above all, you have the opportunity to break new ground; you don't have to patch up other people's mistakes and blunders, you will only have to patch up your own; think of that and be happy.[94]

The potential isolation of such work was compensated to some degree by the camaraderie fostered in nursing homes. Urban staff nurses usually lived together, wore the same distinctive uniform style, took turns on night duty, and sometimes travelled to remote districts together. Perhaps the most significant advantage of public health nurses was the third-party payment. Even when, as in the case of the VON, nurses were instructed to collect nominal fees for services, if patients could not or would not pay, public health nurses still provided care and still drew their salary.[95]

For all these advantages, public health nurses did face several limitations. After the first few years of operation, agencies began to require specialized postgraduate training (up to six months) and those who acquired that training had to compete for a small number of jobs. As late as 1923 only 54 public health nurses were registered with the Ontario Graduate Nurses' Association, while at agencies such as the Margaret Scott Mission the few paid staff nurses were aided by apprenticing students gaining experience in public health nursing as part of their hospital training course.[96] Moreover, although public health nurses enjoyed considerable autonomy in their daily labours, public health work none the less brought graduate nurses back under the control of a permanent supervisor. Medical officers of health, nursing superintendents, or voluntary boards monitored the behaviour of public health nurses on and off duty.

Jurisdictional conflicts with local doctors over the parameters of nursing work could prove equally frustrating. As Meryn Stuart's study of Ontario's child welfare program has revealed, the public health nurses assigned to rural northern towns in 1920 realized they had to 'go very gingerly' because it would be 'most difficult to recover from any friction or upset with these doctors. . . .'[97] In Halifax, Nurse Inglis, anticipating medical opposition to the MHHC program, spent much of October 1920 'proceeding systematically through the city, calling on each physician and soliciting his co-operation and trying to make each familiar with the work being undertaken by this Commission.'[98] While these delicate negotiations were proceeding, other public health nurses confronted the limitations inherent in public health work. Frustrated with the persistently high maternal mortality rates in the Canadian west, the general superintendent of the VON, Charlotte Hannington, tried in the post-World War I years to import midwives from England. Her efforts at improving women's health services were undermined by opposition from the medical and nursing professions, which refused to sanction any scheme that promised further competition in the medical marketplace.[99]

There is some debate among nursing historians as to whether all these organizations truly qualify as public health agencies. The VON in particular has been identified as a visiting nurse service dedicated to providing free bedside care, thus having more in common with private-duty nursing than with government-sponsored programs committed to 'prevention, education and reform'.[100] Certainly the philanthropic origins of groups like the VON differentiated them from state services and their progressive-era confidence in the social application of scientific knowledge. However significant their origins, differentiating too forcefully between curative visiting nurse services and preventative public health programs underestimates the commonalities that nurses working for all these organizations shared. First, whether VON, Gouttes de lait, or school health, agencies all relied on female nurses to provide front-line contact with clients. These nurses were all paid by third-party employers and unsuccessful fee collection did not affect nurses' salaries. Nor were curative and preventative services neatly divided. In addition to the bedside care they offered, Victorian Order nurses implemented measures such as prenatal visits and clean milk stations, while provincial and municipal nurses often found themselves performing bedside nursing for patients well beyond the preventive phase.[101] When the Metropolitan Life Insurance Company subcontracted the VON to provide visiting nurse service for its policyholders it did so because of the preventive impact rendered by improved access to skilled attendance.[102]

Furthermore, all organizations legitimated nurses' community work in terms of missionary zeal and social reform. The 'gospel of health' was constructed not by theology but by bacteriology and epidemiology serving not God but the public good. Even the image of public health workers—nurses wrapped in blue capes, carrying black bags, travelling through working-class neighbourhoods and isolated rural districts to care for the poor and needy—relied on evangelical symbolism. When public health nurses described their daily labours to the public and their co-workers they often focused on their interactions with new Canadians, the poor, or Native people.[103] Mariana Valverde's conclusion that, in the case of the social purity movement, voluntary organizations and the state were mutually reinforcing agents of moral regulation seems applicable to the realm of public health.[104] When in 1909 Halifax VON representative Agnes Dennis reported on her agency's work, she signalled the key role played by visiting nurses in the 'age of light, soap and water': 'The lessons of the value of light, sunshine, fresh air, and cleanliness given by the nurses are most important. . . . Trained nurses open up a new world as regards cleanliness. Their very presence is an object lesson, and many improve by their instruction.'[105]

Because voluntary agencies and state programs alike shared in the evangelism of public health reform, and because they assumed financial responsibility for nurses' salaries, public health nurses occupied a distinct place within the health-care hierarchy. Unlike private-duty nurses, who were at best their patients' social equals, public health nurses assumed a superior social position *vis-à-vis* their patients. The status differential between public health worker and patient reflected the fact that public health services were aimed at members of the working class and/or ethnic minorities. At the same time that nurses represented the middle-class and British or northern European values of the state, nurses were also employees of government health departments or private agencies. As such they were obliged to conform to the rules, regulations, and discipline of their superiors, much as other workers were. In the words of historian Kari Delhi, public health nurses were 'both products and producers of social and state regulation'.[106] Occupying a class position in between the working-class and ethnic minority clientele and the bourgeois state, nurses' position was complicated further by their gender. Public health agencies hired nurses, in part, because as women nurses were assumed to be better equipped to communicate with women in the community and household in a way that male servants of the medical system could not.[107] State and private agencies alike were encouraged in this assumption by women's groups such as the Women's Institutes and the IODE that provided financial and volunteer support.[108] For the front-line nurses, gender could bridge the class hierarchy between nurse and client, thereby pitting nurse against her agency supervisor. Halifax VON nurse Margaret Jones contravened her supervisor's sense of work ethic, but while 'inclined to be lazy' Margaret was 'liked by patients and doctors'. Mae Hamilton was 'very popular with her patients but not very thorough when giving bedside care'. Georgina Mills was assessed as 'generally speaking a very valuable nurse' who was 'always willing to give extra time and effort when necessary'. The fact that Georgina was 'careless about routine but extremely good to her patients' exempted her from censure.[109] Like the family caseworkers studied by Linda Gordon, individual nurses were able to break from procedure to provide services required by clients. If, then, clients were helped by social service workers it was because, according to Gordon, 'individual caseworkers were usually better (although sometimes worse) than the official agency policies they were supposed to follow'.[110]

Examining the common experiences of nurses employed by private agencies and by government programs thus points to the broader ramifications of nurses as social service workers. While VON nurses may indeed have played slightly different roles within the health-care system than did municipal school nurses or rural public health nurses, together nurses working for public health agencies constituted one of the first groups of social welfare workers. Their experiences remind us of the significance of women's labours to pre-welfare state social services, but they also suggest that analyses of social control and class domination were complicated and contradicted by gender relations. As front-line representatives of the social élite and the state, public health nurses remained employees whose gender and class interests did not precisely or completely coincide either with those running social reform agencies or with those of their patients.[111]

'Trade Unionism of the Worst Type'[112]

Like many working women of their day, the second generation of Canadian nurses used a variety of individual forms of resistance to improve their working conditions. Nurses confronted patients, doctors, and administrators and allied with the same groups to play off one against the other, or all. Nurses left jobs, they left town, they left the occupation. But, unlike most working women of their day, nurses also developed strong collective voices to articulate their needs. The organizations Canadian nurses created and sustained reflected the structure of their work and the occupational identity born of it. Borrowing from the organizational strategies of professionals, trade unions, and women's groups, nurses established a unique series of corporate vehicles that have survived the dramatic transformation of health services in the twentieth century.

In the first decades of the twentieth century, nurses joined in the tide of women's organizations being created across the continent. From the international to the local, five levels of associational activity existed to unite graduates of Canadian training programs and to defend their interests. The first nursing organization to which Canadian nurses belonged was the American Society for Superintendents of Training Schools for Nurses (ASSTSN). Conceived at a meeting of the 'Hospital, Dispensaries, and Nursing Section' of the International Congress of Charities, Corrections, and Philanthropy held during the 1893 Chicago World's Fair, the Society united Canadian and American administrators under the slogan celebrated by many feminists: 'organization is the power of the age, without it nothing great is accomplished'.[113] In 1907, Canadian superintendents formed an autonomous organization of superintendents, the CSSTSN (later named the Canadian Association of Nursing Education, CANE), which one year later created the Canadian Association of Trained Nurses (CATN) to promote the interests of all trained or graduate nurses. These organizations would unite in the 1920s to establish the Canadian Nurses' Association (CNA).

At the same time that international affiliation was prompting the formation of national associations, grassroots activity was inspiring local assemblies. Hospital alumnae associations, such as the Toronto General Hospital Alumnae Association founded in 1894, and urban-based groups served as foundations for the national bodies.[114] The original members of the CATN included the national society for superintendents, CSSTSN, two provincial bodies, Manitoba and Ontario, six local groups, ranging from Calgary to Montreal, and seven hospital alumnae associations.[115] The significance of the alumnae groups was suggested in 1907 when the Toronto General Hospital Alumnae Association *Journal* was transformed into the national publication, *Canadian Nurse*.[116]

Initial organizing was not always easy. Ethel Johns recalled the formative years of the Winnipeg General Hospital alumnae group. Her impression 'that there was something gallant about the attitude of these women, who met month after month only to find that few were interested enough to put in an appearance', prompted Johns to join her alumnae association.[117] The involvement of such new graduates contributed to the success of alumnae endeavours and the momentum carried. Each year a new executive was elected and active involvement of the hospital's nursing superintendent guaranteed direct communication to the hospital administration, as well as a source of information about hospital developments.[118] By 1920 alumnae associations existed for all large, and most small, hospital nursing programs in the Dominion, and new schools almost always followed suit. For an annual fee, graduates secured memberships in their alumnae society and with it the right to participate in the social, educational, political, historical, and economic activities of the association. Large numbers of active and inactive nurses contributed funds and enthusiasm for projects as diverse as sick-benefit funds, furnishings for the nurses' residence, receptions for incoming nursing superintendents, scholarships, nursing missionaries in India and China, memorials for nursing's wartime casualties, cards and flowers to sick members and their families, drama and choral groups, bedding and supplies to poor families, archival collections, and bandages and supplies for the Red Cross.[119] At monthly and annual meetings, various committees reported on their assigned projects, followed by some kind of social or educational event.

Members not in attendance at alumnae meetings were apprised of the activities of both their association and their peers through various publications. Alumnae newsletters, journals, and magazines served as important communication points for nurses working on all continents. 'Class reps' were responsible for establishing updated mailing lists of their peers and much of the alumnae energy went into recruiting and maintaining members. Recruiting began well before prospective members had completed their apprenticeships. Most alumnae associations hosted a graduation event for their school and publicized their work among the student population, hoping to generate interest before the new alumnae scattered to the four winds. Banquets held at elegant hotels such as the Hotel Vancouver or Winnipeg's Royal Alexander brought old and new graduates together to reinforce old ties and create new ones.[120]

For their part, instructors ensured that students received apprenticeship training in the system of nursing organization as well as nursing work. To provide experience in collective activities, administrators and organizational leaders endorsed the concept of student representation. Student councils were established in all major training schools, while *Canadian Nurse* reserved space for contributions devoted to descriptions of student activities. The Vancouver General student council, formed in 1918, was one of the first of such groups. Elected representatives from each class of student nurses met with the director of nursing and her supervisors to discuss the interests and needs of the nursing staff.[121]

As nurses moved away from the town or city of their Alma Mater, they benefited from fewer of the services alumnae groups offered. Thus, to unite nurses regardless of educational background, graduate nurse associations or clubs emerged in many urban areas. These groups provided services similar to those of the alumnae associations, followed the same organizational structure, and, along with many alumnae groups, were some of the earliest affiliates of the CATN.[122] Like the alumnae bodies, local graduate nurses' organizations enjoyed grassroot support from active and inactive nurses, and from local nursing administrators. The Graduate Nurses' Association of Montreal, for example, was formed in 1917 under the presidency of Grace M. Fairley, superintendent of the city's Alexandra Hospital, and secretary Mabel F. Hersey, superintendent at the Royal Victoria Hospital.[123] Local organizations continued to flourish, playing particularly important roles for women in small and remote centres.[124]

Among the earliest initiatives taken to organize provincially were those taken by Ontario nurses. Mrs Agnes Pafford, a pioneer of nursing's first generation, has been credited with forming the Graduate Nurses' Association of Ontario (later the Registered Nurses'

Association of Ontario, RNAO). According to official RNAO history, Pafford worked as a nurse only a short time before retiring into marriage, but maintained a strong interest in her occupation. Inspired by the 1901 International Council of Nurses meeting in Buffalo, New York, Pafford 'wrote personally to the Superintendent of every training school in [Ontario] on the subject of Registration, urging Alumnae organization as a necessary preliminary step, and asking for a list of graduates with whom she also communicated.'[125] Her enthusiasm prompted the inception of many alumnae associations, and in 1904 a provincial organization was 'attempted'. Its success led to chapters in regional centres, first in Hamilton (1908), and then in Brantford, Kingston, Ottawa, Owen Sound, Peterborough, and Toronto.[126]

Meanwhile, similar agitation in other regions resulted in the formation by 1920 of nine provincial bodies, each with strong ties to smaller units operating at the local level. The Graduate Nurses' Association of Nova Scotia (later Registered Nurses' Association of Nova Scotia, RNANS) was conceived in 1909. The Graduate Nurses' Association of British Columbia (RNABC) was established in 1912 by members of the Graduate Nurses' Association of Vancouver, the Victoria Nurses Club, the Graduate Nurses' Association of New Westminster, and representatives from Kamloops. In Manitoba, local groups in Winnipeg, Brandon, and, later, Flin Flon worked together to maintain the Manitoba Association of Graduate Nurses (later Manitoba Association of Registered Nurses, MARN). The Montreal group succeeded in establishing a provincial body in 1920, prompting a series of negotiations with a parallel and competing organization operating out of Quebec City.[127]

The internal structure of nurses' representational framework reflected the structure of their workplace experiences. Membership was inclusive and egalitarian. Nurses working in all three sectors of the health-care system joined associations as equals. Nursing associations recognized the fluidity of women's working lives and thus employment status was not a criterion for membership and participation. The many women who did not actively practise, either because of occupational change or marriage, and yet continued to consider themselves trained nurses, were welcomed. Alumnae associations in particular drew on the organizational skills of married women who no longer nursed for pay but who none the less remained vocal advocates of nurses' needs.[128] Whether she was engaged in a private, public, hospital, military, or industrial position, was unemployed or had retired, as long as appropriate credentials could be demonstrated, any nurse could actively participate and throughout her life share in a powerful professional and sentimental community.

Within these organizations hospital superintendents often capitalized on their institutional resources and their predictable work schedules to assume leadership positions, thereby serving as benefactresses to the nursing community. The first members of the RNANS included two private-duty nurses, two wives of prominent Halifax physicians, the superintendent of Victoria General, the superintendent of the Halifax VON, and Eveline Pemberton, owner of Restholme.[129] So, too, the 1918 RNABC council benefited from the leadership of local nursing superintendents.[130] Many hospital administrators donated their time and office space as headquarters for associational registries and meetings.[131] Conversely, rank-and-file nurses played proportionally lesser roles than their numbers suggested. Many, especially those in private duty, found that their erratic work schedules made regular attendance at monthly meetings difficult. It is also possible that some rank-and-file members felt intimidated serving as equals in organizations where their former superintendent enjoyed such prestige. Yet, despite the difference in status and influence, working nurses remained a critical power base within nursing organizations. For their part, nursing leaders recognized that rank-and-file support was necessary if their collective voice was going to carry any meaning in the broader political and economic spheres.

If nurses' organizational structure reflected the reality of the nursing work-force, so, too, did nurses' organizations struggle to shape the conditions under which those nurses laboured. Services that nursing organizations provided drew on the strategies of professional bodies such as the medical associations, on trade unions and working-class fraternal orders, and on women's organizations. Much nursing history focuses on the first of these three, in particular the efforts of leaders to win legal status for trained nurses via 'professional' registration legislation. Between 1910 and 1922, nurses in all nine provinces managed to insert some form of nursing legislation into the provincial acts, although the quality of that legislation varied significantly. Nova Scotia enacted the first nursing legislation, but that bill did not guarantee the RNANS a monopoly over establishing registries or the right to determine educational standards for schools training graduate nurses.[132] In Manitoba, the 1913 act did entrust MARN to set educational standards, but the required minimum of five beds per training institution was so low that any hospital could qualify.[133] Both Manitoba and Nova Scotia would have to wait for further amendments in the 1920s before minimum standards would be increased. Even then, registration acts in those and other provinces only empowered associations to set standards for membership in the

provincial body, and did not make membership or registration mandatory or prevent unqualified practitioners from plying their trade.
Instead, the legislation prohibited nurses who did not meet the criteria
from advertising themselves as graduate or, later, registered nurses.[134]
Provincial legislators would not permit nursing organizations puni-
tive authority over unqualified personnel 'practising nursing', such as
that granted medical associations to limit who had the right to 'practise medicine'.[135]

Second-generation nurses were not unaware that their efforts at
legislative control had fallen short. Despite their assurances that registration legislation would protect the medical profession and the
public, and despite the support of some physicians, nursing activists
confronted male medical and political élites who believed that their
patients and constituents would be better served by an unregulated
nursing marketplace. Some doctors worried that nurses were becoming 'too institutional—too mechanical'. A 1906 contributor to the
Maritime Medical News asserted that 'The "scientific study" of cases
is replacing the gentle touch, the sympathetic interest and the kindly
ministration, and the independent patient demands more heart and
less head in the woman who is to be his nurse than the hospitals of
today are supplying.' To that medical observer, granting nurses legislative authority would only exacerbate the 'problem'.

> The whole question is this: Is nursing a subordinate profession to
> medicine, or is it a separate distinct and independent profession
> which when it gets old enough, is going to sever every connection
> with medicine and set up an entirely separate science or art? We
> will state this proposition less classically: Is the tail going to wag
> the dog?[136]

Given the medical profession's representation in early twentieth-century politics, it soon became clear that the 'dog' was firmly in control.
After extensive debate, a 1919 amendment to the RNANS act was
defeated by the vote of Dr Reid, a medical doctor and MPP for Hants
County. Reid argued that the amendment, which among other things
provided for the registration of nurses who had graduated from hospital training schools of not less than thirty beds, would be a 'hardship
to the smaller training schools in Nova Scotia'.[137] Similar opposition
from 'rural legislators who felt that their small hospitals would be
adversely affected' stalled the legislative campaigns in both BC and
Ontario, while local physicians, including BC's provincial secretary,
Dr H.E. Young, lobbied to have medical doctors represented on
nurses' governing bodies.[138]

Nursing responses to these critiques reveal that leaders understood the class and gender dimension of their struggle. The 1906 RNAO bill was abandoned when proposed revisions threatened to impose masculine control. Nurses complained that 'the Council, instead of being composed of a majority of nurses, would consist of four male medical practitioners, four male members of hospital boards and seven nurses, and that all decisions whatsoever of the Council, might be annulled by the Provincial Secretary.'[139] High-profile nurses such as the VON's general superintendent, Margaret MacKenzie, tried to allay fears:

> Misunderstanding is the cause of much opposition. State registration conveys to many the idea of a trade union, a band of selfish women desiring to exclude all untrained nurses from practicing. It had been asserted on one occasion that if this act were passed a woman would be debarred from nursing her own mother if she were ill. (Laughter).[140]

This effort to dismiss with humour the monopolistic essence of nurses' legislation failed to admit that to many Canadians any limitation on womanly caring constituted, as an Ontario critic put it, 'trade unionism of the worst type'.[141] Attempting to control the market in caring for the sick contradicted the gender-typing of nursing work that characterized it as essentially feminine. Rather than winning professional privilege, nurses' campaigns resulted in class derogation.

Historians of nursing have devoted much attention to assessing, celebrating, and criticizing these early efforts at legislative authority, but they have spent considerably less energy analysing the many ways in which nursing organizations did, in fact, function like working-class organizations. To maintain membership, associations had to do more than draft legislative packages; they had to provide the kind of services that trade unions and fraternal orders offered their members. Occupational associations organized sick benefit funds and pension plans. Registries, through which nurses working in private duty could get jobs and through which nurses could establish and publicize uniform rates and hours, were also essential to working nurses' daily survival. Registrars sought to present a positive occupational image to the public and, in fact, encouraged dissatisfied clients to report poor service to the nurses' association rather than to the press or other members of the community. In addition to mediating between paying clients and graduate nurses, registrars and the associations they represented attempted to bring into their sphere of influence those unqualified nurses competing in the private health-care market. While nursing organizations sought to control who would call themselves trained or graduate nurses, most recognized that they could not eliminate informally trained or untrained practitioners from plying their trade. Instead, graduate nursing groups in the early twentieth century made provisions for unlicensed practitioners to list themselves on nurses' registries, with the hope that the distinctions between trained and untrained would become clear to the paying public.[142]

While services such as sick benefit funds and registries had parallels in working-class organizations, the means by which many of the services were carried out drew on the organizational approach of early twentieth-century women's organizations. Associations sent flowers and condolences or congratulations to members during times of family and personal tragedy or joy. Monthly meetings also provided forums for socializing with other working women, which was particularly important for private-duty nurses who often laboured in isolation, lived alone, and spent their time off work remaining available should the registrar call. When the RNANS needed to raise money for its sick benefit fund, it held a nurses' fair at the Victoria General nurses' home. The fair offered innocent entertainment appropriate to respectable, working women, including a display of dolls dressed in the various hospital uniforms, a stall of 'plain and fancy work', a fortune-teller, and a tea room, while '"Mrs Wiggs", very cleverly represented by Miss M. McDonald of the Victoria General Hospital, with her inexhaustible supply of wit and humour, and seemingly inexhaustible cabbage market, afforded endless amusement.'[143] Associations also mixed business with pleasure at their monthly meetings, but whereas trade unionists might wind up a meeting at the local tavern or a professional group at a private club, nurses brewed a pot of tea:

> After the business of the evening has been concluded there is usually a paper or talk on some subject of common interest or something of an entertaining nature planned. Then, over the cups, a colloquial few minutes are spent. In this way the busy nurse meets her sister workers, which, perhaps would happen no other way.[144]

Be it volunteerism or afternoon tea, nurses drew on aspects of women's culture in their organizational format.

Created in the era of 'first-wave feminism', when the power of women's organizations was being tested and proven on a variety of social and political issues, nursing associations built not only on elements of women's culture but also on the women's movement. Nursing's original leadership élite often came from women trained in the late nineteenth century who brought with them the strong influence of pre-suffrage feminism. National leaders like Ethel Johns credited the

'great upward surge of the woman's movement . . . dragging me unre-
sistingly into its current' for her initial involvement in nursing organizations.[145] Nursing associations generally supported, and were
supported by, feminist groups such as Local and National Councils of
Women, the YWCA, the Professional and Business Women's Club, the
University Women's Clubs of Canada, and the United Farm
Women.[146] For many such female activists nursing pioneers symbolized their goals of female independence, authority, and dedication.[147]
Nurses drew on such sympathies for support when they campaigned
to improve their status. Early nursing organizers viewed their own
activities as part of the larger feminist agenda and recognized the
need for collective empowerment of women. The concept of self-government, central to nurses' own organizations, was perfectly consistent with the larger program of reform endorsed by Canadian
feminists, who enjoyed material and political support from their sisters in nursing. The close connection between political and legislative
reform was revealed by a 1917 resolution from the RNANS recom-
mending that the Maritime group:

> . . . put themselves on record and approve of the advisability of
> granting the franchise to women of the Province of Nova Scotia.
> Knowing that this is a work in which women and men, whether
> organized for suffrage or the moral and social welfare of the peo-
> ple are interested, we decided not to dissipate our energies trying
> to form new societies, but to work as far as possible through exist-
> ing nursing organizations and other organizations of women and
> men favourable to the cause and that this committee do earnestly
> strive to bring about the cause of suffrage by working along the
> line of political education.[148]

These broader social and political campaigns for gender equity
fostered the gender consciousness of nurses within their own organizations and made nursing administrators the logical spokeswomen
for nursing issues. As such, the differential access to leadership
within nursing organizations provoked little dissent, or at least comment, from the general membership in private duty. The lessons
learned from the lengthy campaigns for provincial nursing legislation, and its attendant social legitimacy, reinforced the conclusion that
opposition to nursing self-regulation on the part of male politicians
demanded all the collective strength nurses could muster.[149] If they
wished to gain legislative self-government, nurses and their organizations could not afford to let divisions among different kinds of practitioners get out of control.

Conclusion: The Question of Occupational Identity

The apprenticeship system of hospital staffing and nursing education, the dominance of private-duty work for graduate nurses, and the network of collective forums nurses created, combined in the early twentieth century to forge a distinctive occupational identity. Nurses' sense of commonality was informed by their position within the health-care hierarchy as skilled workers subordinate to the medical profession but privileged compared to lesser-trained nurses or domestic servants. That position was strengthened by the common bond of gender, in terms of the specific legitimation of nursing as 'naturally' women's work, the standards of bourgeois femininity inculcated in apprenticeship programs, the political struggles with male doctors and legislators, and the broader gender socialization that the predominantly female nursing work-force shared. Ethnic homogeneity reinforced this common bond. As White, Anglo-Saxon or French-Canadian, and often Canadian-born women, nurses shared ethnic backgrounds that often underscored their superiority over public ward patients and public health clients.

At the same time, tensions between the occupation's élite and ordinary practitioners revealed significant differences in experience, priorities, and vision that divided nursing administrators and professional leaders from the rank-and-file. While élite members focused on improving the occupation's status through educational improvements, greater emphasis on academic credentials, and achieving 'professional' legislation, working nurses valued the skills they brought to the bedside, fair employment practices and working conditions, and the equality among practitioners that, as graduates of approved training programs, all nurses were expected to enjoy. In the American context, Melosh has characterized these distinct visions for nursing as 'professional ideology' of the élite versus 'work culture' of ordinary practitioners.

> Leaders looked outward, beyond the work experience to its social context and implications . . . and sought to improve nurses' positions within the medical division of labor. . . . Nurses on the job were . . . absorbed in the exigencies and rewards of daily work. . . . work culture includes adaptations or resistance to constraints imposed by managers, employers, or the work itself . . . [it] embodies workers' own definition of a good day's work, their own measures of satisfying and competent performance.[150]

Canadian evidence suggests that the divisions between the two groups were never as complete as Melosh discovered among

American nurses. In Canada, rank-and-file nurses signed suffrage petitions and nursing administrators fought for improved working conditions for private-duty nurses. Nonetheless, the concept of work culture shifts the historical attention away from a narrow focus on professionalizing strategies and provides a window on the experiences and attitudes of nurses on the job.

Competing visions for nursing were evident among Canada's second generation of trained nurses, but they were not, in this era, powerful enough to rupture the common occupational identity. In the buoyant health-care economy of the early twentieth century, differences among nurses were muted by the strength of gender and occupational solidarity. Gender, class, and ethnicity combined to create complex sets of loyalties and tensions at the bedside and on the ward, but the 'safety valve' of private-duty work, and the equality among graduates that it entailed, served to prevent sustained collective antagonisms from crystallizing among nurses. The occupation and its organizations were able to accommodate the two visions and to focus instead on the boundaries between trained nurses and untrained female caregivers and male medical practitioners. Only in the interwar decades, when the market in private duty reversed, would third-generation nurses have to confront growing divisions within the ranks. Even then, fundamental differences of status and experience would be tempered by nurses' shared skills and knowledge that were developed by and for second- and third-generation nurses.

3

Rituals and Resistance:
The Content of Nurses' Work,
1900–1942

Central to nurses' collective sense of self were the skills they brought to sick room, ward, and clinic. Learned by apprentices during their three years on the wards and perfected or adapted by graduates on duty as staff or private-duty nurses, the many rituals and routines that constituted nursing practice shaped nurses' workplace experiences and their position in the community. The various components of nursing work were designed by doctors, hospital administrators, and nursing educators to meet the needs of the evolving hospital and medical care system, and this they did. But nursing practice was not only a reflection of medical priorities and needs. It was also forged by working nurses themselves, for whom the precise protocols and detailed approaches that comprised nursing 'technique' helped define and defend their position within the workplace and the labour force.

The content of nursing work was not static. Over the 1900–42 years, specific therapies and procedures changed, reflecting shifts in medical science and societal expectations, but the overall approach to nursing practice remained consistent throughout. The factors influencing nursing practice that emerged in the pre-World War I years continued to inform the content of bedside care throughout the inter-war years; thus, the content of nurses' work in the first half of the twentieth century is best understood in terms of continuity rather than change. Re-evaluating the content of nurses' work from the point of view of ordinary practitioners elucidates the complex relations negotiated by patients and patient-care providers, but also offers some new insights into the broader questions of nurses' relationships to science and how historians have interpreted that relationship.

Paradigms of Practice

Historians of nursing have devoted much intellectual energy to exploring and explaining nurses' structural position within the Canadian health-care system and the organizational efforts aimed at improving that position. Much less analysis has been devoted to understanding what nurses did within that structural position. Nurses' daily practice is either addressed in terms of prescriptive educational and curricular reforms or receives cursory summary in introductory paragraphs.[1] Existing discussions do acknowledge that in the early twentieth century, nursing work was informed by four paradigms: domestic nurturing; religious devotion, especially to the Christian concept of helping the poor and suffering; military duty and discipline; and scientific medicine. Most agree, or at least infer, that the images of mother, nun, soldier, and 'the physician's hand' combined to create a subordinate occupation. According to most scholars, only in the post-World War II years have nurses gained access to the significant scientific skills needed to break their connection to domestic service, selfless religious calling, mindless adherence to military discipline, and professional subordination to medicine. Whether writing from within the occupation itself, or within women's or labour history, few authors have addressed seriously the theoretical basis of nursing work in the first four decades of the twentieth century.

Traditional histories of nursing work, often written by nursing educators or leaders, have echoed the assessment of medical history in emphasizing the close relationship between medical science and nursing. Within this 'whig' interpretation of progress, scholars have suggested that as medical science developed new strategies and weapons against disease and debility, so, too, did nurses participate in increasingly effective, technological procedures.[2] Predictably, then, authors such as Edith Kathleen Russell, the driving force behind the establishment of the University of Toronto School of Nursing, argued that nursing work in the early twentieth century was predominantly custodial and of limited therapeutic efficacy.[3] In her 1951 essay 'A half century of progress in nursing', the distinguished nursing leader characterized pre-Nightingale nursing as 'despised domestic service' and concluded that for all the dramatic changes in late nineteenth-century medicine, 'By 1900 this content had settled quickly into much domestic work, fairly simple technical skills, and even the appearance in district nursing of some social significance when the individual nurse sensed her opportunity to add this.'[4] Subsequent historical commentators concurred. As they celebrated the introduction *greater emphasis on Science of nursing after 1942 which propelled nursing from "art" to science*

of the 'wonder drugs' of the 1940s, authors such as Tony Cashman characterized the natural processes over which nurses presided in earlier decades as 'slow and inefficient'. Thus, 'the art of the nurse who would sit with a pneumonia patient for ten days, nursing him through his illness', was made 'obsolete' by the advent of scientific nursing in the post-World War II years.[5]

This distinction between the 'art' of previous eras and the 'science' of modern nursing continues to inform the analysis of nursing educators and scholars. The widely used nursing textbook *Canadian Nursing Faces the Future: Development and Change* recognized the significance of early twentieth-century health-care practice, claiming 'most of the lifesaving treatment carried out in hospitals consisted of basic nursing interventions'. But the authors were careful to differentiate nursing interventions, such as the tepid sponge or the mustard plaster, from the 'major advances in medical care which began to change nursing practice in the 1930s and 1940s'. Here the phrasing is critical. Nursing practice, such as plasters, was changed by medical advances, an analysis that distinguishes nursing from medicine but also characterizes the pre-sulfa drug era as non-scientific.[6] The 1940s and 1950s are seen as the decades in which graduate nurses took their rightful place in the curing end of the caring/curing dichotomy.

Even scholars who have examined closely the work of nurses in the pre-1940 era continue to be hesitant to claim scientific status for nurses' work 'before the age of miracles'.[7] Barbara Keddy and her colleagues at Dalhousie University posed the question, was nursing work in the inter-war decades 'scientific or was it "womanly ministering"?' They concluded that 'because of the limited amount of medical knowledge of the 1920s and 1930s . . . nursing's hand's-on technique . . . would have been considered to have been appropriately scientific for the era.'[8] According to these authors, the absence of technical apparatus during the inter-war decades handicapped the scientific practice of both doctors and nurses alike. As the 'physician's hand', nurses brought as little science to the bedside as did medical practitioners. While this analysis correctly identifies the limited technical apparatus employed by either doctors or nurses, it unfortunately conflates scientific theories, upon which modern medical practice rests, with the technological interventions that have characterized post-World War II health care. By confusing technology with science, scholarship generated within the nursing world has defined nursing practice out of the realm of the scientific and thereby failed to examine seriously the theoretical basis of nurses' work in the 1900–42 era.

More recently, women's historians have considered the question of nurses' relationship to science and confirmed the conclusions presented in the nursing literature.[9] Feminist authors have emphasized the modern health-care system's division of labour between caring and curing: doctors cure, nurses care. This 'rigid distinction', claims English historian Margaret Versluysen, was enforced in the late nineteenth century when the medical profession monopolized the 'heroic saving of the sick' and nurses were allocated 'mundane housekeeping chores'.[10] Others have stressed the devaluing of nursing work that coincided with the devaluation of women's work generally. As Canadian scholar Judi Coburn has argued, 'a certain class of men . . . took the more prestigious function of "curing" away from women, leaving them with "caring" (often indistinguishable from domestic work).'[11] According to this approach, the caring part of work should really be seen as domestic drudgery. Nurses were not ladies with the lamp, but domestic servants, performing devalued and demeaned tasks involved with maternal care, albeit in a jazzed-up uniform. Given these analyses it is not surprising that nursing has been excluded by researchers investigating the larger issue of women's relationship to science. For example, Marianne Ainley's edited collection, *Despite the Odds: Essays on Canadian Women and Science*, considers a wide range of women's 'scientific' activity ranging from botany and photography to sociology. Yet, despite this impressive effort at inclusiveness, the collection does not consider nurses, the largest single group of women who, in the twentieth century, have been mostly closely involved in scientific pursuits.[12]

Ironically, while feminist scholars have considered nursing not scientific enough, labour historians have viewed nursing as too scientific. Burdened by the assumption that until recent years claims to scientific status placed nurses in a 'professional' rather than 'worker' category, labour historians have been slow to take seriously nurses' work as work. Because nurses were relatively late in joining the labour movement and public health nurses, especially, appeared to be agents of the state devoted to detecting 'defects' in working-class children, labour historians perceived nurses, like doctors, to be citizens whose middle-class status was shaped by their control over scientific knowledge.[13] Significant exceptions to this trend are American historians Barbara Melosh and Susan Reverby, who have applied the concepts of class analysis to nursing work. Those authors have probed the contradictory effects of scientific thought on nursing practice, showing how scientific medical practice differentiated nursing skills from those of laywomen but also how the quest for standardized procedures exposed nursing to intense managerial control over daily work. Both authors emphasize the loss of control rank-and-file nurses experienced when hospital managers and nursing administrators sought to apply the principles of scientific management to American nursing.[14]

Canadian evidence substantiates that rank-and-file nurses' relationship to science was as contradictory as Melosh and Reverby claim and substantially more complex than the 'nursing as domestic caring' paradigm would have it. This complex relationship is made clear when the historical focus is shifted away from élite, and often prescriptive, sources, such as curriculum guides, textbooks, and records of nursing educators, to consider instead the records left by working nurses. Student assessment books, ward records of service, lecture notes, hand-printed notebooks, student yearbooks, and oral testimony reveal that in the first half of the twentieth century, a craft culture, fostered in apprenticeship training and nurtured by graduate nurses on the job, served to define second- and third-generation nurses in Canada. Science, in terms of both scientific medicine and scientific management and the rationalization of nurses' work, was a critical determinant in locating nurses in a subordinate position within the health-care hierarchy. Yet the very rituals and standardized protocols demanded by administrators and doctors could also be turned to working nurses' advantage, providing a set of discrete skills through which nurses could differentiate themselves from other practitioners and negotiate complex relations at the bedside.

Categories of Nursing Work[15]

The skills that all nurses were expected to possess were learned during their three-year apprenticeship on the wards of Canadian hospitals. Once acquired, these skills were the cornerstone of graduate nurses' practice, whether in private-duty care, on hospital staffs, or in public health work. During their training, students learned their repertoire of skills first in the classroom, then on the ward, with the level of responsibility and difficulty increasing as the students advanced.[16] Supervision was limited and instruction was often interrupted when external crises such as war or epidemic diverted the attention of medical and nursing lecturers and educators.[17] None the less, throughout their apprenticeship, frequent repetitions of the various routines ensured nurses' mastery of the expedient execution of assigned tasks. Nurses graduating from their training programs were expected to be competent in six categories of work. Successful acquisition of each depended on nurses' acquiring the 'language' of medicine and science as well as demonstrating what supervisors called 'executive' skills needed to organize equipment and patients in limited time and space.

One area of expertise included administrative tasks such as labelling and storing patients' personal possessions when admitted, charting and recording all patient treatment, medication, and tests, and taking stock of hospital supplies.[18] Nurses were required to print neatly all charts and correspondence, and thus the instructors evaluated students' handbooks and lecture notes as much for neatness as for accurate content.[19] Feedback on 1933 Winnipeg General Hospital graduate Violet Erickson's first 99 pages indicated that her work was 'Much improved. Would be neater underlined in red ink. Very Good.'[20] Another Winnipeg graduate, Beryl Seeman, did not expect the nursing superintendent, Kathleen Ellis, to have noticed her among the large student population. Years later, however, when Seeman had advanced into a supervisory position herself and was reintroduced to Ellis, the latter responded: 'I remember you. You had very good printing.'[21] The appreciation administrators like Ellis expressed for simple printing skills was somewhat infantilizing, but also was appropriate within the hospital's non-mechanized record-keeping system. So, too, the detailed system for carefully counting and recording all medication was necessary given the powerful painkillers, such as morphine, that were part of the regular ward-stock of pharmaceuticals.[22]

A second set of responsibilities entrusted to hospital apprentices embraced the various diagnostic tests ordered by medical staff. Tests were performed on the ward and then either sent to the laboratory for analysis or results were transcribed directly onto the patients' charts.[23] All tests required that nurses prepare the necessary equipment, complete the proper documentation identifying the type of sample and to whom it belonged, and record results on the correct chart.

A third area of nursing practice, assisting medical and surgical personnel, involved some of the most precise techniques demanded of nursing staff. Nurses were responsible for preparing patients for treatment and assisting doctors in examinations or procedures performed on a ward, or in a specialty service, like the operating room. To facilitate the efficient use of doctors' time, pre- and postoperative examinations, shavings, dressings, dietary regimens, and patient services were all assigned to nursing staff. For example, 'aspiration', a technique used to remove excess fluid from the pleural cavity, required that the assisting nurse paint with iodine the injection site and then drape the patient so that only the treatment area was visible to the doctor. She then tested the equipment, first in the service room and, once sterilized, again while the doctor was inserting the needle. If all went well neither the patient's dignity and confidence, nor doctor's time and reputation, was lost.

While these patient services were performed in concert with doctors, other tasks were performed by nurses alone. This fourth category, therapeutic nursing duties, was comprised of counterirritants, medications, and the numerous enemas, douches, and lavages designed to 'wash out' various anatomical parts. In this era before the introduction of sulfa drugs, counterirritants—a range of poultices, packs, stupes, and foments placed on the diseased or infected area— were especially important elements of nursing practice. For patients on the medical wards, mustard plasters and linseed poultices were commonly prescribed. On either medical or surgical services, real or threatened sites of infection were usually treated with foments. This latter procedure was a particularly labour-intensive one that entailed placing strips of cloth in a linen holder attached to wooden handles. Nurses lowered everything except the handles into a vat of boiling water and when the fabric was hot enough the nurse carried it to the patient's bedside, placed it on the infected site, and then covered it with more dry cloths. This might be performed up to three or four times an hour and each time the nurse had be careful to avoid burning the patient.[24]

Not all nursing responsibilities had such direct therapeutic value. The fifth area of practice, the maintenance of the ward and equipment, supported the hospital infrastructure. The tasks defined in this category often involved simply cleaning the supply room—a job students on night duty often claimed they were doing when a midnight nap was required—but also included the critical task of sterilizing the many medical appliances used in the era before disposable supplies. Rubber gloves, for instance, had to be soaked in a 2 per cent lysol solution for 20 minutes, washed, rinsed with hot then cold water, and finally dropped in boiling water for three minutes.[25] Glass and rubber items each called for equally detailed regimens for cleaning and storing. If broken or ripped, replacement costs often came out of nurses' small monthly stipend. This equipment was expected to be ready for use when tests or medical or nursing procedures were undertaken.

In addition to maintaining vital hospital supplies, nurses were responsible for cleaning and organizing the ward itself. Every day each patient's bed, nightstand, and chair had to be tidied or washed. Following a patient's discharge a specific routine was followed according to the type of ward and particular case. While nurses themselves were not responsible for laundering bedding, they did have to soak any blood-stained linens before sending them down to the laundry.[26] If the outgoing patient was an 'infectious' rather than 'clean' case, a substantially more elaborate procedure was required to sterilize bed frame, mattress, and linens in order to ready that bed for a new inhabitant.

And finally, nursing work involved the many personal service tasks of bedside care, feeding patients, assisting them with ablutions, and maintaining the cleanliness of bed and patient alike. The skills that constituted this sixth category of nursing practice combined personal and therapeutic functions. For instance, nurses not only assisted patients with morning and evening toilets and with baths, but in addition took responsibility for specific cleaning care of external genitals following a urino-genital operation to prevent post-procedural infections.[27] Of course, instructions for some procedures stressed gentility and decorum more than therapy. When a female patient was getting into the bathtub, the nurse was to give her physical support, so the patient could not slip or fall, but the nurse was not to emphasize the patient's dependency: 'If she is unable to help herself and does not do it, give some excuse and help her.' Patient sensitivities were also considered at mealtime. When feeding patients, nurses learned that 'too full a spoon or one that drips is inexcusable'. Some instructions seemed difficult for even a veteran of international affairs to follow. For example, nurses should 'never argue with a patient concerning her meals, be diplomatic rather than use force', but at the same time they were to be 'very strict and give only food that is ordered by doctor'. Similarly, nurses were told, 'do not discuss food with patient', but were also instructed to 'try and find out patient's likes and dislikes' and to 'encourage patient to masticate food well'.[28]

The degree to which students could negotiate these somewhat contradictory directives depended, in part, on where in the hospital they were working. To be fair, retired nurses insisted that treatment did not differ between private and public wards and that all patients received the same care.[29] None the less, standards of gentility were more easily met on private wards wherein an upper-class domestic decor, complete with silver flatware and china dishes, was replicated, and where the patient/nurse ratio was substantially reduced.[30] As one Winnipeg General administrator stressed, 'the service on the private wards would be generally reflected in the patronage of the Hospital.'[31] Of course, catering to private patients created its own frustrations, as nurses' popular culture revealed. The 1923 Winnipeg yearbook included the poem 'The Training', which proclaimed:

> On private flats she learned to dust,
> To wait and smile, as there you must,
> While patients tell long tales
> On public flats she learned to rush,
> On flying feet some cries to hush
> While answering distant wails[32]

Even if the content of nursing care did not differ between private and public wards, the conditions under which care was dispensed certainly did.

By the end of their three-year apprenticeship, nurses were expected to have mastered the routines and procedures involved in all six categories of work, but when students actually assumed the various responsibilities depended on the status of individual students and the shift to which they were assigned. Twelve-hour shifts dominated hospital work throughout the early twentieth century. Even in the 1920s and 1930s, when many administrators had pledged to institute the eight-hour day, the best most hospitals could achieve was a 7 a.m.–7 p.m. day shift with varying hours off in the morning or afternoon so that pupils could study and rest.[33] Night duty remained a straight twelve hours, although unless an emergency arose this shift usually involved less physically strenuous work. Isolated shifts, like nights, or specialty services, such as the operating room and maternity ward, were reserved for more experienced students. Probationers and juniors, on the other hand, were assigned more routine chores like cleaning supplies or watching patients recovering from anaesthetics. From their first days of training, students learned the value of 'system', as Vancouver General Hospital graduate Jessie Law explained. 'When you came on in the morning, one or two of you would be assigned to the service room and you would do that preliminary sterilizing and cleaning up the service room and [others] were assigned to giving out the mouth washes and wash basins.' Even the simplest of chores could prove daunting to novices. Law recalled:

> I had nightmares about that years afterwards, dumping these darn things, because there was a big wagon that you stocked up with all the wash basins and mouthwash cups and kidney basins and hot water and the mouthwash. . . . You started down the wards—they were great big wards, 25 beds at least—and you gave out all these things and got all the patients washed. And then when you collected it all, you emptied all the slops into a bucket and when you got back to the service room you had this horrendous mess to

clean up. Even panning the patients, getting people to the bathroom [was] done routinely, everybody had to be panned before breakfast and lunch and dinner and this procedure went on again before the evening meal. And of course it was all in addition to the daily bath, that happened after breakfast . . . all the tasks were task oriented like that, instead of one person doing everything you were assigned these certain jobs.[34]

By the end of their apprenticeship, however, students were expected and able to assist demanding medical practitioners with complex surgical and medical procedures.

Within each category of work, the precise skills nurses learned changed over the 1900–42 era to reflect trends and fashions in medical practice. The fate of leeching, one of medical history's more infamous techniques, illustrates the process whereby certain therapeutic procedures faded. Winnipeg General alumna Ethel Johns recalled her efforts in 1900 to manage three recalcitrant leeches:

> One night in the eye and ear ward, I was hurrying down the corridor to do the two o'clock treatments, when, to my horror, on the corrugated matting outside the door of the eye and ear operating room, I saw three leeches approaching in hideous loops. I knew they were to be applied to an incipient mastoid in the morning, and here they were, having escaped from their gauze covered jar, making for the front door and liberty. Now to me a leech is as much to be feared as a boa constrictor. Did I quail? No; I got a long pair of dressing forceps and tried force. The leeches stretched in a sickening manner, but remained adherent, firmly adherent, to the matting. I tempted them with test tubes of milk. They scorned me. At last the house surgeon came along. That dauntless youth moistened his fingers with milk, the leeches twined lovingly round them and allowed themselves to be restored without a struggle to their jar, on the top of which I placed a dinner plate and a ten-pound weight so as to keep them within bounds for the rest of the night. They looked somewhat battered—my efforts with the forceps accounted for that—but their appetite the next morning was unimpaired. True, the attending otologist commented on their scars, but was assured by my brave champion that they had 'probably been fighting during the night.' I have never forgotton that intern. I never will.[35]

Leeches remained a formal part of the hospital therapeutics until at least 1928. One Winnipeg student entered the following instructions in her 1925–8 notebook:

There are two kinds of leeches, American and Swedish. Swedish is the best. It will take 1 z [*sic*] of blood. American will take only zI [*sic*]. Kept in fresh clean water with sand in the bottom of the container. *To apply*—Cleanse skin with unscented soap. Place leech in test tube head uppermost. Place on skin. Do not leave patient as leech may crawl into nostrils or ears. If leech does not bite moisten skin with milk or prick skin till it bleeds a little. Do not handle leech too much or it will not bite. To remove leech before it is finished feeding, sprinkle it with salt. Do not use leech twice.[36]

While some apprentices may have continued to learn the secrets of leeching, by 1930 references to that therapy disappeared from student records and no mate to Johns's humorous tale was recounted in oral testimony of graduates of the 1920s and 1930s. By then, foments and 'antiseptic baths' in saline solution replaced leeching as the standard nursing treatment to relieve inflammation and to check infection.[37]

At the same time that specific therapies were being reformulated, a more fundamental shift was occurring within the paradigm of nursing practice itself. Late nineteenth-century nursing educators emphasized the significance of cleanliness, order, and morality central to nursing care. Convinced that an orderly and disciplined environment was necessary for patients to regain balanced health, nursing administrators implemented strict rules and regulations designed to make life within the hospital walls a 'moral universe'. At Victoria General in Halifax in the 1890s, for example, unless otherwise instructed by the attending physician, all newly admitted patients were immediately bathed, and throughout their stay nurses were expected to 'pay particular attention to the cleanliness of the patients, their clothing and bed clothing'. Patients were separated into male wards on the south side and female wards on the north and were forbidden from crossing into areas designated for the opposite sex or even from conversing with each other. Consuming liquor, indulging in any 'game of hazard', straying from their beds during medical rounds, loitering or 'conjugating' in lavatories or on the grounds, spitting, wearing hats on the wards, making excessive noise, using 'violent, profane or indecent language', and any act of 'insubordination' were all cause for immediate discharge. As the primary patient-care attendants, nurses were expected to enforce this patient code of conduct, as well as supervise the behaviour of all visitors.[38] The cleanliness and neatness nurses maintained on the wards symbolized the values nurses hoped to instil in patients and their families. Together, cleanliness, order, and morality provided the environmental balance necessary for patients to regain good health.[39]

As the nineteenth century drew to a close, this older therapeutic paradigm was supplanted by a new approach to patient care in which the principles of modern scientific thought took priority. In 1901, Halifax students were receiving lectures on 'Sterilization' and 'Theory of Sepsis and Antiseptic Treatment', and soon after Winnipeg General pupils attended lectures on Bacteriology and 'Historical Theories Disease', beginning with Hippocrates and Galen, up through to Pasteur and Lister.[40] By World War I, the scientific treatment of disease was well established so that military nurses were applying modern techniques in surgical care. The memoirs of World War I nurse Wilhelmina Mowat revealed that nursing practice on the front was distinctly modern. On one 'extra busy' day in the operating room at #2 Canadian General Hospital in Le Treport, France, three operations were in progress and scrub nurse Mowat was 'handling a table for two of the cases. Somehow an Officer from up the line walked right in, trench coat and all, and before anyone could get to him with a gown, he hung his cane on my sterile table! I had a complete fresh table fast and we carried on.'[41] Even if the officer corps had yet to appreciate the principles of sterile surgical conditions, the nursing staff certainly did.

From a late twentieth-century perspective, the integration of modern scientific concepts into the nursing curriculum signalled a fundamental transformation in the theoretical underpinning of nursing work. But in practice, the actual process whereby scientific theories were introduced was relatively smooth, since both approaches relied on nurses conforming to standardized method and ritualized practice. Nursing educators were able to graft the new routines demanded by the germ theory and surgical procedures onto the older uniformity and order upon which hospital life had been built. Indeed, as historian of medicine Jim Connor has suggested, the regimes of antisepsis and sterilization wrought by the germ theory and Lister's surgical techniques may have captured the public and medical imaginations precisely because they spoke to social preoccupations with purity and virtue.[42] That modern theories of disease could coexist with older approaches to health was illustrated in a 1924 Montreal General Hospital student assignment on 'Hygiene and Sanitation' that took the form of a letter to Florence Nightingale. The 'letter' expressed an approach to hygiene consistent with Nightingale's environmentalist views. Prescribing for nurses a daily bath, well-cleaned teeth, feet, nails, and hair, and plenty of sleep, sunshine, good food, and pure water, the student maintained: 'It is really necessary that a nurse should pay more attention to her personal hygiene [than] perhaps any other person.' From personal hygiene flowed similarly attentive care of patients. Although the student's prescribed personal and patient hygiene conformed to nineteenth-century approaches to nursing, the student defended her regime using twentieth-century concepts of disease causation. The student explained that 'constantly during the performance of her daily duties she is in close contact with practically all kinds of bacteria or disease germs, and not only is she in great danger of infection herself, but there is the possibility also of others becoming infected through her carrying germs of various diseases.'[43] The integration of theoretical approaches was physically manifest in nurses' uniforms. In the late nineteenth century, the uniform represented the cleanliness and social status of the newly trained nurses. In the early twentieth century, the specific routines demanded by the germ theory and scientific management were symbolized in the regimentation of dress required of apprenticing nurses.

The Germ Theory Meets Scientific Management

Scientific principles of the early twentieth century influenced nursing in two specific ways. First, nursing practice in this era must be defined and described as scientific in that it was based on the theoretical understanding and practical application of the germ theory of disease.[44] The historical and theoretical education students received was accompanied by detailed instruction into the application of antiseptic and aseptic technique. Antiseptic surgical technique, 'a system to fight bacteria already in the wound' developed by Joseph Lister, is the best known of the two.[45] Perhaps more significant was aseptic (or aeseptic) technique, which ensured that the patient did not acquire any new bacteriologically based afflictions after admission for whatever health problem the patient already had. Asepsis was particularly important for the public wards of up to 40 patients, all of whom were suffering from different problems, and all of whom potentially might introduce new and dangerous diseases into the hospital environment. Medical and nursing attendants alike could be confident that if they followed aseptic technique they would not become a source of cross-infection.[46]

For nurses, aseptic technique demanded repeated applications of soap, water, and, to a lesser degree, alcohol. It was also labour intensive. The protocol for assisting with a surgical incision illustrates that any procedure that created a wound, and therefore a potential site of infection, necessitated the 'strictest aeseptic technique' from nursing staff.[47] The anatomical region to receive the incision first had to be washed with 'plenty of hot water and soap' and then a 'sterile bundle' of necessary equipment was taken to the bedside on a sterile tray. The nurse then screened the patient, unfolded the bundle, and, leaving one corner of the cloth over the contents of the bundle, transferred with sterile forceps the equipment from the tray to the table. She then draped the patient's bedding appropriately, scrubbed her own hands for five minutes, returned to the patient, and draped the anatomical area with a sterile drawsheet and towels, all the while taking care not to contaminate her fingers. She scrubbed the anatomical area three times with sponges appended to forceps, first using green soap and water, then ether, then alcohol, and finally applied a sterile towel or dressing and bandaged it in place. By carefully following this procedure nurses created a sterile region in which surgeons made their incision.[48]

To create and preserve aseptic conditions, nurses had to execute a carefully delineated and precise set of steps established for each task. The elaborate procedure for administering a hypodermic needle exemplifies this process. Nurses prepared for hypodermic injections by setting up a small tray with the medication, the alcohol lamp, matches and spoon, and a series of sterile jars containing alcohol, sterile water, sponges, needles, and the syringe. The 17-step process is worth reproducing in its entirety to illustrate the interconnections among the various categories of nursing tasks. Nurses learned to:

1. Have medication ready
2. Test your needle
3. Place needle with stilette in spoon and cover with water
4. Boil over lamp 2 min
5. Place cover over wick
6. Rinse out barrel of syringe
7. Draw amount of water required into syringe
8. Discard water remaining in spoon
9. Attach needle to syringe and remove stilette
10. Place tablets on spoon and dissolve with water in syringe
11. Draw prepared fluid into syringe, taking up last drop
12. Expel air from syringe
13. Pick up sponge on point of needle and replace tray in cupboard
14. Cleanse the area, make a cushion of flesh and insert quickly
15. Withdraw slightly and insert fluid slowly
16. Withdraw needle quickly, massage area gently with a circular motion
17. Chart time, medication and initials immediately after giving drug, and mark off in order book[49]

The hypodermic example demonstrates the relationship between the specific therapeutic technique—injecting a medication into a patient—and the regime for non-therapeutic duties—maintenance of wards and equipment. Not only did nurses depend on the aseptic technique of the injection itself, they also relied on the aseptic preparation of basic ward equipment such as jars and water. Thus, the step-by-step procedures involved in the domestic tasks of ward cleaning and maintenance, usually interpreted by historians as evidence of nurses' subordinate domestic status, take on new importance when seen as part of a larger system of asepsis for which nurses were responsible.

The above example also illustrates the second influence of science on nurses' work: scientific management brought to science itself. Pioneered in the late nineteenth century by Frederick Winslow Taylor, scientific management was designed to establish managerial control over industrial production. Taylor and the 'efficiency experts' who followed him studied particular tasks, broke them down into their component parts, and, with the help of their trusty stopwatches, determined the fastest method of performing each part. Scientific management enhanced employer control over production in several ways. It allowed employers to increase production per worker-hour by assigning one small part of production to a worker who would repeat that task throughout his or her shift. The division of labour ensured that employees could be easily trained and therefore easily replaced. Most important, perhaps, was that by dividing conception from execution scientific management increased employers' knowledge and authority over how goods were made. Appropriating the term 'scientific' for a process that in fact was not rooted in any theory of science served to legitimize managerial control over production, which in turn strengthened employers' position in the struggle over workplace control.[50]

The influence of scientific management on nursing procedures in the inter-war decades is clearly evident. Each feature of nursing practice was subdivided into its component steps, and students were drilled in the precise execution of each step. Conceptual authority over how a particular procedure should be executed remained in the hands of doctors, administrators, and educators, while nursing students and staff remained responsible for executing the prescribed tasks according to the standard curriculum. Thus, the elaborate delineation of precise execution was provided for procedures that did not appear to depend on a 'scientific principle' such as asepsis. For example, bedmaking, a task with which all raw recruits to nursing schools would be familiar, was rationalized. Whatever system students had applied to the chore in their own homes, as probationers they learned that when stripping a bed, the table and chair first had to be moved away from it. The nurse was then instructed to place the pillow on the chair with the closed end of the pillow case towards the door, loosen the linen, and fold it in quarters, beginning at the foot of the bed and working up to the head. Detailed instructions of this kind were provided for the remaining elements of the bedmaking process.[51] So, too, was the art of providing a hot-water bottle turned into a science. Rather than teaching nurses to test the heat of a bottle by touch, instructors insisted that novices measure with a thermometer each bottle and administer it only when it was 130°F.[52]

The establishment of standardized procedures for even the simplest of tasks obviously served other agendas than those necessitated by scientific theories of disease. During this era, rules for hospital nurses, on and off duty, were influenced by several powerful models of social organization, such as the convent and the military.[53] But in the realm of daily practice, the most dynamic influence on the structure and content of nursing work was 'scientific' or rationalized production that had proven so successful in the industrial sector. Even the imagery of the 25- to 40-bed wards, with each bed equidistant, each patient's table and chair placed next to their beds, each patient covered in identical bedding, with all blankets tucked tight at the end and sides, evoked mental images of assembly lines.[54] Not surprisingly, hospital vocabulary matched the interior design in its allusions to industrial production. Institutional administrators invoked the language of 'efficiency', 'standardization', and 'per cent capacity'.[55] In 1921, Winnipeg General Superintendent Stephens included in his annual report 'an analysis of the work of the year, that is, what might be called "the production sheet" of the Hospital'.[56] Like their counterparts in capitalist enterprises of the day, hospital administrators routinized staff procedures to 'produce' healthy patients effectively and efficiently, but also to overcome the institutions' questionable reputation, all while operating on limited budgets.

The reasons why hospital administrators and medical practitioners created and endorsed the rigid, routinized, rationalized set of nursing procedures is obvious. Rationalization of technique ensured that the small staffs of RNs could supervise the large numbers and high turnover of student nurses. The growing numbers of patients could move in and out of the hospital without getting their charts, their diagnoses, their results, their treatments, their personal possessions, or even their babies mixed up or lost. Standardized printing techniques

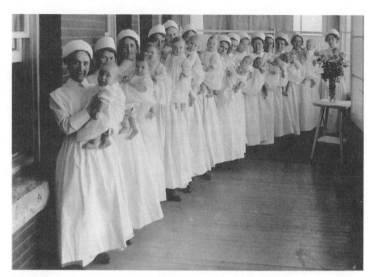

Throughout the early decades of the twentieth century, hospital administrators, confronting dramatic increases in patient demand, often borrowed efficiency techniques of industrial production. Images such as this 1914 photograph of student nurses holding babies born at Winnipeg's Grace Hospital served to remind the public that hospitals were capable of 'mass producing' even reproduction (PAM Foote Collection #1522).

allowed the modern hospital to generate administrative records accounting for patient therapy. Precise procedures for diagnostic tests, for assisting medical staff, and for performing therapeutic nursing duties guaranteed that the institution promoted its reputation as an appropriate location for medical treatment. The maintenance of ward and equipment meant that nurses 'produced' supplies and equipment that were not purchasable. Bedside nursing defended the institutions' reputation of gentility and decorum, which was necessary to attract private, paying patients. Therapeutically, not only did nurses provide doctors with an inexpensive, skilled, and subordinate labour force, but, more importantly, nurses ensured that once patients were admitted to the institution they were safe from possible cross-infections and would leave in better rather than in worse health. That was, after all, the point.

Indeed, the nursing staffs of Canadian hospitals during the 1900–42 era served their masters well. It is for this reason, perhaps, that feminist historians, committed to critiquing gender asymmetry, have been hesitant to examine seriously nurses' relationship to science in this era. Nurses may have assisted the medical profession in its quest for scientific therapy, but scientific management ensured that nurses had little or no control over the content of their work. Yet, when the actions of nurses themselves are examined more closely, they appear to have had greater agency in implementing and enforcing the ritualized system of patient care. Certainly, nursing educators and administrators were key players in reshaping nursing practice to conform to medical and industrial sciences. Occupational leaders, often superintendents of hospital nursing schools, embraced scientific management techniques as part of their larger professionalizing strategy. Precise and standardized methods of executing tasks consolidated nursing's position as critical to efficiently run hospitals while strengthening nurses' claim to a unique 'professional' body of knowledge.[57]

Like nursing élites elsewhere, occupational leaders and educators in Canada paid keen attention to industrial management strategies. In 1927, the International Council of Nurses invited Percy S. Brown, deputy director of Geneva's International Management Institute, to explain the advantages scientific management had to offer the nursing world. His speech, reproduced in *Canadian Nurse* as 'A Few Facts about Scientific Management in Industry', pointed out that nurses 'do a little of everything from scrubbing floors to nursing', whereas in factory production 'we would certainly not use a skilled tool maker who has spent years in acquiring a special technique, and who is compensated very satisfactorily for this skill that he has acquired in scrubbing floors, or doing general janitor work.' He also noted that nurses spend 'confusing, tiring, and wasteful' effort walking around the ward or sick room. Brown suggested that nurses experiment, tracing their movements with coloured string and then 're-routing to shorten the path, using another coloured string for this purpose.' After several different routes had been tried, he suggested, the most efficient use of nurses' time and energy could be obtained.[58]

Brown's strategies for industrial production did not, in fact, translate that easily into the nursing workplace. Nursing educators barely had time to instruct students in the basics of patient care, let alone monitor the flight paths of individual apprentices. And, contrary to Brown's analogy, the nurses performing 'janitorial' duties were junior nurses who were not yet highly paid skilled toolmakers. However unrealistic, the intention of such strategies was appealing to administrators who were trying to meet the seemingly incessant patient demand for services. That demand was intensified by the increased workload aseptic technique required. As Ella Forrest, supervisor of Vancouver General's Infectious Disease Department, reminded her colleagues across the country: 'The one great drawback to medical asepsis is its time-consuming properties and the increased staff, as it requires almost double.' Forrest acknowledged that 'whenever a necessity for "speeding up" occurs, our technique is almost sure to suffer.'[59] Under such conditions, other means of reducing nurses' labour were surely welcome, if not always directly applicable.

If nursing supervisors were not able to benefit from the specific suggestions proposed by efficiency experts such as Brown, they did demand standardized and routinized modes of behaviour from their students and staff. Institutional records of ward service reveal that nursing administrators expected student and staff nurses to demonstrate an aptitude for managing others, and, thus, quality nursing was often equated with quality of administrative and supervisory prowess. Apprentices who 'maintained good order', could 'take serious responsibility', and 'managed the wards well' were judged to have 'superior executive ability'. Accordingly, Victoria General student Margaret Jones was considered a 'very capable nurse, fairly good manager', but paled by comparison to Libby Armstrong, who showed herself to be a 'splendid executive, [who] always maintained good order'. Martha Pritchard had a somewhat checkered career. She was suspended for being 'impertinent' to a head nurse, considered 'temperamental and rather erratic', noted to 'not take criticism very well', and judged 'not fond of doing actual practical work'. None the less, her consistent performance as a 'good executive' prompted her superintendent of nurses to conclude that Martha was 'rather imaginative . . . [and had a] keen sense of humor'. Students like Ruth McCurdy might have made potentially fatal mistakes such as 'opening [the] door to infectious cottages' in her first year, but by the end of her training this 'adaptable and conscientious' nurse was considered of executive quality and 'remained on staff after Graduation'.

By contrast, nurses who did not display managerial talents received fewer accolades and often only begrudging recognition that they provided excellent bedside care. Harriet Ives proved to be a 'most reliable and trustful nurse, but not a good manager of large wards'. Jessie Thurston was assessed as a 'good student' and 'conscientious nurse' and Mary Pollock was recognized as a 'willing worker', but the limited 'executive ability' displayed by those apprentices led the nursing superintendent to conclude they 'would probably be successful on private duty'. Emphasis on executive ability revealed that superintendents of nursing were looking for potential forewomen to join the executive ranks supervising the efficient execution of each new batch of junior nurses. Those without executive responsibility were relegated to the ranks of private duty.[60]

Students were rewarded for demonstrating strong managerial skills on the wards, but they were also expected to internalize the values of industrial work discipline and female submissiveness, to be managed as well as to manage. Halifax pupil Eliza Sellars was evaluated for being a 'very capable nurse' but 'rather difficult to manage at times'. Apparently Miss Sellars had been a 'troublemaker' during the first part of her training, making it 'most unpleasant' for her superintendent of nursing. Classmate Catharine Roddick was accredited with taking 'good care of patients', but character flaws such as showing 'impertinence to night supervisor' led her to be characterized as 'difficult to discipline'. Commentary on Pearl Matheson's work revealed that administrators often saw the ability to manage others as a reflection of internal discipline. Pearl performed poorly in her first two years, but by graduation had proven herself a 'resourceful, industrious rapid worker . . . [with] neat appearance, has a sense of humor, possesses initiative and is quite observing', as well as a nurse possessing 'good executive ability'.[61]

Nursing educators' preoccupation with imposing discipline and conformity on nurses, and through nurses on patients, raises questions about the usefulness of the term 'caring' to describe nursing work. In a controversial article, 'Laying Claim to Caring: Nursing and the Language of Training, 1915–1937', Tom Olson has observed that terms usually associated with caring, such as 'nurturing' or 'comforting', were rarely used by the hospital supervisors he studied. Olson points out that 'the receptive and nurturing qualities associated with caring are considered the natural domain of women generally' and thus nurses are assumed to have placed those values at the core of their work. Instead, the nursing educators Olson studied defined good nursing as '*handling, managing,* and *controlling* individuals, as well as situations.' As a result, argues Olson, in spite of the authority inherent in nurses' management of patients, the 'action, force, and pragmatism' successful nurses required remained hidden, 'obscured by explanations that seem to have a better fit with accepted understandings of work and gender.'[62] Olson's argument is especially apt when considering the priorities of nursing educators and administrators as revealed in records of ward service. When nursing supervisors included on student records comments like 'kind to patient but not capable', the significance of specific skills over more generalized feminine compassion was made clear.[63] It is less clear that rank-and-file practitioners shared the values of their superiors. Many apprentices and graduates chafed under the oppressive regimes established by their superiors, resisting specific rules as well as the standardized protocols more generally. Evaluations for Halifax VON nurses exemplified the tensions over expectations and behaviour that could emerge. Like their institutional counterparts, public health supervisors demanded that staff nurses be dependable, trustworthy, and skilful, but also personally tidy, with 'desirable' manners, disposition, and deportment at work and in the nurses' residence. Accordingly, Marion Hatfield did not receive her VON certificate of postgraduate training because of 'undesirable language . . . [her] general behaviour [was] offensive.' Nurse Curtis considered the night work too strenuous and 'seemed very nervous'. Others were described as 'a good worker, but very sensitive' and as lacking 'enough energy to be a success'. Evelyn Scott resigned her VON position because she was not willing to live in the nurses' home. Nurse Main resigned following her 'insolent correspondence between the boarding house, herself, and the Members of the Committee and the Superintendent.'[64] Resistance was often less direct. Many nurses rejected the conformity and standardization of nursing practice by pursuing careers in private-duty nursing where they faced neither hospital superintendents nor public health supervisors.[65]

Rejecting the constraints of hospital life did not mean, however, that rank-and-file nurses abandoned the scientifically defined practice they learned there. Evidence from nurses who trained and worked in the 1900–42 era suggests just the opposite. While some nurses did resent the lack of creativity their training permitted, by and large the women who constituted the second and third generations of Canadian nurses accepted and endorsed what they termed their 'technique', the various routines invoked for various procedures. Rather than interpret nurses' attitudes as evidence of complicity in their own subordination, or as a reflection of their uncritical acceptance of leaders' professionalizing strategies, detailed examination of nurses' daily work reveals that while science—both in terms of scientific medicine and scientific management—may have served medical authorities well, it also helped nurses define and defend their position in the workplace and the marketplace. The rituals of nursing practice that apprentices learned were the foundation of a distinct approach to patient services that accommodated both caring and curing.

Nurses' Technique and the Parameters of Daily Practice

The specific rituals of their practice empowered nurses to define for themselves what constituted good nursing. Rather than place nurses on one side or another of the care/cure dichotomy, this definition empowered nurses to integrate caring and curing in daily tasks. Domestic and therapeutic functions were embedded in even the simplest of duties, such as making a bed. A carefully made bed promoted the uniformity of ward presentation (highly valued by nursing supervisors) and ensured that patients looked respectable and well attended when receiving their medical or familial visitors. But a carefully made bed also prevented patients from acquiring bedsores, a 'form of ulcer due to pressure', which were cardinal sins in nursing practice.[66] Given the length of time some patients spent at the hospital and the length of time patients stayed in bed following hospital procedures, keeping a patient comfortable was not always easy.[67] Patients might develop bedsores from 'indirect' causes, such as old age or illness, or from 'direct' causes, such as 'wrinkled bed linen, crumbs, lack of proper care and cleanliness, [and] continued pressure', but in either case 'prevention' was the surest treatment.[68] A carefully made bed and an evening massage went a long way towards preventing bedsores and promoting a good night's sleep.[69] Not only did such preventive care aid the patient's recovery, it also guaranteed that nurses did not have to participate in the long and laborious procedures necessary to heal bedsores once they erupted. Given the therapeutic regimens of the day, a well-made bed was central to pre-empting ailments and the accompanying curative labour.

Integrating caring and curing was particularly important to nurses since much of their work entailed performing a number of functions at once. Military nurses in World War I, whose labours were concentrated on surgical care of wounded soldiers, at the same time had to manage the vast number of casualties that at times poured into the front-line medical hospitals. Canadian Medical Army Corps (CMAC) nurse Wilhelmina Mowat recalled: 'We worked hard day and night when there was a big push on. With stretchers on the ground all over the place, one could do very little, give a hypo, light a cigarette or check for any tourniquets that might have been overlooked in the confusion.'[70] In those chaotic circumstances, doing 'very little' in therapeutic terms still required significant nursing labours to ensure that no soldier was overlooked. In private-duty work, nurses had the added responsibility of preparing the patients' meals, a task that often extended into more substantive household chores. A 1932 *Canadian*

Nurse article illustrated the multiplicity of tasks required of nurses by describing the daily labours of a private attending an influenza patient. Having prepared the patient's noon meal, the nurse now faced a sink full of dishes, but before those could be done the coal supply needed replenishing and the nurse descended into the basement to wrestle with the furnace.

> At this time the doctor arrives, and on the way to the front door she must transform herself from a fiend of the lower hell into a ministering angel! In the sickroom she listens politely to the doctor's cheerful remarks, and memorizes his instructions carefully, wondering at the same time if he will go before the things on the stove begin to boil over. He probably leaves two prescriptions to be filled out 'right away,' and she enters into a rapid-fire calculation with the clock and decides that it cannot be done before dinner.[71]

Under such conditions, the nurse assumed the position of surrogate wife, and, like female heads of households, nurses found it difficult to limit the demands placed on them. Such conditions frequently prevailed in rural districts, where ancillary domestic assistance was not available. Whether in town or country, asserting specific routines could, at worst, help nurses get all the tasks asked of them done or, at best, place boundaries on the number of household functions they were willing to assume.[72]

At the same time, the unpredictability of health-care work dictated that nurses had to be prepared to extend well outside the parameters of accepted practice to assume temporarily the duties of medical practitioners, particularly in services such as obstetrics. Under normal circumstances, the nurse assisted the intern or private practitioner to manage the birth and then provided postpartum care for mother and child back on the ward or in the home once the doctor had left. Nursing educators provided students with thorough instructions pertaining to prenatal and postnatal care of mother and child, preparing a sterile area in which the delivery could occur safely and recognizing the various pathologies and difficulties that might occur during labour. What was missing in nurses' education was training in the actual delivery. The 'Confinement Procedure' the Margaret Scott Nursing Mission provided students leapt from the point where the nurse had all the instruments sterile and ready to the point where she diapered and wrapped the newborn. The only reference to the critical intermediate step—delivery—was that 'if time is not limited and patient not too distressed, a sponge bath is advisable.'[73] Yet despite this obvious gap in their education, in both home and hospital births,

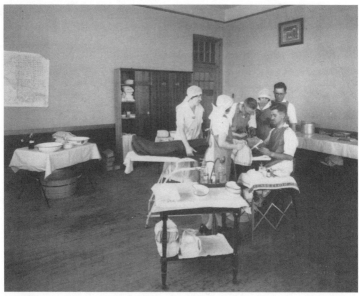

Graduate nurses could expect to practise their technique in a variety of settings, such as the impromptu surgery set up for the travelling medical clinic in 1920s rural Alberta (National Archives of Canada C-029449).

nurses were never certain that medical assistance would arrive on time. For example, enemas were commonly given to parturient women as a natural method to induce labour, a therapy that often had more rapid effects than predicted. Isabel Cameron recalled that doctors expected to be in attendance 'but maternity work is very uncertain' and deliveries would sometimes occur on the ward, rather than in the case room, and before medical staff could be summoned.[74] Even more worrisome were the occasions when attending physicians failed to arrive to preside over home deliveries. One Colchester County, Nova Scotia, nurse learned that lesson when working for a local woman pregnant with her third child. The routine pre-partum enema prompted the unexpected onset of rapid labour: 'It was a regular surprise. I was in a lather of sweat when the doctor got there. . . . if ever I give an [enema] again, should like to be better prepared for surprises.'[75] The frequency with which nurses were required to assume medical duties in such emergencies led some nurses to wish that more substantive obstetrical training had been provided.[76]

Good technique also included a certain degree of innovation to re-create the appropriate conditions of nursing when providing home care. Long-time VON employee Florence Paulson carried with her at all times her black bag. Its contents, including alcohol, forceps, aprons, and rubber gloves, permitted her to create a small sterile field within a client's kitchen and thus execute a specific procedure with-out the threat of infection.[77] Improvisation included making needed equipment, since items like Q-tips and gauze pads were not readily available in many rural areas.[78] In rare instances, nurses went well beyond the creation of everyday supplies to create medical equip-ment. BC nurse Marjorie Leonard was one such innovator who designed and patented several inventions, primarily related to colon health.[79]

As well, nursing technique included functions that extended beyond that of medical therapy and, indeed, beyond the life of the patient. Paradoxically, the 'care of the dead' integrated all the admin-istrative, therapeutic, and proprietary elements of nursing technique. Immediately after a patient ceased to breathe the nurse began an elab-orate set of steps designed to facilitate the smooth transition of the corpse from the hospital to the morgue or funeral home. The nurse first confirmed her unofficial diagnosis with an intern and then noti-fied the attending physician. Once family members had left the bed-side—having been 'treated with kindness and courtesy'—the nurse contacted the admitting office to arrange for removal of the body. Assembling the necessary equipment at the bedside 'as when giving bath', the attendant straightened the body out on the bed and closed the deceased's eyes. Jewellery was removed and the patient's valu-ables were listed on the 'value card'. The nurse then washed the body, hands, and face, using ether to remove any marks, and then redressed any wounds. The nurse, or the orderly if the deceased was male, used gauze to pack the body's orifices and to tie the legs together, the jaw shut, and the arms crossed. If the patient had died from an infectious disease, Lysol was used to wash the body and forceps were used to pack the orifices. As part of the final toilet, the nurse then inserted any false teeth, lubricated lips and eyelids, and arranged the patient's hair, combing and braiding it or 'if in a home do the hair in the usual way'. A tag stating the full name, ward, date, and cause of death was attached with bandages to the wrist and neck, and the body was wrapped in a clean sheet.

At that point an orderly removed the corpse and, when the hall was cleared of any living patients, the deceased was removed from the ward with 'dignity and respect'. The administrative duties of the nurse then continued. The patient's chart was completed with details of the time and cause of death, valuables and value card were sent to the cashier, and the list of clothes and any other belongings were sent to the admitting office together with a bundle containing any possessions. Thus, even in managing deceased patients, nurses laboured to ensure the dignity of the patient, guarantee the bureaucratic efficacy of the hospital, maintain aseptic conditions on the ward, defer to the diagnosis of the doctor, and comfort the survivors.[80] As the protocol for 'care of the dead' illustrates, the scientific underpinning of nurses' work—the many rituals of good technique—did not place nursing on one side or the other of the caring/curing dichotomy, but rather science permitted nurses in the early twentieth century to resolve that dichotomy. For nurses caring was curing.

Good technique not only facilitated self-definition, it also ensured self-protection. Careful adherence to the many steps involved in each procedure protected nurses from exposure to dangerous diseases. In an era when illnesses that are now cured easily were deadly, nursing technique was particularly important to practitioners providing bedside care. Nurses recognized that the most dangerous patients were those being treated for one affliction but also carrying other undiagnosed diseases. Medical and nursing commentators throughout the inter-war decades decried the high frequency of tuberculosis among nursing personnel, while many hospital training schools employed medical and nursing personnel just to treat institutional staff.[81] As part of this preventive strategy, students learned that the study of bacteriology was important for both theoretical and practical reasons. Nurses were expected to understand the 'habits and characteristics of the organisms . . . [that is] the living world of germs around us' not only so that attendants could 'intelligently follow the progress of the disease' but also to 'protect' themselves.[82] Good technique also allowed nurses to prevent accidents such as burns and cuts or orthopedic problems such as strained backs and sore feet.[83]

Students like Myrtle Crawford learned the hard way the value of good technique. Crawford contracted mumps while nursing a mumps victim at the King George, Winnipeg's infectious diseases hospital affiliated with Winnipeg General. As she recalled, 'I'm short and in trying to lift [the woman] I was very close to her and she coughed right in my face.' The young apprentice landed in the hospital for two weeks, during which time her supervisor asked if Crawford would consent to being used as part of a teaching clinic. Crawford agreed, and shortly thereafter the supervisor brought a group of student nurses 'to see this nurse who had gotten mumps'. When asked, 'did you wash your face with soap and water immediately afterwards', Crawford responded that it had not occurred to her, whereupon the supervisor seized the didactic moment and pronounced, 'so you see it's your own fault you got these mumps'.[84] Whether or not the supervisor's unsympathetic analysis would be borne out by a systematic study of cross-infections, such stories signify nurses' shared confidence in the preventive power inherent in standardized procedures. Retired nurses acknowledged the danger of infectious diseases, such as tuberculosis or diphtheria, and often had classmates who fell prey to such ailments, but they also credited their good health to good technique.[85] For their own protection, nurses embraced scientific explanation for the cause of, and the solution for, communicable diseases.

Nursing technique empowered practitioners in a third way. By providing a clear definition of their job technique nurses had some grounds on which to defend themselves against unreasonable demands by doctors, patients, or administrators. Adherence to specific rituals offered nurses one set of limits with which to resist unfair demands or criticisms. Unlike workers in factory production, personnel in service sectors like health care had to contend not only with supervisors but also with an animate 'product', the patient. As Susan Porter Benson has argued in her history of American saleswomen, service work involved social relations distinct from those in industrial work. According to Porter Benson, in department stores 'the two-way interaction between workers and managers became a complex triangle of saleswomen, managers, and customers.' If the managers and customers 'exerted unified pressure' the saleswoman held little workplace authority, 'but when she could play one off against the other she could create new space for herself on the job.'[86] For nurses, similarly complex workplace relations involving worker (nurse), doctor, patient, and administrator demanded an even stronger adherence to occupational boundaries and limits.

Nurturing good relations with patients was critical to nurses' daily work, and practitioners would sometimes bend the rules quite far to facilitate patient comfort. Martha Riggs, a nurse from Halifax's Victoria General, recalled a patient who, contrary to hospital rules, took snuff. Riggs kept the patient out of trouble by hiding the snuff and its symptoms from the head nurse.[87] In return, compliant patients could help nurses get their work done on time or avoid discipline from superiors. For instance, apprentices appreciated the strategy of one patient who could not tolerate the hospital mandate that all covers had to be tucked in on three sides of the bed. The patient would allow the apprentices to make his bed 'to code' and wait until the supervisor had made her rounds before kicking the covers loose, thereby saving the student nurses the extra work of remaking his bed in front of their superior. The registrar of Montreal's Nursing Service Bureau received a letter in 1938 from a satisfied customer. The Bureau had supplied a nurse to a 'frantic father' and 'harassed mother' who were coping with a newborn. The nurse 'arrived at ten or thereabouts, took over the baby, my husband and myself and restored a calm that has been with us ever since in our household.' Central to the nurse's success was 'the wonderful way in which she established our baby's routine'. The letter concluded with a request that the nurse 'gets some good cases. We want her to be available when we're ready for her again. Our baby's a changed being since she came.'[88]

Not all patient-nurse relations were characterized by such reciprocity or goodwill, as some of the most forceful forms of conflict could occur between nurses and uncooperative or unhappy patients. Dissatisfied patients complained directly to hospital administration or nursing associations, demanding that nurses be eliminated from staffs or registries. In 1933, a Kings County, Nova Scotia, man wrote the Registered Nurses Association of Nova Scotia registrar to complain about the treatment his father had received at the hands of a graduate nurse and to petition that the nurse's diploma be revoked.[89] Other times, conflict erupted at the bedside. For example, Winnipeg apprentice Ingibjorg Cross once received instructions to treat a patient with an infection by applying foments to an infected area every 15 minutes during the night. Cross did so, each time being careful not to wake the patient. The next day the doctor mentioned the foments to the patient, who replied that he had received no such treatment. In front of all the other patients, the doctor promptly questioned Cross regarding her alleged negligence. Her defence, that she had followed the prescribed treatment, was corroborated by the other patients who reported that every time they had woken in the night they had witnessed Cross dutifully applying her foments. Somewhat annoyed, the doctor instructed Cross to continue her treatment, but to wake the patient for every procedure. The tactic worked and Cross recalled that the exhausted recipient of her nocturnal care 'begged me to quit. . . . he had [learned] his lesson'.[90]

Some conflicts with patients had more violent resolutions. Myrtle Crawford's father had never been pleased with her decision to enter nursing, so she did not tell him about her experiences of being physically attacked by patients. During one night shift, a deluded patient grabbed her and tried to pull her into bed. She was saved by an orderly, who insisted that she report the incident. Crawford suspected he regretted his advice when the night superintendent '"rewarded him" by telling him that [Crawford] was not to go into that ward again and he had to look after it entirely.' On another occasion, Crawford was patrolling a dimly lit ward during her night shift.

I was just going down the hall and I was carrying my flashlight when he came darting out of his room and grabbed me by the throat and he had me down on my knees by my throat and I couldn't call out or anything, and the orderly happened to come down the hall at that particular time and put him back in his room.[91]

Crawford later determined that the World War I veteran had mistook her flashlight for a gun.

The survivors of such incidents usually considered them humorous in retrospect, and much nursing mythology rests on the bizarre events often occurring on night duty. As an intermediate on night duty, Vancouver General student Cali Dunsmuir was assigned to a patient who was recovering from an anaesthetic. He had been in a bed in the hall before the operation and following it was returned to the ward still anaesthetized. Dunsmuir was carrying out her responsibility of 'watching' him until he safely came out of the anaesthetic. As he did, the groggy patient asked the nurse where he was. Trying not to disturb the other patients on the ward, the nurse whispered: *'You're on the ward.'* The patient sat straight up, looked down the uniform row of sleeping patients on the moonlit ward, and exclaimed: *'In the morgue?!'* and then tried to escape. The nurse leapt up, held him down in his bed, and with the help of the night supervisor managed to convince the patient that he had not been incorrectly proclaimed dead.[92]

Such shared plight and the knowledge that emergency situations would bring rapid assistance from graduate staff bred among apprentices great loyalty to their nursing superiors. Margaret McGillvray, a night supervisor at Winnipeg General Hospital, was a favourite of students because of her calm in the face of such crises, although experiences such as the one recounted by Mary Shepherd must have pushed women like McGillvray to her limits. Shepherd had been assigned night observation on the 'noisy' ward when a patient escaped out the window. Shepherd ran to the door and rushed out after him, but halfway across the street she realized she had left her 24 other patients alone and gave up pursuit. Fortunately, the driver of a passing car caught and returned the errant patient, so while the orderlies, some nurses, and Miss McGillvray united to hold him down, Shepherd prepared the strong sedatives as ordered by the doctor.

He was fighting full force, it was just terrible, and he was swearing at us and threatening that everyone involved was going to be murdered. . . . he was lying perfectly still and Miss McGillvray was helping to hold him and *just* as I went to jab him with the needle he jumped and the needle went into Miss McGillvray's thumb.

The 'excitable' McGillvray asked, 'did you lose any, did you lose any' and, getting a negative response, instructed Shepherd to 'put it into the patient'. In spite of Shepherd's assurance to McGillvray that none of the sedative had been lost, it was not until several hours later when McGillvray was 'still going strong' that Shepherd was sure she had hit the right target.[93]

In other situations students were not as pleased to see their superiors. Assigned to night duty on Winnipeg General's 'D Flat', the soldier's ward, Myrtle Crawford came on duty to take over from the evening duty shift nurse, only to find chaos ruling and her classmate 'walking up and down the corridor wringing her hands [saying] "what'll I do, what'll I do" '. Without waiting to find out what had happened, Crawford 'barged into the men's washroom', broke up the fight occurring there, and ordered the men back to bed. Having restored order, the night nurse discovered that the men had convinced the evening nurse to let them have a birthday party for a patient. As Crawford recalled:

> Their party was booze, and they were all high so I told them to get into bed and to pull the bed cloths up over their heads because the night supervisor was coming around and I didn't want to see one person out of his bed. And there wasn't. By the time she came everybody was quiet in bed, and of course the whole ward reeked of liquor and you can't tell me that the night supervisor didn't know what was going on.

Fortunately, the assistant supervisor, not McGillvray herself, had come to check on D Flat, and Crawford concluded that McGillvray, a nursing sister in World War I, had purposely sent her assistant to the scene: 'you can't be a nurse overseas and not know what went on that night'. Unlike her assistant, who could keep her suspicions quiet, if McGillvray 'knew about it she would have to take action'.[94] Whether McGillvray's absence was intentional or not, Crawford's belief that the veteran supervisor purposely avoided the potentially disastrous scene reflected the admiration and affection felt for such role models. The discipline and confidence women like McGillvray offered the younger generation mediated some of the harsher features of hospital routine.[95]

Allegiances with supervisors were critical during the many seasons when demand for hospital services outstripped available hospital staff. In 1921, the director of nursing at Vancouver General, Ethel Johns, critiqued hospital procedures for night-duty cases. Calling for a reorganization of emergency operation protocol, she reminded the hospital superintendent that 'it is not unusual for [the medical staff] to expect the patient to be in the operating room within a few minutes—forgetting that no matter how quick and efficient the nursing service may be, a sick patient cannot always be hurried in procedures of this kind.' In defence of the night nursing staff in the nursery, Johns recounted the experiences of one nurse 'obliged to give anaesthetics practically throughout the night and was unable to give any supervision or direction to pupils.' Calling for improved staffing on night duty, Johns maintained: 'No woman can administer gas oxygen anaesthesia and at the same time direct the work of inexperienced pupil nurses in two case rooms. . . . Nurses are at present being called upon to perform duties which are properly those of a medical man and at the same time to accept blame because the nursing service is unsatisfactory.'[96]

In other instances, when attending physicians required assistance the institution could not provide, staff and students could use their rituals to negotiate with difficult doctors. Since only a fine line differentiated apprenticing and graduate nurses in the hospital, doctors could distinguish one from the other by their stocking colour—students wore blue, staff wore white. On one occasion, recalls a retired Vancouver General graduate, a doctor demanded that only graduate nurses, not students, 'scrub' for him.

> At night we didn't have that many Graduates on, you see, they'd be students on, so our Supervisor always kept white stockings up there and when any of us had to scrub for this man we took off our black stockings and shoes and she gave us white stockings, because he always looked down to see. If he saw white stockings that was fine he'd go and scrub. . . .[97]

Inverting standard procedure was only possible when the interests of graduate and student nurses coalesced, but when they did, nurses were able to use their own procedures to cope with pressures.

Negotiating the social relations at the bedside was further complicated by the legal ramifications that other women workers rarely had to consider. For hospital nurses, patient health and the nurse's status could be jeopardized through carelessness, even when executing a simple task such as a fomentation. Steam and boiling water presented significant risks for patients and practitioners, but while nurses accepted the occasional minor burns as part of the job, they knew that burning a patient could result in discipline, including suspension. Two Vancouver General nurses confronted the dangers of hot water when they were suspended for '[failing] to take the necessary precautions as applying to operative cases'. The apprentices had been attending a patient who was recovering from a 'slight operation', but when they placed overheated hot-water bottles in the patient's bed the anaesthetized patient received serious burns. The patient sued for earnings lost during her convalescence from hospital negligence and the two nurses were relieved of duty for one and two weeks, respectively. The same fate befell another Vancouver student who made a mistake with a patient's medicine.[98] Nurses soon came to realize that the precision expected of students created a margin of error that protected them once they were expected to assume full responsibility for patient care. Myrtle Crawford concluded 'if you learned how to do it perfectly you wouldn't go too far off if you got careless.'[99]

Once nurses left the hospital school and entered into private practice they were legally responsible for remaining within the parameters of accepted medical and nursing practice. Narcotics such as morphine created particularly difficult issues for practitioners. Although possession of such narcotics was technically illegal, private-duty nurses often had small amounts of narcotics, whether left over from a completed case or kept on hand for emergency or rural patients. In fact, some nurses were compelled to maintain a supply of such drugs because at times 'a physician expected the nurse to have morphine in readiness to carry out a telephone order.' Recognizing the legal grey area this placed nurses in, the RNANS acknowledged in 1936 that 'considerable allowance might be made for a nurse having morphine in her possession for emergency use, but at the same time . . . she might not receive much protection in event of a serious involvement of a patient or doctor.'[100]

The experience of one graduate nurse exemplifies the delicate position that private-duty nurses faced. In June 1937, nurse Mitchell took a job in rural Saskatchewan, providing private care for a male heart patient, for whom strychnine had been prescribed. Concerned about the treatment, the nurse wrote to a medical practitioner she knew from her hospital training. The doctor replied with detailed instructions pertaining to the administration of 'simple Strych. grain' or a hypodermic injection of strychnine tablets if that served to regulate the pulse. The doctor later refined his prescription and recommended a combination of nitroglycerin, strychnine, and digitalin taken orally, and codeine for sleeplessness. Throughout the correspondence the doctor praised the nurse's 'very informative and intelligent' letter and assured her that 'we must depend on the nurse—her judgement and observation, etc.'[101] This correspondence reveals several critical features of doctor-nurse interaction. Certainly, patients and doctors alike relied on nurses to provide intelligent patient care in conditions where access to medical attendance was limited. For nurses working in relatively isolated conditions, medical communication assured the nurse that she was following an appropriate therapeutic regimen, particularly when administering such powerful drugs. Moreover, written documentation such as the doctor's letters also offered legal protection should the nurse require it at the time, or in the future.[102]

Alma Kelly's experience with a dissatisfied patient illustrated the fine line between nursing work and medical work. In July 1928, Nova Scotia's Yarmouth Hospital faced a lawsuit. One of its patients claimed that while dressing a wound Superintendent of Nursing Kelly went beyond nursing procedure and punctured the 'enduration' in the leg. The nurse claimed that she 'merely let the artery clamp slid [*sic*] into the wound to keep the mouth of the wound open to allow the pus to come out with the least difficulty', but the patient insisted that his wound had been further damaged, and was incensed that the nurse had presumed diagnostic authority in suggesting he would need an operation. Kelly's provincial association rallied to her defence, sending two of its more eloquent leaders to Yarmouth to testify on Kelly's behalf, but the judge ruled in the patient's favour. In February 1929, as Kelly was preparing to leave her job in Yarmouth, she wrote to the RNANS to thank association representatives for their support during her court case. Her postscript that 'no judge can make an innocent person guilty' belied the ambiguous legal position nurses occupied.[103] Expected to meet whatever contingency arose in bedside nursing, they were also liable to charges of practising medicine without a licence.

As scientifically informed technique served to define nurses in the workplace and in the law, so, too, did it help distinguish them in the marketplace. Traditional analyses of scientific management have emphasized its significance in 'deskilling' workers and therefore disempowering them *vis à vis* the labour market. In many spheres of secondary production, scientific management ensured that male workers, including clerical workers, lost their jobs to easily replaceable unskilled or semi-skilled workers.[104] On the other hand, women workers came into the world of paid employment from a different direction than did men. Early in the industrialization process, women were defined as low-skilled and were ghettoized in poorly paid and unorganized sectors of production. Thus, for female workers, white-collar jobs, however rationalized, represented an increase in status and superior working conditions, especially those jobs that required mathematical or literacy skills.[105] For nurses, rationalization of production aided in the concrete delineation of their skills and in differentiating them from their 'unskilled' competition in the household/community. Ideologically, science allowed nurses to distinguish their work from maternal caregiving, which is still considered the domain of all women.[106] For nurses at the workplace, claims to specific rituals, all in the name of science, were more useful than abstract professional concepts in elevating trained personnel above the informally or untrained competition in the marketplace.[107] The careful delineation of what was and was not good nursing was particularly important in the crisis-ridden inter-war decades during which nurses struggled daily to win legal and financial recognition of their value.

Popular Culture and Occupational Identity

In private homes and on hospital wards, the rituals of nursing practice represented the expertise that was critical to nurses' survival, economically and physically. For these reasons graduates felt proud of the distinctive skills that their technique represented and incorporated that technique into their occupational identity. Student nurses admired their superiors who could perform particular tasks with ease. One Winnipeg General graduate recalled that 'As a probie I used to envy the junior nurses when they would wring these foments because I thought those forceps were kept there by a neat twist of the wrist you know and I was very disillusioned when I learned that they were just plain clamped on.'[108] Another Winnipeg veteran insisted that she could recall only one postoperative infection, and even then she suspected the surgeon to have been the culprit who 'broke' the sterile field of her dressing tray.[109] A Halifax grad left her training school confident that she could 'tackle everything'.[110]

Popular culture created by nurses themselves in the 1920s and 1930s revealed the centrality of science to daily life in the hospital. For example, student yearbooks, produced annually by graduating classes, were filled with humorous references alluding to features of scientific practice. In one edition, a joke entitled 'Medical Definitions' reinterpreted the term 'aseptic' to mean 'Person not believing in any-thing' and defined toxic as 'Loquacious'.[111] More elaborate parodies of hospital life usually took the form of substantially revised poems or song lyrics. The 1927 Winnipeg General *Blue and White* contained a poem entitled 'The Microbe's Serenade' wherein a 'love lorn microbe met by chance at a swagger bacteroidal dance' a 'bacillian belle'. This 'protoplasmic queen' was the 'microscopical pride and pet of the biological smartest set' who so impressed her microbial suitor that he asked, 'What futile scientific term can well describe their many charms?' Pursuing the germ, he "'neath her window often played this Darwin-Huxley serenade' and, declaring his fidelity, assured the subject of his affection that: 'We'll sit beneath some fungus growth, till dissolution claims us both.'[112]

In the 1928 Vancouver General *Nurses Annual*, the poem 'The Bacteriological Ball' once again personified bacilli. This time a 'gay bacilli' held a party in the laboratory, inviting 'only the cultured'. Referring to the cellular structure of the various organisms, the poem continued:

> The Diplococci came to view
> A trifle late and two by two
> The Streptococci took great pains
> To seat themselves in graceful chains . . .

Playing on the social stigma associated with venereal disease, the poem alluded to a tension between the bacillus causing pneumonia and that causing gonorrhoea:

> The Pneumococci, stern and haughty,
> Declared the Gonococci naught,
> And said they would not come at all
> If the Gonos were present at the ball.

Once the fête began, the potential dangers of laboratory life were forgotten:

> Each germ engaged herself that night
> Without a fear of phagocyte
> T'was getting late and some were loaded,
> When a jar of formaldehyde exploded.

Under assault from such efficient an agent of sterilization:

> Not one survived, they perished all,
> At that bacteriological ball.[113]

While nurses' daily workplace interaction with science most often involved ether, green soap, and boiling water, none the less laboratories, formaldehy̆de, and microscopic organisms all emerged as central characters on the pages of student yearbooks.

Popular verse also served to link the scientific principles of asepsis with the hard work students were expected to do, especially as probationers. In a poem entitled 'Scrubs' senior nurses reminded disgruntled juniors of the value simple cleaning skills could make to patient care and medical practice. The poem began:

> A Probationer stood in a ward one day
> With a brush in hand and a basin tray.
> Her task—beds, tables and chairs to scrub,
> And anything else that needed a rub.
> 'How long will it last?' was the maiden's cry—
> 'I'll be tired out long ere the day goes by.
> Is there never an end to the cleaning that's done?
> Must I still do this when my cap I've won?'

But 'scrub we must' insisted the author, for whether in ward, diet kitchen, or operating room:

> The more germs scrubbed and boiled away
> The better the chances, so they say,
> For wounds to heal in the long, hard fight
> To bring back health. . . .

The rewards of such labour were found when, as seniors, nurses served as operating room 'scrub' nurses. As the last stanza explained:

> To be trusted to share in a surgeon's task
> Is as great a thing as a nurse could ask:
> So cheer up, probationer, do not mind
> The work that tedious now you find
> It will pleasanter be the more you do,
> And the day will come when you'll be through:
> Then, with an understanding smile,
> You'll look back and say, 'It was all worth while.'[114]

That careful adherence to technique would facilitate nurses' maturation from unskilled probationer to highly skilled assistant was elucidated in a Winnipeg General poem from 1923, entitled 'The Training'. It concluded:

> At last she reached the white 'O.R.',
> Where patients coming from afar
> Endure the surgeon's knife:
> And there she learned to sterilize
> And keep her technique in such wise
> She might not lose her life.[115]

Similar themes were echoed in other contributions, such as those entitled 'Routine' and 'Aseptic Technique'.[116] A more elaborate depiction of nurses' technique and the social relations at the bedside was presented in the 1926 yearbook contribution, 'The Hooting of Dan Mackay'. This parody of a Robert Service poem described a local surgeon, the 'dangerous D.S. Mackay', and his treatment of nurses in the operating room. Because 'the staff were all stepping out', a student assumed the role of Mackay's senior scrub nurse. As the operation proceeded, the 'well-masked' apprentice was 'trembling with fear' but 'never batted an eye'.

> So they hacked and slashed and sliced away,
> till the deed was almost done;
> The surgeon, as usual, roared and raged and abused
> each nurse but one.
> The staff nurse, she just carried on, with her technique
> no fault could be found.
> She doled out retractors and forceps and her knowledge
> of suture profound.

In spite of the scrub nurse's competent assistance, the cranky doctor flew into a rage when he discovered that his attendant was not a graduate. The student concluded with a defiant tone:

> We aren't so wise as you Doctor guys, but strictly between us two,
> If you'd only give us a fighting chance, you'd see what we really
> could do.[117]

Yearbook contributions also acknowledged that once outside the regime of the training school, nurses would need to adapt their technique to suit the circumstances of their patients and their jobs. A Misericordia General Hospital yearbook poem, 'Farmyard Sanitation', observed the career of a nurse who 'hied to Hick-Town Junction/Soon after graduation'. Her introduction to 'farm-yard sanitation' included trimming the turkey 'with antiseptic shears'. Her decision to place the hens on a 'rigid diet' resulted in their 'laying eggs in mass production', and she went on to '[souse] the sheep in Kresio Dip' and to sterilize the ducks. The final verse revealed the private's ultimate success:

A permanent wave in bossy's horn—
With bobby-pins it's twisted;
She's getting quite a boyish form
Now that her tummy's lifted.
The little chicks are always fed
On sanitary worms;
The calves and colts fumigated
To keep them free from germs.
And thoroughly to carry out
Her systematic plan,
Next week with germicidal soap
She'll scrub the poor hired man.[118]

Conclusion: Reflections on Gender and Science

These humorous expressions of students' three-year engagement with the germ theory and scientific management reveal the critical intersection of science and nursing practice in defining nurses' workplace experience. Scientific theory of asepsis along with managerial efforts at rationalization combined to define what medical and administrative staffs thought nursing practice should be. But within those parameters, the scientific underpinning of nursing practice also helped nurses to create their own standard of quality care while empowering them to defend themselves economically, legally, and physically. Historical scholarship that concludes that rank-and-file nurses in inter-war Canada were outside or marginal to the dominant scientific concepts of the day fails to capture the essential role those concepts played in nurses' daily lives.

This analysis suggests significant points of revision are needed regarding the place of nursing in the history of medicine. Canadian medical historians have been slow to integrate nursing work into studies of health-care history, often providing only cursory mention of nursing service before going on to detail administrative structures or medical achievements. Yet, close examination of the nursing skills delivered by second- and third-generation practitioners reveals that nurses were active participants in creating the culture of scientific medicine and, as the largest patient-care work-force in the medical system, in establishing the hospital as the dominant location for the delivery of health services in twentieth-century Canada. If we are to account fully for the particular development of the Canadian health-care system, an analysis of nurses' work must be integrated into medical history.

In challenging the interpretation of nurses as non-scientific care-givers, this chapter demonstrates that we cannot characterize nurses as merely victims of science and modern medicine. This does not mean, however, that Canadian nurses in the the pre-World War II era can simply be reclaimed as unrecognized women scientists. Nurses had a fundamentally different relationship to science than did women struggling for equality and recognition in male-dominated fields such as chemistry, botany, or even medicine.[119] Like their counterparts in other scientific pursuits, nurses used science, and within the work-place they used it to gain an element of control in daily practice. But nurses did not generate new scientific knowledge, and in that way cannot be described as scientific practitioners or scientists. Rather, nurses employed concepts generated by non-nurse researchers and used that knowledge under the direction of doctors. In other words, as the 'physicians' hand' it could be argued that nurses merely carried out scientific orders but did not engage critically with scientific knowledge.

It could be argued that practitioners in many fields of science did not generate scientific knowledge either. Medical science is the most obvious example, wherein general practitioners used concepts learned in medical school but did not critically engage with, or develop additions to, that knowledge. Similar observations could be made about occupations such as pharmacy, physiotherapy, or even engineering, but two critical factors differentiated such practitioners from nurses. First, nurses were not trained in scientific investigation, and the pedagogical emphasis on execution and economic efficiency, rather than conceptualization, of various procedures left little time for students to develop scientific research techniques.[120]

Secondly, once licensed to practise, nurses could not generate sci-entific knowledge because they were legally barred from doing so. After all, only doctors were entitled to diagnose and prescribe. Indeed, the cornerstone of medical professionalism lay in the medical monopoly over such conceptual rights. Even public health nurses, who have long boasted greater autonomy than their counterparts in other branches of nursing, were reminded in 1919 that when visiting a sick patient 'treatments must never be suggested nor opinions advanced. . . . Never commit the error of diagnosing.'[121] Realizing the significance of this issue, the 1932 Weir *Survey of Nursing Education in Canada* asked its respondents, 'do nurses prescribe?'[122] Even if nurses did observe repeatable trends in patient response to their care, such knowledge was illicit since that kind of diagnostic skill was reserved for the medical profession. When nurses did perform medical procedures, like delivering babies when doctors were absent, legal imperatives denied nurses the right to claim financial remuneration for that work or any intellectual contribution. This, then, speaks to issues of power and legitimacy more than scientific status. The mind had no sex, but the law did.[123]

Recognizing the gendered nature of women's legal and social authority over scientific knowledge, some feminist scholars have concluded that because of culturally or biologically determined gender roles women 'do science' differently than men. These authors have argued for examining women's 'different voice' and 'feminine science'.[124] Yet the specific experiences of nurses suggests that a concept like feminine science must be applied judiciously, for not all women shared the same relationship to scientific authority. Comparisons between nursing and other female occupations that sought social legitimation through science illustrate this point. Domestic science was one such occupation that, in the early twentieth century, embraced scientific discourse by wedding the germ theory with scientific management in order to transform, largely unsuccessfully, the status of domestic labour.[125] Such a comparison highlights the broad social application of the scientific paradigm in the twentieth century and serves as an important reminder of the many uses to which the word 'science' has been put.[126]

At the same time, too heavy an emphasis on the ideological power of scientific language detracts from the very different successes women had in achieving social and occupational legitimation through science. Nurses' experiences in the hospital, as students, staff, or special-duty attendants, convinced them not just of the discursive importance of science in distinguishing their work from 'untrained' caregivers in the household, but also of the efficacy of treatment that aseptic technique and adherence to the procedural routines ensured. After all, during the pre-'miracle drug' years, hospital wards were not ravaged by cross-infections, nor were surgical patients afflicted with postoperative infections. Indeed, hospital administrators and doctors agreed that nurses' technique 'worked'. Thus, even if science is best understood as a social and intellectual paradigm rather than a distinct and documentable body of knowledge, nurses contributed to the development of that paradigm, and to its legitimation, in a way that occupations like domestic science, or even social science, did not. Nursing practice incorporated scientific thought but also produced a concrete or material body of evidence—that is, the ascent of the hospital as a safe and legitimate venue for health services—which itself was part of the dominant paradigm of knowledge in this century.

Nurses, therefore, occupied a unique place with respect to modern science. Neither victims nor unsung heroines, nurses cannot be categorized as oppressed by science or as liberated by it. This highlights the importance of creating a feminist conceptual framework that can capture the diversity of scientific roles women have assumed in the past. The historically specific conditions under which different groups of women interacted with scientific thought need to be explicated before any general statements about women, gender, and science can be made.

For Canada's second and third generations of trained nurses this means taking into account the particular dynamics of the workplace. Nursing cannot be written directly into the existing literature on women and science because their work was not only about science. As an exclusively female occupation, nursing practice was premised on other 'paradigms', including socially constructed definitions of feminine nurturing and female sexual/social respectability. Science was but one, although a critical one, of the forces that constructed nursing life. Thus, in fulfilling their role as the health-care system's largest patient-care work-force, nurses used science in a manner specific to their relationship to production—to their patients. Positioned between doctors and patients, and between institutional administrators and familial caregivers, nurses were defined by scientific concepts, but also invoked those concepts to define themselves. Required simultaneously to care and cure, nurses in the 1900–42 era used scientific knowledge—both in terms of the contemporary theoretical understanding of infection, but also in terms of the 'rational' rituals of technique—to resolve the contradictions inherent in their daily lives.

4

An Occupation in Crisis: The Third Generation of Graduate Nurses, 1920–1942

The rituals and routines of nursing practice helped second- and third-generation nurses define the parameters of their work and defend their position within the health-care system. The composition of the work-force and the content of nursing practice united practitioners across generations, strengthening the powerful occupational identity that had emerged in the early decades of the century. Yet for all the commonalities in the content of their work, nurses of the inter-war generation plied their trade within a very different political economy of health from that of their predecessors. By the 1920s, nursing and non-nursing commentators were noticing that, in spite of the significant role nurses were playing at the bedside and in spite of the public recognition they were receiving, nurses' own economic health was in peril. Each year hospital training schools across the nation graduated new practitioners into a private health-care market that itself was eroding as more and more patients relied on hospital services provided by new classes of apprenticing nurses. This downward spiral of more nurses and fewer private, paying patients, endemic to the health-care system of the 1920s, was exacerbated by the economic depression of the 1930s. Irregular employment, uncertain pay, and difficult, sometimes dangerous, conditions of work began to tarnish the reputation of the occupation that had seemed to promise so much to Canadian women.

The Third Generation of Graduate Nurses

The crisis affecting Canadian nurses was documented by the many observers monitoring nursing's rapid pulse. As they recorded the signs and symptoms of occupational distress, commentators such as George Weir, professor of education at the University of British Columbia and soon-to-be minister of education and provincial secretary responsible for health in British Columbia's Liberal government, provided a detailed portrait of the third generation of Canadian nurses. Together with data in such sources as Canada's Dominion Bureau of Statistics (DBS) *Census*, comprehensive occupational surveys such as Weir's identified a number of sociological characteristics that third-generation nurses shared. The most obvious was their gender. No more than 227 male nurses ever appeared in the census reports for these years, and none at all in 1931. The remaining practitioners—who by DBS tabulations numbered 21,162 in 1921, 31,898 in 1931, and 38,709 in 1941—were women.[1]

More than 90 per cent of female graduate nurses were single or self-supporting. In the years following World War I, the percentage of nurses who were widowed or divorced stood at 8 per cent, reflecting the large number of women who had lost spouses in the 'Great War'. For the next two decades, widowed and divorced women dropped to 5 and then 1 per cent for graduate nurses.[2] The overwhelming proportion of unmarried nurses was not surprising since nurses, like other female wage-earners, were enjoined to leave paid labour upon marriage.[3] This social taboo was formalized by hospitals, which would employ only women who were divorced or widowed and not accept married students into their training schools.[4] Throughout the 1920s and 1930s most married women who practised their trade did so on an on-call basis, particularly in small communities with a limited pool of trained personnel. Many of these 'inactive' nurses let their association memberships lapse until they returned to more regular employment, thereby escaping classification by Weir or the DBS, though their contributions to community health were verified by local histories and oral interviews.[5]

The formal proscription on employing married nurses shaped the age composition of the third generation of Canadian nurses. Weir's conclusion, that the median age of private-duty and institutional nurses in 1930 was 31 years, confirmed DBS data.[6] The 1931 census reported that the female work-force was distributed over all age categories from 14 to 70 years, with 26 per cent falling in the 20–4 age category and another 27 per cent in the 25–35 age group. Compared to other women workers, a much higher concentration of nurses, 42 per cent, were ages 25 to 34. In all but the older age categories of over 65, a larger percentage of nurses were working than the majority of working women. That the age profile of nursing was occupationally distinct becomes clear when nursing is compared to other white-collar occupations. Because jobs as teachers, stenographers, typists, telephone operators, bookkeepers, and cashiers required relatively short periods of training, women in those occupations began their working lives earlier than did graduate nurses, who had to complete three years of hospital apprenticeship. But a higher proportion of graduate nurses remained in their field of training after age 25 than did those in other white-collar jobs.[7]

The relatively late age at which graduate nurses embarked on their careers was a function of the minimum age requirements for entry into hospital training schools and the three-year apprenticeship.[8] In 1931, few student nurses were under 17 years old and by 1941 the practice of schools accepting anyone under 18 years old had been virtually stopped. This contrasted sharply with teachers, who might well be teaching with a third-class certificate at age 16.[9] Minimum age standards also influenced educational levels. Records for Ontario registered nurses in 1923 calculated that of 675 members, 25 had matriculation, 26 had four years of high school, 58 had three, 146 had two, 162 had one, and 156 had public school only. In addition, 34 had private school preparation, 36 had been educated in a convent, and 32 had 'business training'.[10] Although such credentials pale by comparison to women entering professional university training, relative to the majority of women workers nurses boasted superior educational backgrounds.[11] The 1941 census calculated that of the 832,840 women in non-military occupations, 50 per cent had 9–12 years of education, while another 11 per cent had 13 years or more. By contrast, 60 per cent of graduate nurses claimed they had 9–12 years and 33 per cent boasted 13 years or more.[12]

The gap between minimum education and minimum age requirements meant that many aspiring nurses had to wait a year before entering training, during which time they worked at other jobs or at home. Winnipeg General Hospital grad Mary Shepherd worked in her father's store for a year until she was old enough to begin her nursing education. Determined to become a nurse, Shepherd calculated that her year as a sales clerk would help her 'get used to standing all day' once training began. Other nurses were less sure of their career goals and gained experience in other fields before entering nursing. Teaching in particular lost numerous recruits to nursing, as the testimony from Winnipeg General alumnae revealed. Mabel Lytle and Olive Irwin both preferred nursing over teaching. Ingibjorg Cross convinced her older sister to end her teaching career and become a nurse. Myrtle Crawford followed her father's advice and taught for two years before joining her sister Ruby in nursing's ranks. Some, like Isabel Cameron, Grace Parker, and Anne Ross, attended university before continuing their education in the hospital, while others such as Beryl Seeman stayed at home and helped with farm and home chores before beginning their apprenticeships.[13] Thus nursing capitalized on, rather than competed with, the growing number of girls from all class backgrounds who were earning their high school diploma.

Canadian nurses of the inter-war era also shared nativity. In 1921, 78 per cent of nurses and nurses-in-training were Canadian born, compared to only 17 per cent born in the British Isles, 4 per cent in the United States, and 1.3 per cent in Europe. The latter figures remained constant over the next two decades. The most dramatic change occurred in the presence of British-born women, which by 1941 had dropped to 8 per cent of the graduate nurse work-force and 3 per cent of students. Canadian-born women continued to dominate the ranks of graduate nurses, by 1941 accounting for 88 and 94 per cent of graduate and student nurses respectively. Some of this shift correlated with the restrictions on immigration in the inter-war years, but even then nursing remained more solidly native-born than other women's occupations.[14]

Whether foreign or native-born, most Canadian nurses were White and of Anglo-Saxon descent. In 1931, 76 per cent of graduate nurses claimed British ethnic heritage, 18 per cent stated French, 5.8 per cent listed themselves as of other European ancestry, another .28 per cent were designated as 'Hebrew', and the remaining .06 per cent were of Indian, Japanese, and Chinese origin.[15] The virtual absence of women of colour in nursing's professional ranks was enforced both by federal immigration restrictions and by the racial discrimination practised by hospital nursing schools. Whether Black women in Nova Scotia, Japanese Canadians in British Columbia, or Native women anywhere, women of colour rarely were accepted in training programs on the grounds that White patients could not be entrusted to the care of non-White nurses. When Chinese and Japanese-Canadian women were admitted to the Vancouver General Hospital in the 1930s, their entry was predicated on the assumption that they were needed to work in 'their own' communities, which were poorly serviced by the formal health-care system.[16]

These colour bars were usually unwritten and only received formal articulation when challenged. Yet they were systematically endorsed and enforced by nursing administrators, as the experience of Mavis Hill revealed. In July 1940, the president of the Toronto Colored Liberal Association, Mr G. Roberts, received a letter from Donald Hill.

Not only did Hill consider the concern he was bringing forward 'a very vital matter affecting our race', he also believed that as a 20-year resident of Toronto and a municipal and federal taxpayer, he was 'entitled to that consideration which all citizens should have'. Hill's concern lay with his daughter, Mavis, who had completed four years of high school and now, at age 21, wanted to become a nurse. She had written to the Toronto General Hospital requesting an application for its program, explaining that she was 'coloured'. Instead of an application form, Mavis received a letter from the hospital stating that there were no vacancies at the school. Undeterred, Mavis again wrote the hospital, this time using a pseudonym and another address, and not mentioning skin colour. The reply instructed the applicant to call at the hospital for an interview.

At this point, recognizing that she had been rejected because of her race and 'too embarrassed to go for an interview', Mavis gave up. Her only other option was to apply to an American hospital school, but as her father explained to Mr Roberts, several issues made going south of the border an impossibility. Mavis was not an American citizen and 'the prevailing rate of exchange and the difficulty in getting American money' would have forced Mr Hill 'to spend hard earned Canadian money in the States'. More importantly, Hill concluded, refusing Mavis entrance to a Canadian program on the grounds of her heritage was 'unfair to her and [established] a terrible precedence of discrimination against coloured girls.'[17]

Mr Roberts responded to Hill's request to 'find out what are we to do with our girls who are desirous of taking this course' by contacting Harold Kirby, minister of health for Ontario. He, in turn, passed the matter on to Deputy Minister McGhie, who contacted the registrar of the Registered Nurses' Association of Ontario (RNAO). On behalf of her organization, the registrar replied:

> The negro population of Toronto would hardly justify the establishment of a separate training school. . . . we must keep in mind the reaction of patients to nurses in training, and there would no doubt be many protests from patients and doctors if colored nurses were introduced into the wards. Training schools for colored nurses were established in the United States for this reason. I believe that applicants from Canada would be accepted for training with the understanding that they would return to their own land on completion of the course.[18]

McGhie passed this information on to Roberts and, conveniently distancing himself from any political damage, noted that while the

Nurses Registration Act provided for inspectors of nursing schools, it did not allow for governmental intervention into school admissions policy. McGhie's optimistic advice that Mavis pursue her education at an American hospital school revealed that he neither had paid attention to Hill's explanation nor had the political will to challenge the status quo.[19]

Colour bars, minimum age and educational standards, and the proscription against marriage combined to define the nursing work-force in a particular way. Nurses shared gender, age profile, and marital status, and were privileged by education, nativity, ethnicity, and race. Together, these characteristics suggest that nursing attracted and accepted those Canadian women with significant social and personal resources, women who at least in sociological terms were privileged relative to other working women. But the advantages that nurses collectively possessed were not necessarily the products of élite class backgrounds.

Determining the precise class origins of inter-war nurses is difficult given the limitations of documentary evidence. Unlike American institutional administrators, who regularly recorded the occupation of students' fathers, superintendents of Canadian nursing programs appeared remarkably unconcerned with the class status of new recruits. The same institutional records that cited students' ages, home towns, educational achievements, and religious affiliation were silent about the occupations of male heads of households. This historical silence can be read as evidence that students were so homogeneously bourgeois that no mention of shared class origins was necessary, or can be interpreted to mean that a father's occupation held little significance in determining who could become a nurse. The latter interpretation is borne out by those few sources that do address the question of class. The most thorough was Weir's *Survey of Nursing Education*, which, as the lone study to investigate the occupations of nurses' families, provided invaluable data on this controversial 'variable' in nursing history.

For each of the respondents to his written questionnaire, Weir recorded the occupation of the nurse's father or guardian and then assigned each nurse to one of six categories: unskilled, semi-skilled, skilled, farming, business and clerical, or professional. While Weir's data have some limitations, his investigation into class origins does document the diversity of background that characterized inter-war nursing.[20] As Table 4.1 demonstrates, only 14 per cent of Weir's respondents hailed from professional families and a further 30 per cent had fathers in business or clerical pursuits. The combined figures for the 'unskilled', 'semi-skilled', and 'skilled' categories revealed the marked presence of working-class women in nursing. Few daughters of miners, labourers, lumbermen, teamsters, or loggers made their way into hospital training programs, but those who did enrol shared a broad working-class heritage with over 30 per cent of students and 20 per cent of graduates. Whether the differential between the results for students and graduates was a function of a high dropout rate among working-class students, a lesser tendency among working-class graduates to pursue RN status, working-class women's greater predilection for private-duty work (and therefore less chances of filling out Weir's survey), or the peculiarities of those particular years was not clear.

Table 4.1
Occupation of Nurses' Parents or Guardians, 1929–1930

	Unskilled	Semi-skilled	Skilled	Farmer	Business & Clerical	Professional
Student nurses	2.1%	8.0%	21.1%	38.1%	22.0%	8.7%
Private-duty nurses	1.4%	5.4%	17.2%	39.4%	23.3%	13.3%
Hospital nurses	1.3%	3.1%	14.7%	35.9%	30.6%	14.0%
Superintendents	0%	3.8%	10.6%	32.0%	39.4%	14.4%
Public health nurses	.06%	2.7%	15.6%	28.1%	33.1%	20.0%
Total	.97%	4.6%	15.8%	34.7%	29.7%	14.0%

SOURCE: G. Weir, *Survey of Nursing Education in Canada* (Toronto, 1932).

Weir's figures reflect the diversity of class backgrounds represented in the third generation of nurses. Documentation from other sources substantiates that nurses came from a variety of class backgrounds and from every district of urban centres.[21] Working-class women were well represented in the occupation and at least some received early educations in working-class consciousness and politics. Jean Ewen claimed that when her father became increasingly involved in Communist Party politics she and her siblings became 'of necessity, independent, self-reliant brats'. Ewen took advantage of

Winnipeg's employment options when in 1927 she secured work in the laundry of St Joseph's Hospital. Within two years Jean had taken on a new role in the hospital, as a student nurse.[22] In the early 1930s, Winnipeg graduate nurse Brenda Farmer resided with her family in their Riverview home. Her father, Seymour James Farmer, was a trained chartered accountant who turned his attention to labour politics in the post-World War I years. Farmer was successful in two mayoralty contests and in 1931 was serving his third term as a member of the Legislative Assembly.[23] Across town, graduate nurse Agnes Puttee lived in her family's College Street residence with sister Winnifred, a teacher, and with brothers Arthur, an engineer with Canadian Engineering and Construction, and Harold, an inspector for the Bureau of Labour. Their father, Arthur, well known in the city as a former Labour MP, worked as manager of Printer's Roller Company. Whether these women shared their fathers' left-wing political beliefs is not clear, but the significant presence of women from working-class households does challenge the stereotype that only middle-class women became nurses.[24]

The occupation of male household members appears a less significant determinant than the occupation of nurses' sisters. Very few graduate nurses lived in households with sisters working in the industrial or blue-collar occupations. Rather, those nurses who returned home after graduation to live with their families resided with sisters working in clerical, sales, or teaching jobs. Evidence from Winnipeg's *Henderson's Directory* illustrates this point. Of the 204 unmarried nurses living with their families, 108 of the nurses listed employed sisters. Only four of those nurses had sisters working in occupations that might have been industrial production, at Picardies, the stockyards, a printshop, and as a packer. As well, Julia Taylor lived with her mother Anna, an operator at Ladies Kraft Manufacturing.[25] Seventy-one per cent of nurses' sisters worked in white-collar jobs as clerical staff (36 per cent), salesclerks (4 per cent), teachers (20 per cent), librarians (3 per cent), nurses (8 per cent), or telephone/telegraph operators (3 per cent). For instance, a Winnipeg General graduate, Violet Crone, grew up in the working-class district of Elmwood. Her father Frank was an employee of Priestley's grocery store, sisters Ada and Lily were clerks at Eaton's department store, while a third sister, Nellie, was on staff at Stovel's Printing Company, and her brother Albert was employed by Brown and Rutherford's Lumber Company. Hailing from a very different family background, nurse Elizabeth Parker and her sister Frances, an assistant at the Winnipeg Public Library, lived in the north River Heights home owned by their father, University of Manitoba Professor M.A. Parker.[26] Such individuals exemplify the larger pattern that occupational options for women cut across class lines established for their male siblings. While it is possible that industrially employed women and their nurse sisters simply did not live together, a more likely explanation lies in the process whereby families endorsed certain kinds of training and employment for their daughters. Regardless of occupational background of nurses' families, whether unskilled, skilled, professional, or business, certain households decided that they valued and could afford skilled training for women.

Reconceptualizing class and gender in this way aids in understanding the many rural and agricultural families who sent their daughters into nursing training. Nearly 35 per cent of nurses who completed Weir's questionnaire claimed that their fathers were farmers. Hospital records revealed that an even greater proportion of nursing students originated in rural communities. In the years 1924–9 and 1931–9, 37 per cent of Winnipeg General graduates hailed from Manitoba districts and towns other than Winnipeg or Brandon and a further 22 per cent listed townships in rural Saskatchewan other than Saskatoon and Regina as their homes. Almost one-third claimed urban residence: 29 per cent had families in Winnipeg, but very few Brandonites, only 1 per cent, had chosen the Winnipeg hospital over the Brandon General program. The small number of women from western Ontario towns such as Keewatin, Fort Francis, and Port Arthur-Fort William (the Lakehead) demonstrated the continued importance of Winnipeg as a regional centre for Canadians living west of Lake Superior.[27] Winnipeg's second largest hospital, the Misericordia General, also relied disproportionately on rural applicants to its school of nursing. Between 1921 and 1933, 180 nurses graduated from Misericordia. Of that number, 54 per cent came from rural areas of Manitoba and Saskatchewan, while only 29 per cent were from Winnipeg homes.[28]

Documentation from the east and west coasts verified that the Manitoba pattern was not anomalous. Between 1925 and 1942, the percentage of Vancouver General graduate nurses claiming Vancouver as their home ranged from 20 to 45 per cent. Over those same years women from other regions of British Columbia and Canada migrated to Vancouver for their training, with a marked increase in the migration of women from the prairie provinces over the 1933–42 years. This was particularly true for immigrants from rural Saskatchewan, which at the peak in 1939 accounted for nearly one-quarter of Vancouver graduates.[29] At Halifax's Victoria General Hospital women from rural and small-town Nova Scotia outnumbered those from the Halifax area more than five to one. Of the 144 graduates from the classes of 1934–8 and 1940–1, 85 per cent had left their homes in the Nova Scotia countryside to apprentice at the Victoria General.[30]

Like their urban counterparts, the rural women who journeyed to local or regional hospital schools were those whose labours in the family economy were replaceable. Even some 'home children', British orphans and abandoned children from agencies like the Barnardo homes who were fostered out to families in rural Canada, managed the transition from their apprenticeships on Canadian farms to apprenticeships in Canadian hospitals, although as Joy Parr has demonstrated, such transitions were often difficult and reserved for 'bright, adventurous daughters from prosperous farm families'.[31] Hospital schools offered room and board, and skilled training and certification—all the elements necessary for secure passage out of the agricultural economies and their limited roles for women.[32] Such opportunities were especially significant in the 1930s when the agricultural crises of droughts, plagues, and low grain prices displaced many rural dwellers.[33] While their brothers rode the rails looking for work and handouts, rural women went to nursing school.

Not all these women came off the farm. Many were residents of small towns that offered little waged work and even fewer eligible men. Mary Duncan, Mary Shepherd, and Harriet Pentland grew up in the towns of Glenlyon, Beulah, and Boissevain, Manitoba, where their fathers operated dry and 'fancy' goods stores.[34] To these women, inheriting the family enterprise was not an option. As long as a son existed, rural women, whether living on a farm or in a small town, were unlikely inheritors of family property, and once a brother married the labour of his sister was made redundant by that of his wife. Urban hospitals were thus the unintended benefactors of inheritance patterns that dispossessed the daughters of the countryside. For working-class and farm women alike, familial finances as well as family ambitions for their daughters and sisters, rather than absolute class status, influenced accessibility to nursing training.

Regional economies also served to influence which women entered nursing. Certainly the limited industrial base in the three prairie provinces shaped the profile of the nursing work-force in that region. According to Weir's data, only 17 per cent of nurses from the prairie provinces came from working-class backgrounds as compared to percentages of 20.5 in Ontario, 26.2 in BC, and 24.4 for the Maritimes. More puzzling was Weir's tally for Quebec's nursing work-force, which cited that only 11.5 per cent were of working-class background. It is possible that working-class women in Quebec may have viewed options in that province's industrial sector as more appealing than white-collar jobs such as nursing. At the same time, because Weir was less successful in involving French-speaking nurses in his survey, his calculations for Quebec may also have under-represented Quebec women from working-class backgrounds. The higher returns in the 'Business and Clerical and Professional' categories for Quebec may have reflected a high occurrence of daughters of that class entering the field or may be a product of a high return rate from the urban and white-collar English sector.[35]

Whatever limitations on data, the portrait of the occupation that emerges is of a group of working women who were relatively privileged compared to their sisters in other sectors. While remaining the domain of single women, nursing permitted a significant percentage of its members to continue working later into their lives. On average, nurses were thus slightly older than other working women, boasted higher educational credentials, and were more likely to be Canadian-born. Like most working women tabulated by the DBS, nurses were almost all White. But the women who comprised the third generation of Canadian nurses did not all come from middle-class families; they claimed a range of class origins. What appeared a more critical determinant than male head of household was the gendered configuration of household resources. Nurses came from families who were willing and able to make do without their daughters' incomes for the years necessary for the women to complete the requisite high school education and the three-year hospital apprenticeship. At the very least, families had to be able to afford to let their daughters save their pre-training earnings to cover the small but significant educational costs. As such, the third generation of Canadian nurses occupied a privileged position at the pinnacle of a hierarchy of jobs that welcomed women workers.

Like their counterparts in previous generations, inter-war nurses chose their occupation from a narrow range of options designated as 'female'. Retired nurses from the 1920s and 1930s concurred that 'in those days, women only had three choices, teaching, secretarial work and nursing' and, like teaching and secretarial work, nursing required skills that could be acquired with relatively little expense and translated into paid work relatively quickly.[36] Such assessments of women's occupational choices must be interpreted carefully. True, service jobs did employ more than half of Canada's working women in 1931, but within the service category domestic service remained the single largest source of employment throughout the inter-war years. As well, some areas of the manufacturing sector employed large numbers of women.[37] Claims that the educational and clerical sectors were nurses' only other occupational choices must therefore be understood not in absolute but in relative terms. Nursing, teaching, office work, and even salesclerking were pursued by women who were privileged enough to be able to avoid domestic service.[38] Certainly there were some opportunities for women of élite backgrounds in the male-dominated professions of law, medicine, and architecture, but the limited numbers of female professionals in those fields (203 women doctors, 54 women lawyers, and 2 architects nationally) continued to reflect both the sexism within the professions and the few women who possessed the financial means to acquire professional educations.[39] When universities did establish female faculties such as University of British Columbia's School of Nursing, which constituted more welcome environments for women than did the male-dominated faculties, most aspiring nurses could afford neither the tuition, board, and room or the extra years out of the work-force that university education demanded.[40]

Within the range of available options, women's reasons for choosing nursing over pursuits such as teaching varied. Ingibjorg Cross, Mary Shepherd, Josephine Mann, and Helen Smith all credit their decision to enter nursing to a local nurse whom they admired.[41] Some nursing students followed their siblings and mothers to their Alma Maters. Isabel Cameron's mother had graduated from Winnipeg General; Myrtle Crawford joined her sister at Winnipeg, while Beth Purdy and her sister Nan both left McConnell, Manitoba, for training at the Brandon hospital. Others chose hospitals considered prestigious or that offered specialty services, like pediatrics. Mabel Lytle just remembers 'always wanting to nurse', while others were conscious that nursing was second choice. One retired Winnipeg nurse considered other educational options but pursued nursing when it became clear that her family did not have enough money to finance higher education for both her and her brother.[42]

Some new recruits pursued nursing against the wishes of their families. Olive Irwin, raised in a farming district near Holland, Manitoba, left teaching in 1918 to train as a nurse contrary to her mother's advice. Myrtle Crawford's father decided that she should become a teacher because that occupation was 'more genteel' than nursing. Crawford disagreed. Ingibjorg Cross's father had been a patient in the Virden, Manitoba, hospital, an experience that led him to conclude that nursing was not a fit occupation for young women. When Ingibjorg informed him of her plan to enter the Winnipeg General program, he refused to finance her training. She raised the money for the $25 tuition fee and her uniform by helping neighbours with their harvest and from her winnings at rural sports days.[43] Similar conflicts erupted between Canadian families and the 'home children' they had adopted over releasing trust fund money so that the young women could pursue nursing training.[44]

Whether their decision was endorsed by parents or not, many women recognized that acquiring marketable skills was a necessary alternative to matrimony. Jo Mann left her home community of Hillside, Manitoba, to train at Winnipeg. Mann's mother had impressed upon her daughter that skilled training was essential if women were to enjoy personal autonomy and financial security.

> My mother felt every woman should have something to do. She had been left with dad having lost his leg and running a farm and they told her he would never be able to work again and [that] he would be more or less an invalid. She suddenly realized she didn't have anything to fall back on. How could she earn a living for so many of us, for four children? She felt we should go to school and have a profession of some kind.

Mann left nursing upon marriage, but resumed her career when her husband's illness made her the family's lone breadwinner.[45] The numerous examples of women from earlier generations whose nursing salaries supported themselves and their dependants were substantiated throughout nurses' careers by the experiences of their peers. Jo Mann's roommate had entered training when her newlywed husband died suddenly.[46] Vera Chapman returned to private-duty nursing when her husband of five weeks passed away.[47] Chapman's friend and classmate, Violet McMillan, also re-entered paid nursing work when she was widowed and left to support her three children.[48] Nursing permitted these women and many others to assume economic responsibility for their families when the husband's death, disability, or financial difficulties required that they do so.[49]

And, of course, many women never married, while others worked for many years before choosing a marital partner. Table 4.2 presents available documentation on marriage patterns for Winnipeg General graduates of the 1920s. Of this sample, nearly one-third never married, while another one-fourth did not marry until at least ten years after graduation. Records from Victoria General in Halifax reveal a similar pattern, with more than two-thirds of graduates of the 1924–7 years still self-supporting by 1930.[50] For those who did marry, the experiences of older women and of their peers reinforced the importance of

Table 4.2
Winnipeg General Hospital Graduates, 1920–1928: Never Married, and Married Within 1, 3, 5, 10 Years, and More Than 10 Years of Graduation

Year of Graduation	Never Married	%	Within 1 Year	Within 3 Years	Within 5 Years	Within 10 Years	After 10 Years	%	Total
1920	15	39%	5	6	4	5	3	8%	38
1922	13	30%	1	7	2	12	9	20%	44
1924	19	35%	1	2	5	7	20	37%	54
1926	19	29%	4	12	4	10	17	26%	66
1928	26	27%	16	18	2	9	26	27%	97
Total	92	31%	27	45	17	43	75	25%	299

SOURCE: *WGH Alumnae Journal/Annual*, 1921–45, 1963, 1974.

possessing skilled training should circumstances necessitate a return to the work-force. Skill took on new meaning for this generation. In a world of work that continued to deny women equality and valued work according to its sex typing, skilled training held out the possibility of economic self-sufficiency, if not complete autonomy.

'Far too much time spent "waiting" for cases':[51] The Economic Crisis of the Inter-war Years

The composition of the third generation of Canadian nurses, combined with the apprenticeship system of training and the content of nursing practice, united a work-force that was otherwise geographically dispersed and divided among different subsectors of the health-care system. At the same time, that occupational unity was being threatened by an economic crisis that beset nursing in the inter-war years. While the crisis affected all sectors of the occupation, private-duty nurses experienced the earliest and most devastating effects of nursing's economic dislocation.

The distribution of practitioners among the three subsectors—hospital, public health, and private-duty nursing—remained roughly the same in the inter-war period as it had in the 1900–20 years. So, too, mobility among subsectors and out of the occupation and back to active practice continued to make precise numerical descriptions difficult. Census data for 1931 reported that 8,795 nurses, or 43 per cent, were privately employed, while 5,257, or 26 per cent, worked in the institutional sector. Another 4,500 practitioners were salaried employees working for public health agencies, as industrial nurses for corporations, or in doctors' offices. Weir's investigation discovered slightly different ratios. He found only 15 per cent of RNs were employed in hospitals compared to the 35 per cent working in private duty. The 42.1 per cent of RNs who were 'inactive' were most likely, according to Weir, nurses who would return to the private market when and if they returned to nursing. Records from local associations depict slightly different ratios again, suggesting the fluidity of the distribution of practitioners as well as the regional variation that existed.[52]

The distribution of nurses was also characterized by an urban-rural differential. National figures for 1931 established that 5,267, or 26 per cent of the total nursing population, were employed by institutions. Yet census data indicated that in cities of over 30,000 people only 22.2 per cent of nurses worked in hospitals. Cities attracted and supported slightly greater concentrations of private-duty and public health nurses than did the countryside.[53] Nova Scotia evidence substantiated the rural/urban distribution. As of January 1924, Halifax and Dartmouth accounted for 75 of 204 RNs registered in Nova Scotia, while 26 lived in other parts of Canada, in the United States, and abroad. The remaining 103 were distributed in small towns throughout Nova Scotia.[54]

The numerical dominance of private-duty nurses was a function of graduate nurses' persisting preference for non-institutional work. Like previous generations, third-generation practitioners celebrated the autonomy, independence, and variety of the private market, making private-duty work a welcome change from their training years. As one Alberta nurse advised: 'After finishing those three spin-curving, chest-cramping, foot-twinging, memory-testing, ether-scented years of hospital training, it is well for every nurse who dons her candy-box cap to go out into the world to fight her battles alone, to enter the field of private work. . . .'[55] While a case could last several months, others lasted only a few days. A testimonial from a Victoria General nurse suggested her cases averaged less than two weeks each:

> The private duty branch of nursing offers untold opportunities for coming in contact with all that is interesting in the nursing profession. . . . Each of fifty-four cases I have had since graduating two years ago has been of a totally different nature, so that to one new in the field they were a constant source of interest.[56]

Cases varied in length, location, and activity according to whether the patient and doctor requested 12- or 24-hour attendance for days, weeks, or months, whether the patient was admitted to hospital or treated at home, whether the family employed other domestic assistance or relied solely on the nurse, whether the patient resided in city or countryside, and whether the illness was chronic, acute, contagious, or psychiatric.

Despite allegations as to 'the high-handed manner in which [the private nurse] picks and chooses the cases she is disposed to accept', nurses accepted the flexibility and variety of assignments, and only a small proportion of nurses, less than 20 per cent nationally, consistently refused certain types of patients or locations.[57] Weir reported that 24-hour duty and country cases were the most frequently rejected, while domestic work was performed by only 55 per cent of Weir's respondents. Where nurses lived influenced their ability to reject certain kinds of tasks. For example, the fact that practitioners in the prairie provinces accepted country cases and domestic tasks with far greater frequency than did their peers in other regions reflected the vast expanses of rural districts that nurses serviced and

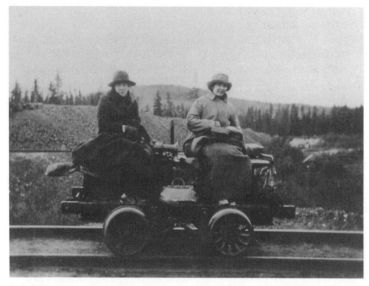

Public health work often promised nurses adventure that took them far from the world of urban hospitals. These public health nurses were photographed using a railway cart for transportation in northern Ontario (Archives of Ontario S15530).

the absence of any other domestic assistance in those isolated farm communities.[58]

In a *Canadian Nurse* bragging session between nurses in eastern and western Canada, the author of 'Nursing in Rural Ontario' assured readers that 'even in our older settled Ontario, the private nurse has ample scope to exercise her every talent.' The author agreed with her western counterpart on the preferential conditions of countryside over cityscape. 'It seems to me that rural nursing is far more satisfactory than in the city, even though hours are longer and the hardships greater. A good nurse makes a reputation for herself and retains it—she has full scope for her own individuality.'[59] Working in Canada's geographic centre, Manitoba RN Catherine De Nully Fraser spoke for all private practitioners when she emphasized the rewards felt by a job well done. Speaking from her 'experience having "specialed" 140 to 150 patients, many of them in their own homes, where hospital conveniences are lacking', Fraser argued that it was a nurse's privilege to determine the amount of domestic work performed for patients.

Nurses sometimes feel that they are imposed upon, or are expected to do what lies outside their province when nursing in patients' homes. . . . No hard and fast rules and regulations can be laid down as to the duties of a private nurse. She is more or less free to make her own arrangements with the family and to use her own initiative in a way she cannot do in institutional work.[60]

Most nurses agreed that the 'personal freedom' inherent in private practice contrasted sharply with the 'regimen and disciplines of institutional nursing' they had encountered as students.[61]

Of course, the private market was not without its pitfalls, chief among them the problem of collecting fees. For such practitioners, the growing demand for special-duty nurses represented the ideal compromise. As a variation on private work, special nursing of patients in hospitals involved the one-to-one care student and staff in institutions rarely encountered, but, as Mary Catton of Ottawa's Protestant General Hospital explained, it also accorded nurses some protection from the vicissitudes of the unregulated market. 'Special nursing in a hospital may not be all sunshine and roses, but nevertheless has many favourable features in comparison with private nursing in general in that the nurse gets a certain amount of protection from the hospital.' Protection came in the form of fee collection. Catton believed 'the hospital should . . . assist in securing the payment of bills', but since institutions often found it difficult to get their own charges covered, the likelihood that they would also take on the special nurse's financial cause was slim. None the less, knowing that discharged patients had to pay doctor and hospital bills made it somewhat easier for special nurses also to demand their fee.[62]

As the urban middle class grew and public demand for institutional surgical services increased, the availability of hospital-based special-duty cases expanded apace. Yet that same institutional growth also undermined the private health-care market. Hospitals continued to rely on the apprenticeship system of staffing and therefore the construction of new hospital wards was accompanied by increases in student enrolments. Increased enrolments meant that three years later the nursing work-force received large infusions of new practitioners all competing for cases and staff positions. But the percentage of Canadians who could afford private nursing care did not grow proportionally. The difficulty of making wages cover the cost of living, which many Canadians faced in the economically unstable 1920s, maintained a ceiling on the patient population commanding the resources necessary to purchase skilled attendance.[63] As the 1920s progressed, the downward spiral of increased reliance on hospital services, growth in the graduate nurse population, and reduced demand for domestic health care sent conventional nursing into a tailspin. One 1921 observer bleakly summarized the fate of the average hospital graduate: 'Her work is uncertain, she must frequently be idle whether she can afford it or not, [and] years of faithful labour win no recognition.'[64] The still more generalized economic depression of the 1930s accentuated, but did not cause, the crisis that began taking form soon after World War I.

Local registry records confirm that the nursing crisis had begun well before the stock market crash of 1929. In the Maritime region, which never fully regained economic stability after World War I, nurses struggled with the impact of recession throughout the 1920s. The president of the RNANS, Sibella Barrington, explained the problems faced by Nova Scotia's private nurses in her September 1924 *CN* report.

So many industries have closed, people have left the Province and general depression is at present responsible for the slow growth in many lines, nursing included. . . . Private duty nurses are kept fairly busy, but it is very seldom that the demand is greater than the supply.[65]

Available statistics for the Manitoba Association of Registered Nurses directory suggest that while the absolute number of calls filled by the registry rose dramatically during the 1920s, these jobs were shared by growing numbers of nurses. Between 1922 and 1929 the registrar of MARN's Nurses' Central Directory fielded an annual average of 3,833 requests for graduate nurses. By 1929 this trend peaked at 5,848 calls, an increase of 65 per cent. Between 1924 and 1929, however, the Winnipeg General alone had added a possible 395 RNs to this pool, representing a 78 per cent increase from just one institution.[66]

Despite efforts by some training schools to reduce their student work-forces during the 1930s, the imbalance between trained attendants and paying patients actually deteriorated as patient requests for nurses declined.[67] In the words of the MARN registrar: 'As you remember, prior to 1929, hospitals all over the Continent were graduating such increasingly larger classes of nurses that a serious over-production was bound to result. The situation was suddenly made acute by the on-set of the depression in the fall of that year . . . .'[68] The 6 January 1933 report of MARN's registrar explained:

The year 1932 has indeed been a very slack year for the private duty nurses. It would appear that some of the reasons for the lack of work is that the health of the community is good, but the greatest factor is the severe financial strain that the whole community is suffering from and is now undergoing.[69]

Winnipeg graduate Helen Smith recalled being unemployed up to four weeks between private-duty jobs. During those weeks Smith stayed 'close to the phone', waiting for the registry to call. Fellow alumna Violet McMillan received so little work during the early 1930s that she was forced to go on relief, during which time she awaited calls from the registry.[70] By 1936, conditions had not improved. That year, of the eight occupations recording the greatest numbers of unemployed women, the highest percentage, over 22 per cent, was among graduate nurses.[71] When in 1942 MARN's registrar was asked if enough nurses were available to meet any emergency, she reported that in 1938, 1939, and 1940, averages of only 16, 17, and 21 nurses were called to work per day of 145, 141, and 106 available, respectively.

Table 4.3
Average Weeks Spent Employed, Unemployed, Ill,
and on Vacation, 1929–1930, Canada

Sector	Employed	Unemployed	Ill	Vacation
Private-duty nurses	29.9	14.3	4.5	3.3
Institutional nurses	46.3	.7	.8	4.2
Public health nurses	47.1	0	.9	4.0
Superintendents of nursing	45.0	0	2.7	4.3

SOURCE: G. Weir, *Survey of Nursing Education in Canada* (Toronto, 1932).

The impact of unemployment was most pronounced within the private health-care market. Table 4.3 lists how the respondents to Weir's survey spent the twelve months prior to his investigation. As early as 1930, private-duty nurses were having trouble getting enough weeks of work to keep them financially solvent, whereas hospital and public health positions guaranteed more regular employment. Averaging less than 30 weeks on duty, Weir's private-duty participants booked off for fewer weeks of vacation than did their peers in public health or institutional work, and they sat idle for over three months. Weir's figures may have masked unemployment in the institutional and public health sectors in that nurses who lost their positions with hospitals or agencies may have returned to the private-duty pool rather than call themselves unemployed institutional or public health nurses. Before long, however, unemployment in all branches of nursing became apparent, especially when financially strained provincial and municipal governments began reducing their public health commitments. For instance, in 1933 the Manitoba Public Health Nursing Service laid off 30 staff nurses when many rural districts could not maintain their part of the municipal/provincial funding arrangements.[72]

Hospital nurses faced a slightly different set of circumstances. Throughout the 1920s, institutional staff, graduate and student alike, faced growing patient demand on already overcrowded hospital facilities, especially publicly financed beds and wards. The following decade the number of hospital jobs and the number of positions available for apprentices began to erode, leaving the remaining staff to cope with heavy patient loads. As the pace of work intensified, the health of hospital staff and the ability of institutions to recruit replacement staff suffered. As early as 1928, Kathleen Ellis was suggesting that graduate nurses would have to supplement student staff if standards of care were to be maintained. Complaints from patients about the inadequacy of care included 'inability to get nurses when needed', 'lack of skill of students', 'nurses tired and apparently overworked', 'inattention and indifference to disturbing noises', and 'too many different nurses, none of whom seem informed of what the others have done'. Such complaints reflected the chronic problem of overwork for those institutional nurses who kept their positions.[73] A 1937 letter to the editor of the *Vancouver Daily Province*, written in the aftermath of a debate in the BC legislature over a CCF private member's bill proposing to regulate the hours worked by hospital nurses, demonstrated that working nurses were painfully aware of the penalties hospital staffs were paying. A nurse from Comox wrote: '[In] almost every hospital in the province nurses are being seriously overworked, and [are] leaving hospital service with ambition crushed and health broken.'[74] While their sisters in private duty waited for their next paying patient, institutional nurses endured 12-hour duty and a seemingly endless supply of dependent patients to tend.

Related to the differential pattern of unemployment among the three sectors was a sectoral difference in the annual salaries commanded by Canadian nurses. Weir calculated that the annual average income for private-duty nurses in 1929–30 was only $1,022,

Figure 4.1
Annual Income, by Province, 1929–1930

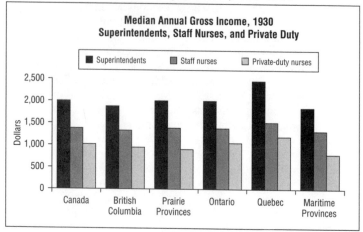

SOURCE: G. Weir, *Survey of Nursing Education in Canada* (Toronto, 1932).

compared to $1,385 for institutional staff and $1,574 for public health workers. Superintendents averaged over $2,000 that year. Figure 4.1 provides a regional comparison of annual income. The slight economic advantage staff nurses enjoyed in the late 1920s waned the following decade. Rural institutions especially had tried to attract staff in the 1920s by offering slightly higher wages than paid to urban hospital nurses. A decade later, many small hospitals struggled to pay their staff at all.[75] At Pine Falls, Manitoba, the hospital continued to function in the mid-1930s thanks to one regular paying customer, the federal government, which took financial responsibility for First Nations patients. Still, the hospital reduced nurses' wages from $90 to $60, dropping the staff salary below that of Winnipeg General nurses. Even superintendents felt the effects of fiscal restraint. In 1934–5, Jo Mann accepted a new position as superintendent of Weyburn's mental hospital, only to discover that after one month the provincial government unilaterally reduced her salary by $50 per month.[76]

Private-duty nurses found individual families even more difficult employers to deal with. In addition to the lost wages that resulted from being unemployed, on average, more than three months of the year, private-duty nurses faced the additional burden of being underpaid, or unpaid, for their labour. Mary Catton's *CN* article included the story of

... a recent graduate ... [who] spent her first case of three weeks on a farm. At the end of her case the farmer offered her a 'fatted calf' in payment of her fee, as an alternative to waiting until the following fall for payment. On the spur of the moment, with the problems of transportation and final disposal of the animal looming ahead, she elected to wait.[77]

In 1954 Vera Chapman received a letter from a former patient containing the $10 the patient had owed for work Chapman performed in 1933.[78] Like Chapman, many nurses could find jobs, but they had trouble getting paid. A survey conducted between 1933 and 1935 among Manitoba private-duty nurses revealed that 'thirty-two per cent of the nurses in the province of Manitoba have not received the full fee for one case during the past two years', and 231 cases were nursed with no remuneration.[79] Such documentation flew in the face of the standard fees established by provincial nursing associations of $5 for 12-hour duty, $6 for 24-hour duty, and travelling expenses for out-of-town work.[80]

On this irregular income, private-duty nurses had to meet the constant costs of board and room that most institutions and many organizations provided. Private-duty nurses arranged for their own accommodation, which they had to maintain even when lodging temporarily at a patient's residence. Having to pay rent substantially raised the cost of living for these nurses over their peers 'living in'.[81] Weir illustrated this additional complication in private-duty work by preparing two 'typical budgets of the average private duty nurse', that of 'Nurse A', whose familial support saved her from being 'entirely dependent on her earnings to provide for the future', and one for the self-supporting prototype, 'Nurse B'. As Table 4.4 illustrates, the former required nearly $1,400 to cover her expenses, while the latter had to earn $1,600 per year, but in both scenarios costs far outstripped the annual average income of $1,022 his private-duty survey respondents reported.

While living with their families was one way many nurses could financially survive in the private sphere, Weir reminded his readership that nurses in all subfields faced responsibilities for 'family or personal obligations which consumed their last dollar above bare living expenses' and that nurses' wages were by no means 'pin money'.[82] Whether falling into Weir's categories of 'A' or 'B', most private nurses averaged well below the standard of living Weir deemed necessary for them to remain 'a member, and probably a leader in the community'.[83]

Table 4.4
Estimated Cost of Living, Canada, 1929–1930

| | Annual Expenditure in $ | |
Item	Nurse 'A'	Nurse 'B'
Rent and board	325.00	444.00
Clothing	250.00	300.00
Uniforms	60.85	91.05*
Laundry	105.00	144.00
Fees	21.00	21.00
Car fare	45.60	45.60
Insurance	166.30	132.00
Charity	60.00	60.00
Recreation	60.00	60.00
Dentist	43.00	40.00
Dry cleaning, etc.	12.00	36.00
Health, beauty parlor, etc.	12.00	36.00
Presents, gratuities, and subscriptions	75.00	75.00
Sundries	30.00	30.00
Holidays	120.00	100.00
Total	$1,386.15	$1,590.65

*'This includes two pair of shoes, white polish, six blouses, three skirts, eight aprons, eight bibs, six pair cuffs, six collars, eight pair stockings, three caps, and misc repairs to uniforms.'

SOURCE: G. Weir, *Survey of Nursing Education in Canada* (Toronto, 1932).

The disparity between annual income and cost of living and what that disparity meant for women workers was manifest in the relative abilities of nurses to save for the future. Financial advice such as that offered by Kathleen Snowdon, thrift adviser for the T. Eaton Company, appeared periodically in nursing publications and optimistically declared that 'haphazard, thoughtless spending is certain to deprive us of much that the same income well administered would provide'.[84] Wise budgeting alone, however, could not prevent the disillusionment that many graduates experienced as their income failed to stabilize after several years. As a 1926 *CN* reprint of an *American Journal of Nursing* article confessed:

When you have come to the end of three financially lean years in a school for nurses and find yourself a full-fledged nurse, privileged to write RN after your name, and have temporarily placed in your pocketbook the cheque for your first case, you are entitled to feel, for a few days at least, that you are in the near-millionaire class. Perhaps the cheque is for $168, for it was a four-week case. Oh Girl! What a delirious time you will have spending those dollars for things you were forced to do without when your hospital allowance was $10 a month!

Enthusiasm for the financial independence that pay cheques represented wore thin as the memories of student life began to fade.

But perhaps you have been writing RN after your name for some time, possibly for several years, and have grown accustomed to fairly frequently pocketing cheques of three figures and yet for some reason or other your bank account fluctuates sadly. . . . You have learned, too, that your income is not as magnificent as you thought it would be until you discovered that you cannot be on duty every day in the year. . . . There are forced periods of waiting . . . .[85]

In a reprint from the Federation of Women Teachers' Association of Canada *Bulletin*, Flora Stewart alerted *CN* readers that economic marginality was a dilemma facing many working women.

Sad to relate, the basis of remuneration still rests in masculine hands, with the result that the average professional and business woman has none too large a margin between necessary expenditure and income. Having chosen a career . . . the thrills of independence in youth, the delightful freedom which independence brings in middle age, carry in their train the dire necessity of independence in old age.[86]

The inability of private-duty or institutional sectors to implement a system of experience-based pay increments made cumulated savings a rarity. The opinion of the average public health nurse 'that she is 10 per cent better off financially than when she first began her career nearly 9 years earlier' was shared by very few private-duty or institutional nurses.[87]

Approximately half of the private-duty nurses Weir consulted had saved nothing from their year's labour and a further 40 per cent had saved an average of only $240 over the previous year. Fifty per cent of hospital nurses had no savings to show at the end of the 1929–30 work year, whereas 45 per cent had averaged $314 of surplus wages. Public health nurses enjoyed greater financial security, with 40 per cent banking an average of $400 that year.[88] Weir found that only 3 per cent of the public health respondents had saved nothing over their careers, whereas 47 per cent of hospital and 54 per cent of private-duty nurses showed no career savings. The remaining 46 per cent of private practitioners claimed a surplus of less than $600. Even the superintendents Weir consulted, who as a group saved a median figure of $2,078 since embarking on their careers, worried about their economic future. Savings could only stretch so far if unemployment or sickness struck.[89]

The solution for many lay in insurance and annuities, which would, in the opinion of one veteran private-duty practitioner, 'help [nurses] remove from their lives that sordid financial anxiety which must sap peace and pleasure from their existence.'[90] Over 50 per cent of private-duty nurses owned insurance or annuities, as did 58 per cent of superintendents, 68 per cent of hospital employees, and 80 per cent of public health workers. Unfortunately, annual payments into insurance or pension plans, however judicious for the long term, once purchased were hard to maintain, especially given the very real health hazards faced by working nurses. Lamenting the lack of 'financial protection' for many private-duty nurses, Weir concluded: 'Were their health to give out at any time, or when they become too old to work— and the life of a nurse is especially hard and exacting after the average woman reaches about 50 years of age—there appears no alternative but economic ruin'.[91] Other commentators agreed that the threat of disease intensified nurses' economic perils. In a polemic endorsing superannuation, M. Judson Eaton argued in *CN*:

> In almost every other occupation the fact is recognized that it is impossible for people to work seven days in the week—not to mention twelve hours out of twenty four. . . . Not so with the nurse. Every day's rest or recreation she takes represents a loss greater than any gain possible on a day 'on duty'. She may, and often does, work overtime and risks her own health recklessly when the life or welfare of her patient is at stake, and when, after the battle is won, she is obliged to spend a week, a month—or sometimes longer— recuperating from the effects of the strain. . . .[92]

In a similar vein, Montreal private nurse Agnes Jamieson used her position on the CNA Publication Committee to condemn the extreme length of nurses' working days. Jamieson called for the abolition of 24-hour duty and the exploitation of nurses that around-the-clock attendance involved: 'If patients are not sick enough to have [and hire] night nurses they are well enough to stay alone', wrote Jamieson. Even 12-hour shifts—'actually fourteen hours from the time [the nurse's] alarm goes off in the morning until she arrives home at night, weary and ready for bed'—were debilitating when worked consecutively.[93] Despite efforts to the contrary, throughout the 1920s and 1930s these hours continued to prevail in domestic and special-duty service, and private nurses faced double indemnity: they needed steady work to exist, but steady work undermined their health and threatened their ability to work steadily.

Institutional nursing promised more reliable volume and hours of work, and thus more reliable income, but no real relief from long shifts. Graduate nurses were all too familiar with the day-duty/night-duty schedule that had dominated their lives during training and often attributed their survival as apprentices to their initial good health. Martha Riggs, a 1925 graduate of Halifax's Victoria General, recalled:

> We'd come off duty in the morning . . . we had to give the report and everything, we'd stand there just dead after twelve hours running, practically running up and down . . . it was work, work . . . we must have been very smart . . . not only smart but we must have been very healthy coming from the country because we just worked like dogs.[94]

Not all nurses avoided the health risks inherent in institutional work. Investigations into the alarming rate with which nurses appeared among the clientele of tuberculosis sanatoriums suggested the rigours of hospital work could be dangerous to students and staff alike. In her article 'Increase of Tuberculosis Among Nurses', the lady superintendent of the Queen Alexandra Sanatorium in London, Ontario, Ann M. Forrest, pointed out the bitter irony of tuberculosis increasing 'among one of the valuable groups of workers in the campaign for better health.' Citing a study of 13 Canadian tuberculosis facilities, with 1,514 women in residence, Forrest noted that 99, or over 6 per cent, were nurses. 'As many nurses were under treatment as school teachers, stenographers and university women taken together.'[95] Another study of 60 nurses admitted to Manitoba's Ninette Sanatorium discovered that 40 had developed symptoms during their hospital training.[96] Weir's calculation that hospital and public health staff suffered from less than one week of sick days per year, compared to the four weeks private-duty nurses missed work due to ill health, may have masked the degree to which staff nurses with long-term health problems had to give up their hospital or public health jobs and retreat to the more flexible private market. This option could only be exercised for the short term, however, for in the long term economic exigencies demanded steady employment for all nurses.[97] The words of one veteran highlighted the double-edged dilemma confronting nursing's majority: 'I am very fond of my work, but consider the irregularity and long hours impair my health.'[98]

Issues of financial and physical health influenced the relative ease with which nurses in each type of work could support themselves throughout their careers. Only 7 per cent of Weir's private-duty respondents and 5 per cent of hospital staff nurses were over age 50, compared to 10 per cent of public health nurses in that age category. Superintendents were older still and the fact that nearly 20 per cent of those included in Weir's study were employed after their fiftieth birthday served as mute testimony to the career potential realized within the administrative sector.[99] The average age of private-duty and hospital nurses that Weir consulted was 31 years, whereas public health nurses were 37.4 years on average and superintendents 42.5 years. This age differential correlated to the difference in years of experience accumulated by nurses working in the various subsectors. Private-duty and hospital nurses claimed less than six years of work experience. With an average of 8.8 years' experience, public health nurses were, like their peers on hospital staffs and in private practice, predominantly graduates of the 1920s.[100]

Not so with superintendents. Only 26 per cent of the 150 administrators Weir contacted had graduated since 1920. Over two-thirds had completed their training before the end of World War I and in 1929 they averaged 14.5 years work experience. Thus the age gap between administrators and the graduate nurses working in hospitals either as staff nurses or as specials signified substantially different generational experiences.[101] Several factors reinforced the age and experience differential. First, by the 1920s most hospital expansion had ceased, so that the opportunities for promotion were limited to those second-generation nurses who had gained valuable supervisory experience during the earlier decades of growth. Occupational leaders like Grace Fairley, Kathleen Ellis, Ethel Johns, Christina MacLeod, and Mabel Gray launched successful administrative careers in the 1910s that spanned the inter-war decades.[102]

A second factor was movement within the occupation. Most new graduates entered active practice providing one-to-one care to individual patients in the private market. As financial difficulties mounted, many private-duty nurses tried to improve their lot by shifting into one of the more stable areas of employment. Of the more than 50 per cent of institutional nurses who, in 1930, cited experience in other sectors of the occupation, 89 per cent had worked as private-duty nurses for an average of 1.3 years. Only 11 per cent had transferred from public health employment. Public health positions required at least six months of postgraduate training, and only those new graduates with financial capabilities and a passion for public health work pursued these positions immediately. Over 70 per cent of public health nurses who responded to Weir's survey worked for more than a year in another subsector before pursuing their public health careers, with averages of two years in private duty work and 2.5 years in institutional service.[103] Mobility between the occupation's subsectors kept the average age of the private-duty work-force low, especially compared to the more stable administrative sector.

The data from Weir's *Survey of Nursing Education in Canada* verified that by 1932 many nurses had already moved out of the private market and many others planned to follow suit. Of those actively practising only 55 per cent of private nurses were satisfied with their branch of the profession, as compared to 71 per cent of institutional nurses and 87 per cent of public health workers. Many private nurses were sadly disappointed in the 'material satisfactions' their work offered and the limited opportunities for 'leisure' that uncertain employment caused. By the time Weir began his nationwide tour, economic strain was forcing many private nurses to consider seriously the occupational options they had earlier rejected. In the words of Weir's respondents:

I enjoy my work very much but I would not advise any one else to join the profession on account of uncertain employment—not enough leisure and unprofitable in comparison with other professions, e.g. stenography, teaching.

If there was anything other than nursing that I knew how to do, I think I would do that.

More than one-third of the private-duty group were undecided as to their future plans, and they pondered whether to continue doing the work they preferred or to seek employment, nursing or otherwise, that would improve their financial status. Claimed one woman, 'I intend to remain in private duty nursing unless I find an ideal husband.'[104]

As the 1930s progressed, pressure on all three subsectors increased, prompting large numbers of graduates to abandon active practice in Canada. The size of the student nurse population remained fairly constant over the 1931–41 period, with 11,436 in 1931 as opposed to 11,822 a decade later.[105] Weir's numbers for 1931 were comparable. Yet if 11,436 students were enrolled in nursing schools in 1931, then by 1934, when all the potential graduates would have been added to the active nursing population, 31,898 graduate nurses should have been in the work-force in 1934 alone, with the graduating classes of 1935 through 1940 swelling the ranks further. The fact that by 1941 the work-force only measured 26,887 indicates the substantial departure from active practice through retirement, marriage, occupational change, or death.

An alternative solution to leaving active practice was outmigration, particularly to the United States. The high wages and plentiful work in both private and institutional nursing had been attracting Maritime nurses to New England since the early years of the century. As Martha Riggs explained: 'The reason most nurses went to the US, Boston in particular, Boston was *the* place, was money . . . because the middle class in Nova Scotia like myself in those days they didn't have that kind of money.'[106] In 1936 MARN's registrar speculated that unemployment among nurses was being kept in check by the 'exodus' of 40–50 nurses to Minnesota.[107] This analysis was confirmed in 1939 when she explained:

> [a shortage in the US] was precipitated in the fall of 1936, when, under the Works Program Administration, a vast sum of money was voted for Public Health work. This field of employment attracted so many nurses that many of their hospitals were almost depleted of their general duty staff. They consequently turned to Canada for help. During the following ten months, over three hundred passports were issued by the American Immigration authorities in Winnipeg alone to nurses. . . . One hundred of those being to nurses registered at the Nurses' Central Directory in Winnipeg. What a relief it was to our local situation is shown by the fact that instead of fifty on call per day from [one] hospital, as in November 1936, the same month the following year there were but twenty.[108]

Within three years wartime nursing shortages were causing nursing leaders to view this outmigration with less enthusiasm, but in the meantime it was viewed as a temporary solution to a problem that local leaders had, for a decade, been unable to solve.

Outmigration could not, however, resolve the larger issue that economic dislocation was damaging nursing's position as a privileged occupation for working women. In the early 1920s, apprenticing nurses looked forward to the personal and fiscal freedom that life as a graduate nurse would bring. A poem published in Vancouver General's 1926 yearbook, entitled 'Finance', bemoaned the poverty of student life, concluding that:

> I'll have to work on for a year or two
> Before my dreams can all come true—
> But the joy of living will just be great
> When I've become a graduate.[109]

But by the end of the decade the 'joy of living' appeared as elusive as ever. In the words of a 1934 Winnipeg graduate:

> It is with a feeling of secret shame and remorse as well as a good deal of foreboding that training schools of today send their young graduates out, for they know only too well what a barren future awaits them. And the young graduate herself, no longer is she serenely confident: it is rather with a shrinking feeling of fear that the '34 nurse must face the future.[110]

Nurses' impoverished state became a common theme in the occupational popular culture of the 1930s. The Vancouver General *Nurses' Annual* of 1937 included student M. Barton's reworking of a Robert Chambers poem. Barton's verse proclaimed:

> And by that sea, that quiet sea,
> Beyond the farthest line,
> Where all the foments I have burned,
> Where all the things I might have learned,
> and all the cash I should have earned,
> I'll find![111]

The implication that economic self-sufficiency could be found only in some future paradise was more forcefully articulated in a drawing of a nurse whose uniform was patched and pinned together together. Once again the nurses' uniform stood as an occupational symbol, but now as a signifier of all that was wrong with the occupation that had promised so much to working women.

The erosion of rank-and-file confidence in their occupational choice was echoed by commentators like Weir, who questioned whether the economic status of the third generation of Canadian nurses could allow the practitioner to be 'a member, and probably a leader in the community'. Weir's consternation over nurses' community status revealed the deeper meaning signified by unemployment and wages. Although they continued to earn more than many working women, the precarious financial conditions nurses faced jeopardized the ideal of economic and social independence for women. Nurses were supposed to be economically self-sufficient; nursing was supposed to offer a viable economic option to marriage. For those who

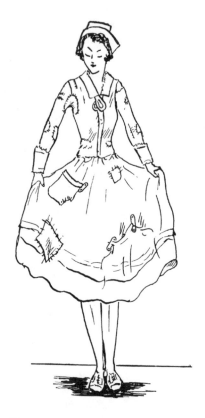

'Two more payments and she's mine!'

SOURCE: Vancouver General Hospital, *Nurses' Annual*, 1937.

hoped the 'new day' had arrived, nurses' experiences confirmed their worst fears.[112] If nursing, an occupation privileged by a relatively long period of institutional apprenticeship, could not offer women financial stability over their lifetimes, then the entire concept of women's economic independence was called into question.

Collective Responses to the Economic Crisis

The economic crisis of the inter-war decades threatened not only the livelihoods of women relying on nursing skills for economic sustenance but also the image and reputation that first- and second-generation nurses had struggled to build. As the crisis of employment intensified and as proposed solutions proved difficult to implement, internal differences among the occupation's subsectors appeared and the occupational cohesion that shaped nurses' associational structures began to crumble. In their efforts to maintain unity within the occupation and within established organizations, association leaders debated the appropriate actions to be taken. Hospital employment of graduate nurses to provide 'general duty' bedside patient care emerged as a temporary solution for the unemployment crisis. In the short term, that strategy prevented the immediate fragmenting of nursing's occupational cohesion, but in the long run it served to highlight differences among nurses, reassert a permanent hierarchy among them, and open the door for alternative modes of organizational activity.

By the early 1920s, Canadian nurses had established organizational structures at six levels. Student councils and alumnae associations represented the interests of apprentices and graduates of individual schools; local and provincial organizations united trained nurses working within local and regional health-care markets; and national and international bodies addressed issues that transcended provincial and national borders. Relations among these organizational levels were characterized by co-operation and practitioners were encouraged to maintain membership in their alumnae, local, and provincial associations. At the national level, in 1924 the Canadian National Association of Trained Nurses merged with the Canadian Association of Nursing Education to form the Canadian Nurses' Association (CNA). Throughout the 1920s the CNA worked to streamline the structure of affiliation among nursing organizations and create a strict vertical integration maintained by careful adherence to jurisdictional powers of each level. When French-language nursing journals were established in Quebec, *La Veilleuse* in 1924 followed by *La Garde-Malade canadienne-française* in 1928, *Canadian Nurse* treated them as complementary, not competing, publications. In an effort to facilitate good relations with their Quebec sisters, *CN* published excerpts from the Quebec journals and reports of the activities of French-speaking nurses.[113] Thus, unlike their American counterparts, Canadian associations overlapped but did not compete for recruits and loyalty.[114]

This did not mean that difference was not recognized within nursing associations. Provincial and national bodies in particular acknowledged the diverse experiences of nurses working in various contexts and thus in the early 1920s established 'sections' for private duty, public health, and nurse education designed to deal with issues unique to each kind of nursing work. Each section had its own convenor, and at each meeting—monthly, annual, or biennial—the convenor reported on that section's activities and concerns. Policy proposals generated within each section were brought before the general membership for discussion and endorsement. In this way private-duty nurses, who because of their mobility and independence were all too easy to lose contact with or to alienate, had a separate and formal voice designed to ensure their representation, while nursing educators could maintain their traditional focus but within the broader collective endeavour. In accommodating the various kind of practitioners, nursing organizations maintained their monopoly of representation, at the same time reasserting a belief in the equality of members.

The structural equality did not, in itself, ensure that all members had equal access to participation in associational life. Most private-duty nurses, working within the erratic and unpredictable private market, lacked the resources necessary to volunteer for associational responsibilities. In contrast, those with salaried positions in training schools or public health agencies could depend on scheduled time off. Indeed, institutions and agencies often encouraged their nursing staff to attend professional events. This produced unequal representation in leadership positions, with hospital training school staff and public health nurses filling more than their share of positions on executives and boards.[115] Counterbalancing the fact that private-duty sections attracted fewer delegates and generated fewer associational leaders was the numerical superiority of private practitioners. With the majority of members behind them, private-duty representatives insisted that only practising private-duty nurses could represent their interests. In this way, the rough equality among graduate nurses was reinforced within nursing organizations.

The balance between the dominance of hospital and public health nurses in leadership positions and private-duty nurses' numerical superiority was challenged by the economic crisis of the inter-war years. Nursing's organizational structure was jeopardized by the threat of loss of membership, by conflict from within existing organizations, and by the possibility of alternative organizational forms. To maintain organizational and occupational unity, nursing leaders experimented with a number of strategies to cure nursing's ills, but the solutions proposed often provoked new problems and exposed fresh cracks in the occupational and organizational cohesion.

Associational cohesion was directly threatened when underemployment and unemployment reduced the membership base of local bodies. Provincial and alumnae associations depended on a large base of support to secure membership fees, to lobby provincial governments regarding legislative concerns, and to assert collective control over issues such as wage scales and unlicensed competition. The potential membership base had already been eroded in many places by outmigration from the occupation and/or region. For nurses who remained in the Canadian nursing markets, if the registry was not providing work then there was little reason for the ordinary nurse, living on precarious income, to spend $1 or $2 per year on membership fees and a further $10 per year to be listed on the registry. The MARN registrar was not alone among women of her position when she reported in 1931 that of 267 nurses registered 133 were in arrears, some up to two years. Organizations embraced various strategies for consolidating their membership base. In an effort to facilitate financial support from working members, MARN reduced the directory fee in 1932 from $10 to $8, but by 1935 the ongoing problem of collecting fees convinced the Manitoba association to write off dues unpaid from January 1930 to July 1934.[116] Elsewhere, registrars removed errant members from the registry file.

To convince existing members that the local organizations were in fact defending the interests of local nurses, associations took further steps to consolidate membership. As unemployment worsened, local associations tried to stem the inward flow of new practitioners. In July of 1930, the registrar of the Vancouver Graduate Nurses' Association informed the readership of CN that the 'oversupply' of graduate nurses, caused in part by the recent influx of nurses 'from outside points' and in part by the large classes of graduating students, had forced the association to decide 'that our first duty is to these nurses already resident here'. Prospective migrants to the west coast were warned: 'So in all fairness to the profession at large, we wish the nurses to understand that anyone coming to Vancouver at this stage takes the responsibility of long periods of unemployment.' The BC decision to deny newcomers access to the registry appears to have been unique, but elsewhere hospitals were pressed to hire only their own graduates, and health agencies were encouraged to employ only locally trained nurses.[117] When Winnipeg General Hospital graduate Sadie Thorvaldson applied in 1939 to Winnipeg's Margaret Scott Mission, she explained that she had left her public health job in Edmonton because 'I find myself, along with other "outside" graduates asked to find employment elsewhere.'[118] Protecting locally trained practitioners did allow alumnae and city associations to act on behalf of their members, but the long-term effect of such policies was a balkanization of the Canadian nursing work-force. Increased dependence on local agencies and employers contradicted provincial and national policies of reciprocity and, perhaps more seriously, undermined the portability of nursing certification, which had been one of the positive features of RN status.

As local associations struggled with questions of membership and mobility, a second challenge to the existing organizational framework emerged, the creation of competing representative bodies and more militant strategies for change. In 1928 national nursing attention focused on student nurses at Guelph's General Hospital when they walked off the job. The unenthusiastic report in *Canadian Nurse* of the event was contributed by a former hospital director. Blaming the 'meddling of a sensation-seeking city press', the author lamented that 'the recent regrettable discord has attracted far more attention than it deserved.' The *CN* commentator sympathized with the difficult situations faced by many superintendents and reminded disgruntled apprentices that 'when she feels aggrieved at the superintendent: she may be a superintendent herself some day.' Allusions to the possibilities awaiting graduate nurses could not erase the fact that nurses might look outside their occupationally specific vehicles to improve their working conditions.

> Had not outside meddling and publicity fanned the embers into a fierce flame the sparks of trouble would in all probability soon have been quenched. I am confident that the nurses have been badly advised, probably by well-meaning friends, and that in cooler moments they will regret sincerely having taken part in an organized and decidedly unprofessional walk-out.[119]

Yet the possibility of invoking external support remained a real option for nurses confronting poor working conditions and an unstable market. In the late 1930s, complaints lodged by individual nurses to the provincial government resulted in Fraudina Eaton's 1938 study of labour conditions in British Columbia's hospitals. The RNABC later confessed that it had not initiated such a study. Nursing organizations were concerned about the negative effect that other kinds of lobbying groups might have on the traditional basis of associational strength. In 1938, the CNA General Assembly was reminded:

> If the Nursing Profession does nothing toward furthering a plan for an eight hour duty for nurses then it can be expected that labour groups will compel action by legislation. In nearly every province, legislation has been enacted to protect every type of

person connected with the hospital except the nurse. If the Profession is not going to take a definite stand then organized nursing might as well stop talking about eight hour duty nurses.[120]

This concern about losing authority over their occupation was well placed in a decade of radical solutions. Given the dramatic class struggles occurring in the inter-war years, labour leaders were perhaps too preoccupied to unionize nurses, but there were signs that radicalism was in nurses' midst.[121] In 1934 newly graduated Annie Glaz suggested to the Winnipeg General alumnae that temporary solutions to nurses' economic problems would no longer suffice. Acknowledging the efforts made by 'those occupying high positions who, by virtue of their posts and their wide influence have carried their share of the burden', Glaz declared:

> we feel it is not fair to them to do more than their share. Nor is it fair to us, for we will naturally become dependent and clinging, all initiative will be nipped in the bud and we will remain dormant, devoid of any fighting stamina. . . . We alone can alleviate our present deplorable situation.

Her conclusion was that 'in unity there is strength. Let us show that youth, unconquered and undaunted shall march to victory.' This was suitably ambiguous, and could have been interpreted as a call to associational unity. Although Glaz's later efforts to transform Manitoba's provincial association into a union failed, the effort did suggest that her call for a march to victory included using tactics outside the usual repertoire of nursing organizations.[122]

When in April 1939 the nursing staff at St Joseph's Hospital in Comox, BC, struck for improved conditions, the conventional nursing organizations had to conclude that the possibility of radical action was real indeed. The previous month the nurses had presented to the hospital board a list of demands that included the adoption of the eight-hour day, two weeks' annual vacation plus an allowance for two weeks' sick leave with pay, improved meals, and a monthly laundry allowance of $2.50. Several of these demands were granted by the board, but as the Vancouver press reported:

> No allowances were made for the undergraduate nurses who have been receiving less consideration than the maids. Feeling that rest was the most important, it was decided to forego all demands if we could have one day a week off duty, which would still leave a minimum 54 hour week day shift and 70 hour week night shift.

When this request was refused and no counter-proposal made, nine graduates and undergraduates, out of a staff of 12, walked off the job. After a week of substantial political and media attention, the hospital board agreed to the nurses' demands and the eight-hour day, six-day week, and two weeks' paid vacation were won.[123]

In the context of these two threats to the existing organizational framework—loss of membership or the possibility of new more radical forms of collective action—nursing organizations confronted a third challenge, that of internal conflict among members. As nursing commentators struggled to make sense of economic instability, many were tempted to blame private-duty nurses for their own lack of work. A 1939 MARN report stated:

> The hospitals have graduated too many of whom they are not anxious to call back on cases, and is the Registry justified in sending on a case a nurse whom her own hospital refuses to call, as we are responsible to the patient and to the Doctor for the service we can give them in this respect—but of course we have to use what the hospitals graduate.[124]

Graduate nurses' preference for private-duty work caused tension among nurses, as the following words of the MARN registrar revealed:

> While we have a surplus of nurses, we have not a surplus of *good* nurses, and we certainly have too many of a mediocre calibre. The private duty field is over crowded, not because of the real private duty nurse, the competent nurse who likes that work and intends to keep at it and has worked up a good practice, but because it is the place to which all flock who are unable to find what they want to do elsewhere.[125]

Blaming the unemployed for unemployment was not unique to nursing, but as an undercurrent that bubbled through nursing politics of the inter-war years it demonstrated the divisive potential that instability in the private market encouraged. When private-duty nurses turned to their collective representatives for solutions to dangerous working conditions and debilitating unemployment, the spectre of criticism and conflict was raised, as the debates within the CNA revealed.

Notes of discord could be heard within the CNA as early as 1921. Ironically, they were struck by Ethel Johns, one of Canada's most politically conscious practitioners.[126] In February of that year Johns presented a paper claiming that private nurses 'had nothing to say for themselves'. Given that Johns considered herself a private-duty nurse at the time, her words were meant as a challenge to nursing's majority to articulate their experiences and opinions. One did. In March 1921 a letter to *CN* from an anonymous 'Private Nurse' responded to Johns, directing her and other superintendents to 'clean their own steps. Never have I seen such mean unprincipled things done as I have known to be done by superintendents. . . .' Citing a tale wherein a student nurse had been expelled from a training program two months before her graduation, the anonymous critic went on to discredit the nursing experiences of most superintendents.

> At our conventions I have had ample opportunity to see how little the self-promoters really knew about the actual work. . . . No wonder you [Johns] allude to the pathos and bathos you passed through [in the past year of nursing] no doubt, you had all of half-a-dozen patients, five mild and one serious. What thrills you must still have. Now do tell us something about it at the next convention, and then we privates will be able to say, it truly is a nurses' convention, for some one did say a word about nursing this year.[127]

This letter, the most blatant criticism of anything or anyone to be printed in the first fifty years of the journal, highlighted the tensions between generations that conflict between nursing administrators and the rank and file provoked. While some working nurses, like the author, resented the position of occupational authority assumed by hospital superintendents, others continued to view institutional management as logical leaders and allies. A number of responses demanded a signed apology from the author and the end to anonymous contributions. Private nurse Annie Kennedy of Vancouver, BC, was among those most incensed that 'anything pertaining to the subject of private nursing, so remote from the work, so misleading, so petty and so utterly crude, should have found its way in among the regular thought-toned articles of our National Nursing Journal.'[128] When *CN* editor Miss Helen Randal, herself a former lady superintendent at Vancouver General, refused to publish the anonymous author's name, Kennedy ended her 12-year subscription to the journal.[129]

While the rough-and-tumble over professional ethics and public criticism raged, a more measured voice of dissent arose.[130] That voice belonged to a Toronto nurse, Miss A. Gaskell. The 1920 convention had been Gaskell's first. She and her four private-duty companions had eagerly anticipated an inspirational message, but instead found that 'the private duty nurse was the butt of the meeting'. Comments such as those made by Johns that 'many private duty nurses remained on cases much longer than required in order to draw large fees' (Gaskell

reminded the CNA that the length of tenure on a job was 'usually not settled by the nurse') prompted Gaskell to become involved in CNA sectional politics. The following year Gaskell returned to the national
meeting, this time as convenor of the Private Duty Nursing Section, and
immediately raised the question, '[is] there not a little tendency to criticize the private duty nurse?' Acknowledging that members of her section were too often 'inarticulate', an understated Gaskell began:

> It will . . . not be unfitting that a humble, private duty nurse of long
> experience, speaking for her sisters in the profession, on the neces-
> sity, desirability and utility of organization, should ask you to
> consider for a little while the reasons for the silence and in-
> effectiveness of the private duty nurse.

Gathering steam, she insisted that private nurses' inactivity was a
direct result of their conditions of work:

> The reasons are very clear to the nurse herself and should be easily
> comprehended by others. Long hours of labour of the most exact-
> ing and exhausting nature are disastrous to clearness and original-
> ity of thought, and the absolute lack of time for much-needed
> recreation, proper reading, religious exercises and social inter-
> course, which privileges the other branches of the profession enjoy
> to a far greater extent than does the private duty nurse, are not
> calculated to be productive of any very valuable or enlightening
> assistance from a body so handicapped.

No wonder, Gaskell observed, that 'with so many other occupations
offering easier conditions of work', nursing was waning in its popularity as a career choice. Whether or not Gaskell intended to touch the
nerve of nursing educators, who themselves worried over the recruiting potential of their schools, her final assessment that 'the opinion of
the five thousand private duty nurses of the Dominion has never been
sought in any matter of real moment to their profession' was a direct
challenge to the national body to take seriously the problems confronting the private-duty practitioners.[131]

Invited or not, private-duty nurses continued to voice their discontent through their national section and their national journal. Continued references to the 'inarticulate' majority of nurses working in the
private field reflected anxiety over the dominance of the CNA executive positions by nursing superintendents and recognition of the trou-
bles facing private-duty nurses. Johns risked further attack in 1930
when she offered her 'first-hand impression' of the 1930 CNA convention to the *CN* readership. 'One of the happiest features of the

convention', wrote Johns, 'was the active participation of the younger group of nurses. They not only had the courage of their convictions, but also the ability to express them clearly and well.' Amid veiled allusions to conflicts that arose at the meeting, Johns addressed the issues confronted by the Private Duty Section:

> The nursing profession as a whole is passing through a difficult phase, and this group more than any of the others had had to bear the brunt both of criticism and of economic stress. Its members discussed their special problems not only with frankness and good sense, but with a complete absence of the bitterness which might well have been held excusable in their difficult circumstances. . . . Watch the private duty nurses during the coming year. They not only know where they are going; they are on their way.

For all the difficulties inherent in pulling together such a dispersed group of private practitioners, policies presented by the Private Duty Section revealed that their members knew what they wanted to achieve—a solution to the employment problems vexing the private market. Implementing such policies was another matter. Johns's prediction that 'constructive suggestions were put forward [by the private-duty representatives] which, if carried into action, ought to show definite results before long', soon proved overly optimistic as the CNA's ability to defend the interests of its rank and file was tested.[132]

Under the leadership of articulate Private Duty Section chairs like Gaskell, three sets of solutions dominated national and local strategies for alleviating employment problems. The first focused on hours of labour, the 10-hour and later 8-hour day, which nurses hoped would not only improve their conditions of work but also create more employment for more nurses.[133] At the CNA's 1924 biennial meeting, the Private Duty Section presented a resolution to the General Assembly endorsing the abolition of 12-hour duty. Arguing that no other occupation demanded such long hours and that 'the undue length of the working day' was driving nurses out of private-duty work, the resolution asserted:

> . . . whereas the continued overweariness due to long hours of the most exacting labour must inevitably result in a much poorer quality of service rendered to the sick. . . . And whereas the private duty nurse knows that even a ten-hour day is too long for the kind of work she has to perform, yet because she realizes the difficulties under which hospitals carry on and because her desire is to disturb hospital management as little as possible . . .

Therefore be it resolved that the hours of duty for private duty Nurses in hospitals be from 8 a.m. to 6 p.m., and 8 p.m. to 6 a.m. The same hours to obtain in private homes where possible, at the discretion of the nurse.[134]

Responses to the resolution were mixed. Some members, like Miss McLelland of Montreal's Royal Victoria Hospital, informed the assembly that 'a similar plan was working out satisfactorily' at her institution. Miss Jean Gunn, superintendent of the Toronto General Hospital and a veteran CNA leader, was less enthused about private nurses controlling work within the hospital and disagreed with the hours of duty being 'so definitely stated'. Asserting the institution's ultimate responsibility for nursing services, Gunn was willing only to agree to 'some arrangements . . . whereby shorter hours could be planned'. To gain support from the nursing educators, Gaskell reminded her audience that at base what private nurses wanted was the 10-hour day. Her amended resolution, that nurses work 'ten consecutive hours, beginning preferably at 8 a.m. or 8 p.m.', was successful.[135]

Having agreed on the policy, a further motion determined its implementation. The Private Duty Section was empowered to send copies of the resolution to superintendents of nursing across the country. Boards of directors were deliberately overlooked since it was feared that 'this motion presented to hospital boards would cause considerable criticism, possibly of an adverse nature, but by presenting the resolution to superintendents of nurses the latter could quietly put the experiment into effect.'[136] This decision placed the responsibility for negotiating the 10-hour day on the shoulders of nursing rather than medical or lay administrators, but it also reflected the confidence of the CNA in the institutional authority of nursing superintendents. For their part, private-duty nurses believed that in the hospital private patients and their physicians would respect such a policy, whereas in the physician's office or the patient's home, asserting the 10-hour day would be virtually impossible for individual private nurses.

Some superintendents tried to accomplish this goal, but generally speaking, the 10-hour day continued to elude most private nurses during 1924 and 1925.[137] Correspondence in 1925 between the new national Private Duty convenor, Miss McElroy, and RNANS chair Jane Wakins revealed the former's scepticism regarding private nurses' ability to enforce 10-hour duty and her belief that each hospital would adopt a different plan. None the less, advocates were undeterred. Resolutions endorsing reduced hours were presented at biennial meetings in 1926 and again in 1928, embarrassing the Nursing Education

Section whose members were clearly unable or unwilling to implement the change. In 1928, the CNA chair intervened in the stalemate by ruling 'that as identical resolutions were passed at the 1926 meeting . . . the resolutions of the Private Duty Section as presented today, July 7th, 1928, be deleted.'[138] But the prospect of sectional conflict worried members of the Nursing Education Section and plans were made to rectify the 'lack of communication' between the sections. The result was seen at the next convention when Grace Fairley, a career superintendent and active participant in the Nursing Education Section, moved that year's 10-hour-day resolution.[139]

Meanwhile, McElroy's prediction that achieving a national standard would be difficult proved correct. While some institutions were struggling to abolish 12-hour shifts, others were experimenting with the more radical reduction of hours. In 1934 the CNA Private Duty Section discussed the introduction of 8-hour shifts in BC hospitals and soon the 8-hour day became the rallying cry within the Private Duty Section. But as late as 1938 CNA representatives were still lamenting that few institutions had implemented any change in nurses' shifts: 'The question of shorter hours for nurses has been considered at practically every hospital and nursing meeting during the past twenty-five years, yet the majority of schools have been unable to put shorter hours into effect.'[140]

For private-duty nurses, the 10- and later 8-hour day represented not just an improvement in working conditions, but also a system whereby the number of jobs per nurse could increase. Many also realized that a more radical reorganization of the private market would be needed to turn the tide of underemployment. To this end nursing organizations explored a second set of strategies, group and hourly nursing. Both were aimed at the clientele who were neither wealthy enough to hire private-duty nurses nor impoverished enough to rely on public ward or charity care. Calculations that this 'middle class' included 80 per cent of the population were substantially inflated, but the establishment of 'semi-private' hospital wards indicated that a medical service between private and public was in fact needed. Recognizing that patients such as these could not afford round-the-clock nursing attendance, private practitioners experimented with ways to offer patients part of a nurse. Hourly nursing could simply be added to existing registry services. Patients or their doctors could request daily attendance from the registry, which would assign a nurse to provide domestic nursing care on an hourly basis.[141] In spite of reports that hourly nursing had been implemented in many American cities, it seemed to have limited appeal for Canadian nurses. Registries may not have been willing to assume the responsibility for collecting patients' fees and distributing them among participating nurses or perhaps the VON, which provided a similar but subsidized service, could accommodate the existing demand for hourly nursing care.[142] In either case, hourly nursing received less attention than group nursing, the other strategy for bringing patient and nurse together.

Group nursing was a system whereby private hospital patients were grouped and assigned to several nurses. First raised at the 1926 CNA meetings, papers on the subject by Dr A.L. Lockwood of Toronto's Lockwood Clinic and Miss Gray, superintendent of the Colonial Hospital in Rochester, Minnesota, sparked extensive discussion at the 1928 CNA conference.[143] Group nursing was tested in 1931 when the alumnae association of the Winnipeg General Hospital established a 'Graduate Nurses Trust Fund'. Winnipeg graduates working in and around the city were asked to make monthly donations to a fund designed to create more work for their unemployed sisters. The $2,402.85 collected in the first year of the fund's operation provided 587 days of group nursing work for 74 nurses.

> In the majority of cases nurses have been put on group nursing for ten days at a time, two patients each with the same hours off duty and paid on the same basis as group nurses on the Hospital Staff. This gives each nurse $31.50 for ten days, laundry and meals provided by the Hospital. On several occasions nurses have been put on with our own graduates who were ill.[144]

Pearl Brownell, private-duty representative from the MARN to the CNA, was the Winnipeg alumnae association member in charge of the fund. During the second and third years of operation, the fund grew to $4,487.95, and between 1933 and 1934 $1,104.25 subsidized 357 days of work for 42 practitioners.[145] However, the program relied for funding on the very work-force that was in need of work, and thus by 1935, contributions decreased markedly to less than $400.[146] By 1936 one graduate had concluded that:

> We must face with equanimity the fact that this situation abounds—there are hundreds of experienced nurses needing work, and vast numbers of sick requiring expert care, but to bring the two together is the problem engaging the attention of hospitals and governments everywhere. . . . We are unable to solve this problem. It must work itself out of this vicious circle of No Money, No Work; No Work, No Money.[147]

After four years the 'emergency' measure of the alumnae association had run dry.[148]

Elsewhere in the nation, group nursing was also being te
1935 survey of unemployment conditions in Nova Scotia reveale
East Kings Memorial Hospital in Wolfville was using group nursin
a method to curb unemployment among nurses in the Annapolis V
ley.[149] In all instances, group nursing, like hourly nursing, relied on the
institution to ensure a concentration of patients. Recognizing this fact,
the CNA's Private Duty Section proposed in 1930 that a joint committee between it and the Nursing Education Section be struck to address
ways in which group nursing could be established. In 1932, the Private
Duty Section nurses again emphasized the importance of co-operation
between themselves and the hospital administrators in implementing
groups and hourly nursing 'schemes'. Little came of these proposals,
and for all the enthusiasm that group nursing engendered in the Private
Duty Section, within the Nursing Education Section of the CNA the
subject was barely mentioned.

Instead, nursing educators focused on the third solution to the economic crisis, the reduction of the number of student nurses enrolled at
training schools. Overproduction of nurses, it was argued, was a critical element in creating unemployment for all. In 1930, the following
recommendation was presented to the CNA:

> Whereas there exists marked and increasing unemployment
> among nurses in all parts of Canada
>
> Be it therefore resolved that the Nursing Education Section
> request the CNA to send a communication to all hospitals in Canada
> conducting schools for nurses, asking the boards of these hospitals
> to seriously consider the question of the supply and demand for
> graduate nurses within the boundaries of Canada before increasing
> the number of student nurses to meet additional nursing needs of
> the hospital, and that the policy of the employment of graduate
> nurses to meet these demands be adopted until such time as the
> unemployment conditions have been readjusted.[150]

Two years later, with the full recommendations of Dr Weir in hand,
the General Assembly of the CNA convention took a much stronger
stand. Sessions on 'The Approved Training School', 'Analysis of the
Cost of Nursing Education', and 'The Distribution of Nursing Services' resulted in a series of resolutions empowering the CNA to contact hospital school boards of directors with two requests: a reduction
in student nursing personnel and a concomitant increase in graduate
nurse staffs in hospitals where such moves would be economically
efficient. Institutions intimidated by the potential economic strain of a
new staffing system were urged to undertake cost analyses of the
apprenticeship model.[151]

...mendation were critical. Firstly, while
...d within the Private Duty Section, it
...resented it to the General Assembly.
...their failure to show leadership on the
...y a response to unemployment of their own
...s an act of good faith to the private nurses in their
...y, while questions of hours and group nursing contin-
...discussed in the Private Duty Section, only the proposed
...ction in the student population received any serious attention by
the rest of the CNA representatives throughout the 1930s. Private
health services received only limited attention, while replacing hospital apprentices with graduate nurses emerged as the main strategy for
solving the employment crisis.[152] The 1935 RNANS survey of Nova
Scotia hospitals asked, 'what is being done . . . to relieve nurses'
unemployment'? Some superintendents of nursing had reduced the
student work-force, hiring more graduate nurses for general duty,
while institutions like the Halifax Infirmary reported that a program
whereby 'we employ grads on general duty when needed at a
minimum wage leaving them free to take a private duty case when
available' had been instituted.[153]

Conclusion: Professionalization, Proletarianization, and the Meaning of General-Duty Nursing

After the initial experiments with graduate staffing of hospitals in the
1930s, in the early 1940s a new political economy of health prompted
wide-scale institutional reliance on the bedside care provided by general-duty practitioners. The CNA estimated that in 1943 over 14,000 of
its members were employed by hospitals and public health agencies,
as compared to only 6,000 in private health services.[154] Historians of
nursing have posited the rise of general-duty nursing as a critical shift
in the transformation of nursing services. Those scholars who emphasize the exploitive nature of apprenticeship training applaud nursing
educators for using the crisis of the inter-war years to break the chain
of dependency between hospital labour and nursing education. In
doing so, these historians claim, nursing superintendents took a crucial step towards professional autonomy and control over the educational process. Conversely, those researchers who recognize
private-duty nurses' long-standing antipathy to institutional labour
interpret nursing educators' efforts to employ graduate nurses as part
of the larger process whereby nursing was proletarianized. According
to those authors, the employment crisis of the inter-war years

provided the economic leverage necessary to force graduate nurses to abandon private duty and accept hospital employment.[155] Both the professionalization and proletarianization analyses overestimate the inevitability of graduate staffing systems. Canadian evidence suggests that graduate staffing of hospitals was neither linear nor preordained. Rather, nursing administrators used their limited institutional resources to create one of the few solutions not only to the economic crisis but also to the potential fragmentation of their organizations. As proud defenders of nursing's autonomous organizational structures, nursing educators and administrators recognized that if the existing associations could not respond to the economic crisis, then members would turn elsewhere for support, whether to other occupations, to other locales, or to other organizational forums. The conflict that developed within nursing organizations, combined with loss of membership and flirtations with radicalism, served to remind nursing leaders of the fragility of their organizational structure.

Although alternative strategies, like group nursing or hourly nursing, never received enthusiastic support from educators and administrators as did solutions that reshaped the educational process, it was also the case that nursing superintendents did not immediately seize the opportunity to revamp completely the apprenticeship system of staffing. When graduate nurses were introduced as general-duty staff providing bedside patient care, their presence was often explained as a temporary measure, not as a permanent staffing change. In 1933 Vancouver General Director of Nursing Grace Fairley explained to the hospital community:

> In an effort to lessen the effect of long periods of unemployment [on young graduate nurses] the policy of the hospital during the past two years has been, not to fill the junior staff positions permanently, but to rotate the available graduates giving as many as possible short terms of duty. While this is not stabilizing the staff to its greatest efficiency it has given that opportunity of work and experience that is so vital in keeping up the morale of young graduates.[156]

Fairley's words were hardly those of an administrator devoted to the proletarianization of her occupation, as some theorists would suggest.

In fact, many large hospitals did not substantially alter their staffing arrangements at all. Smaller institutions, facing expensive renovations to student residences and elaborate affiliation with larger educational institutions, turned to graduate staffing in the 1920s and early 1930s. The large urban hospitals, which might reasonably have been expected to take the lead in breaking institutional reliance on student labour, were often the last to introduce staffs of general-duty nurses. Leading training schools continued to produce large numbers of students every year. Victoria General Hospital, Nova Scotia's largest institution, exemplified this broader trend. When asked in 1935 what her program was doing to alleviate unemployment, Superintendent Gladys Strum replied 'nothing special'. Her school had actually graduated more students in 1934 than in 1933.[157]

Graduate nurse staffing of hospital wards, whether on a temporary basis or as a permanent reorganization of patient-care services, did allow some practitioners to survive the economic dislocations of the inter-war years, but in doing so it initiated two sets of changes that would fundamentally alter relations among nurses. First, as institutional administrators attempted to aid their unemployed graduates, the ability of nursing superintendents to serve as benefactresses for the occupation was challenged. For an occupation that commanded little authority in universities or in law, hospitals and the important role nursing educators and administrators played in them represented one source of institutional and social power. Through their leadership positions in nursing organizations and through their administrative positions in hospitals, nursing superintendents held power over the fortunes of their graduates, but that power base proved limited. The lack of will, or resources, exhibited by superintendents of large hospitals, many of whom were CNA Nursing Education Section leaders, raised new problems for hospital/nurse relations, for not only were private-duty nurses beholden to their benefactresses in the institution, those benefactresses seemed unable to provide much patronage.

Grace Fairley's efforts throughout the 1930s to improve the working and living conditions of Vancouver General students illustrated this tension. Frustrated with the ongoing shortage of personnel and resources, Fairley used the institution's annual reports to lobby the hospital community for improved funding. In 1932, the newly appointed Fairley wrote: 'The continued overcrowding of wards, beds down the middle of the wards and in corridors, is markedly handicapping efficiency. Lack of supervision and working continually in congested conditions appear to be responsible for the majority of nursing errors.' In 1937 Fairley was still arguing the same case: 'The overcrowding of the general wards has become a chronic or permanent picture rather than an unusual one. . . . This creates an environment for the graduate and student that does not permit of professional poise or the calm thinking that is essential to GOOD NURSING.'[158] Fairley's direct and public critiques of the working conditions in her hospital were striking in their force. Perhaps because Fairley had served as senior nursing administrator in the largest institutions in Canada, or perhaps because she was at her wit's end, hers were the most public and direct critiques to be published by a nursing superintendent. For all her efforts, the director of nursing seemed powerless in negating the effects of overwork and ill health that plagued Vancouver General's nurses in the 1930s. Funding for a new residence was not approved until 14 years after Fairley had begun her campaign for improved housing. Fairley's inability to protect her staff from exploitive conditions placed her in a difficult position, for while she continued to enforce the discipline of the apprenticeship system, she could no longer adequately serve as its benefactress.

The hospital-based strategies to cure nursing's ills had a second long-term effect. Private-duty nurses learned that solutions to their economic problems were contingent on institutional resources. For those nurses who returned to the institutional sphere as waged employees of hospitals, the system of general-duty staffing created a two-tiered nursing structure that divided bedside nurses, or nurse-workers, from administrators, or nurse-managers. This shattered the possibility of a rough equality among practitioners that work in the private market had permitted. Indeed, differences between administrative and rank-and-file nurses, and between generations, which had been reconciled with increasing difficulty throughout the third generation of nurses, would begin to crystallize within the fourth. The great irony of leaders' experiments in general-duty staffing was that through this attempt to prevent the fracturing of nursing organizations, graduates were brought back into the institutional hierarchy wherein the conditions that would foster the creation of alternative organizational forms—unions—were created.

5

'The Case of the Kissing Nurse': Femininity, Sociability, and Sexuality, 1920–1968

Throughout the economic and political dislocation of the inter-war years, the bonds of gender bridged the gulf developing between nursing leaders and the occupation's rank-and-file and bolstered leaders' efforts to maintain occupational unity. Just as their experiences as disenfranchised women had united nurses during the early twentieth-century battles for registration legislation and suffrage, in the inter-war years a particular sexual and social image of femininity, created and endorsed by nurses, was critical to their self-definition and public profiles as respectable working women. As the political economy of health was reorganized in the years after 1942, nurses' occupational image was realigned to bring it closer to that being advocated for all women. Like their attitudes towards science and to the economy, occupational leaders and working nurses in both the third and fourth generations did not always agree about what defined respectability. The standards of appropriate feminine behaviour inculcated by nursing educators and designed to meet institutional needs frequently clashed with apprentice and staff visions of modern femininity. This chapter explores the tensions surrounding nursing and gender by tracing the shifting definitions of appropriate social and sexual behaviour for nurses prescribed for third- and fourth-generation nurses and by placing nurses' gendered roles in the context of the broader social definition of femininity, which itself was not static.

Nurses and Flappers

In the years after 1900, the apprenticeship model of hospital staffing was adopted by Canadian hospitals trying to meet the growing patient demand for hospital services. Throughout the second generation of trained nurses, nursing administrators in private and public, religious and secular institutions, who were responsible for recruiting young women into their schools and occupation, grappled with the contradictions of femininity and sexuality. Senior staff had to convince apprentices to adhere to the demeanour and deportment of Victorian femininity, but also insisted that their genteel staff acquire intimate knowledge of the bodies of strangers. To maintain the reputation of their schools and occupation, the professional élite clearly had to distinguish professional from carnal knowledge. To accomplish this, nursing educators, administrators, and association leaders created an elaborate set of rules and regulations, what Gary Kinsman has termed a regulatory regime, to shape the behaviour of apprenticing staff. Nursing leaders assumed that over the course of the three-year apprenticeship, students would come to appreciate the virtues of this socio-sexual norm and continue to uphold it when they graduated into private practice. Nursing leaders were also aware that in the private market the pressures from doctors and middle-class patients would reinforce the feminine ideal that nursing schools had emphasized.[1]

The feminine vision that nursing leaders created was an exaggerated version of Victorian social deference, sexual passivity, disinterest or ignorance, and ladylike gentility. The schools accomplished this end by establishing strict rules of behaviour and decorum that students ignored at their peril. The key element of ladylike behaviour was restraint. Students were expected to restrain from making too much noise, not only on duty but also during their off-duty hours in the nurses' residence. Smoking and drinking were taboo. Nurses were particularly encouraged to refrain from gossip about their patients or colleagues. Most important, nurses were to avoid insubordination or other emotions that put them out of control. Failure to demonstrate the necessary internal discipline was rewarded with punishment.

This definition of femininity hinged on a particular vision of sexual behaviour. Like their deportment in other personal relations, nurses' sexuality was to be constrained and contained, for while their position within the health-care system was premised on a heterosexual complementariness, as the partners or mates to the male doctors, that partnership was supposed to be asexual. The entire system of regulation developed by hospitals was designed to constrain female sexuality off duty and to neutralize it completely on the wards. In addition to the strict hours regulating residence life, students could only entertain visitors in the reception room and could not have visitors, other than perhaps mothers and sisters, in their own rooms.

Permission had to be sought if nurses wanted to receive a male patient or ex-patient at the residence.[2] At some institutions a student could be dismissed for having her name 'linked' with that of a patient. Nurses were not expected to become romantically involved with men in the hospital and at some institutions explicit rules were established making it illicit for nurses and orderlies to go out together.[3] Nursing leaders were slightly more relaxed about nurses' developing relations with doctors. Even there, however, student nurses were warned not to flirt or 'pose' when on the wards. These various elements of social and sexual restraint were considered as a single goal, together ensuring that students would be as well chaperoned in nursing school as they were assumed to be at home. As late as 1935 one superintendent of nursing heard reports that some of her students had been smoking in a restaurant. The errant apprentices lost their free evenings for more than six weeks but also received a warning that 'smoking leads to alcohol and progresses to promiscuity'.[4]

The strict parameters of this regulatory regime were part of the broader 'moral regulation' of the day. Like the moral reformers studied by Mariana Valverde, nursing leaders sought to reformulate what Valverde terms the 'ethical subjectivity' of their apprentices, not merely repressing desire but redefining it.[5] Nursing leaders did not expect apprentices to avoid heterosexual relations altogether but to contain those relations to limited off-duty hours. For this reason, residences were not designed to cloister their inhabitants completely. Weekly late leaves, provisions for receiving guests in the residence lobby, and school-sponsored dances all accommodated heterosexual activity within strict limits. Nor did nursing commentators deny the importance of heterosexual femininity in creating a good nurse. Ellen Knox's 1919 publication, *The Girl of the New Day*, reviewed the job options facing women in post-war Canada. Knox's chapter 'The Joy of Nursing' began: 'Nursing touches the mother instinct, which is alive in every true woman, from the oldest and ugliest spinster driving geese over the common, to the merriest-hearted school girl playing hockey in the field.'[6] Proclamations such as Knox's echoed Nightingale's famous phrase that 'every woman is a nurse', but like Nightingale, Knox was careful to note that while nursing drew on feminine attributes and might prepare women well for marriage and motherhood, nurses themselves were not expected to pursue both paid work and maternity. As with other white-collar women, marriage precluded active pursuit of a nursing career.

Despite the public celebration of nursing's bourgeois femininity, not all student nurses embraced the institutional regulations with equal enthusiasm. Hospital records indicate that nursing administrators were regularly admonishing their students for failure to conform to the behavioural norm. Students who chose not to limit their sexual and social behaviour resigned, sometimes because of marriage but in other cases from conflict over the hospital schedule or rules. But surprisingly few apprenticing nurses abandoned their training, in part because in the years before World War I, the Victorian image of respectable femininity did not appear old-fashioned or outmoded compared to that being prescribed for other women. If anything, the model devised within nursing reinforced Victorian notions of bourgeois femininity, so that nurses simply experienced a more intense and extreme version of the model of femininity and sexuality being advocated for all women, especially those of the middle class.

By the 1920s, however, nursing's vision of respectable sexuality began to stand in contrast with the liberated sexual mores being advocated for the new woman. Christina Simmons has examined how in the 1920s the 'Myth of Victorian Repression' was constructed by experts such as sexologists to signal what was wrong with American gender relations and why a sexual revolution was needed to revise them. The new woman of the 1920s was to be sexually liberated, actively pursuing heterosexual relations. By condemning the repression of pre-World War I gender relations, these commentators indicated that healthy sexual lives demanded expression, not repression. Within this context, nursing appeared anomalous. The feminine persona reinforced by nursing leaders and educators in the inter-war years was in fact emblematic of Victorian sexual restraint, which by the 1920s experts considered outmoded and dangerous.[7]

The most obvious symbol of this disparity was nurses' dress. Throughout the 1920s and 1930s, nursing schools across the country retained the uniform style of the second generation, with all its similarities to the dress of late nineteenth-century domestic servants. As in the previous generation, student progress through the ranks as probationer, junior, intermediate, and then senior nurse was accompanied by some new addition to the uniform to signify the maturation process. Upon graduation, practitioners were permitted to wear an entirely white costume—dress, cap, stockings, and shoes. The symbolic inversion of traditional female imagery, wherein the colour white signified nurses' workplace experience rather than a bride's sexual inexperience, was reinforced by the elaborate graduation ceremonies (modelled after wedding ceremonies) sponsored by training schools and alumnae across the country.[8] Such symbolism also reaffirmed the asexual status of trained nurses: they graduated out of the cloistered world of hospital life sexually and socially pure, driven by vocation and profession, not by marriage or sexuality.[9]

Given the power of the symbolism, it was logical that nursing administrators vigorously defended the dress code they had established. Only on the question of hair did supervisors fail to impose their standards. As bobbed hair became all the rage with North American women, superintendents of nursing resisted the fashion, punishing students who took the plunge and bobbed their locks, and insisting that students wear their hair long, in a bun on the back of their head, with their cap perched on top. One apprentice at Halifax's Victoria General Hospital decided to use her day off to acquire a bob. When she returned to the ward, the nursing superintendent demanded that the student retrieve her shorn hair and pin it back onto her head so that she might continue to conform to the conventional style.[10] In this battle the older generation lost and bobbed hair became the standard coiffure, but on other issues the old guard held fast. In the fashion world of the flapper, hemlines were rising and waistlines dropping, but within nursing the uniform remained pinched at the waist, and seven inches off the floor.[11]

Nursing leaders were not unaware of the differential that had developed between their staffs and the dress and ethos of other women. In an address to the Winnipeg General Hospital Alumnae Association in 1927, the hospital's superintendent of nurses took the opportunity to '[defend] the young nurse of the present day' to her audience of older women. The superintendent insisted that 'in spite of the criticism given the so-called "flapper" of today . . . there is a large proportion amongst our pupils who measure up to the best in the past not only of our own school but of the nursing world in general, even including those whom we revere as having made our profession what it is today.'[12] Whatever flapperish impulse was present in nursing, nursing's leadership felt confident that it presented no threat to the carefully nourished sexual, social, and personal restraint that dominated the occupational definition of femininity. The occupational élite was emboldened in its position by the economic realities of inter-war Canada. Despite the economic dislocation of the era, nursing remained one of the few skilled and respectable occupations available to working women, one that offered board and room during training and, especially for rural women, a safe point of entry into urban job markets.

Resistance and Critique

The labour market advantage that inter-war nursing held did not deter the development of resistance to, or critique of, nursing's conventional image. Occasionally, non-nursing commentators depicted nurses in a negative light. Arthur Stringer's 1920 novel, *The Prairie Mother*, was one of the few Canadian fictional works to use the nurse as a symbol for unappealing femininity. In the first few pages of the novel Stringer's heroine was contrasted with the unattractive obstetrical nurse who, in spite of her skilled assistance in the successful delivery of the heroine's twins, was portrayed as repulsive. One of the last things the prairie mother remembered before succumbing to anaesthetic was the 'loganberry Pimple on the nose of the red-headed surgical nurse who'd been sent into the labor room to help.' The nurse never acquired a name. When the heroine's labour was over and she regained consciousness, the first thing she saw was 'a face bending over mine, seeming to float in space. It was the color of a half-grown cucumber, and it made me think of a tropical fish in an aquarium when the water needed changing.' The patient's confusion was erased when she 'finally observed and identified the loganberry pimple . . . and remembered that I was still in the land of the living and that the red-headed surgical nurse was holding my wrist.'[13]

Stringer's unflattering depiction of the working nurse was underscored by the psychological and social distance he created between the heterosexual heroine and her single female attendants. Rather than seeing the nurses as allies, Stringer's protagonist considered herself abandoned by her absent husband, and believed the doctor and three nurses were laughing at her. Nor did the prairie mother's relationship with her private-duty nurse develop into a meaningful or intimate one. Such portrayals in popular fiction clearly delineated between the modern mother and the unattractive, unmodern, working nurse.

Occasionally, other commentators turned a critical eye to the sexual personae of Canadian nurses. In 1928, the national journal *Canadian Nurse* published an article by Leslie Bell (occupation unstated) on 'Nurses and their Attitude Toward Sex'. Bell argued that in order for nurses to respond adequately to patients' sex-related problems, the practising nurse must adopt 'modern' attitudes towards sexuality. Calling for a more open and frank approach to discussing sexuality, Bell advised nurses to divorce emotion from sex: 'Why should the whole matter of sex be bound up with such intensity of feeling? We do not treat our other "instinctive drives" in the same way? We do not, generally speaking, fear or conceal our perfectly legitimate desire for food and drink.' Bell acknowledged that the rational and open-minded approach might be difficult for some nurses to adopt. 'For those brought up in the "old school" of thought, where reticence and modesty were considered all important, it *does* require courage to change one's point of view and discuss frankly and comfortably the problems of sex.' Bell's gentle admonishment to the occupation for its prudery differed in tone, but not intention, from another *CN* article published five years later. In it, Dr Atlee, professor of gynecology and obstetrics at Dalhousie University, pronounced on the subject of 'Uniforms and Stereotyped Minds'. Demanding that nurses 'wake up to the fact that they are living in a freer, more modern age', Atlee criticized the standard nursing uniform for its lack of utility and beauty. Arguing that, as women, nurses' confidence would be damaged by wearing an unattractive uniform, he suggested: '[The uniform] should follow the natural lines of the body, but not so closely that it is tight anywhere to discomfort. Surely if it has become necessary that automobile builders make their automobiles with graceful lines—a nurse might have a stream-lined, graceful tonneau.' Atlee acknowledged the nineteenth-century tradition that the conventional uniform represented: 'We have a lot to thank that autocratic Victorian lady for. . . . But Florence Nightingale is dead, and the century that bore her is dead, and this is another age.'[14]

With the exception of these occasional critiques of the occupational image, nursing received surprisingly little negative public commentary in the inter-war years.[15] Unlike American popular fiction, which regularly presented a range of nursing images, Canadian writing tended to support the traditional nursing persona.[16] The CNA defended this traditional image. Concerned that their occupational symbol was being misappropriated by the business world, in 1936 the national body struck a committee to investigate 'the Use of the Figure of a Nurse in Commercial Advertising'.[17] Rather, resistance to the conventions of the Victorian sexually constrained femininity came from within nursing, from the apprenticing and graduate nurses who chafed under the strict regime their superiors imposed.

One obvious point of resistance emerged when freshly graduated nurses rejected the prescribed femininity of their student days. Advertisements in student yearbooks revealed that local businesses, like the intrepid T. Eaton Company, were anxious to capitalize on the market for modern uniforms. The 1928 Misericordia General Hospital yearbook included an advertisement showing uniforms with dropped waists, short skirts, and no bib or hat, much more in keeping with contemporary 'flapperish' fashions. The caption read: 'Are Uniforms all Alike? Indeed no, says the experienced Nurse who always buys hers at Eaton's.'[18] Other images also depicted graduate nurses in substantially more fashionable dress. The Misericordia yearbook for 1929 included a cartoon/sketch entitled 'Contribution from Obstetrical Department', which depicted a slim, composed woman sitting in a

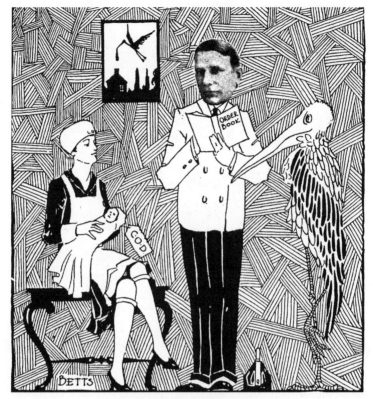

Contribution from
OBSTETRICAL DEPARTMENT

SOURCE: Misericordia General Hospital, *Blue and Gold*, 1929.

chair holding a baby. The figure appeared to have little interest in the baby, but instead was looking away while the viewer saw the straight, thin dress and, most telling, stockings rolled down at the tops revealing her knees. Recognizing that many nurses desired more up-to-date costume, some employers provided uniforms that, like the images in the Eaton's advertisements and the yearbook cartoons, were distinctly modern. The VON uniform, for example, included a drop-waisted dress, a tie, and a cloche hat.[19]

The promise of stylish dress upon graduation did not change the fact that within nursing schools themselves, overt criticism of dress

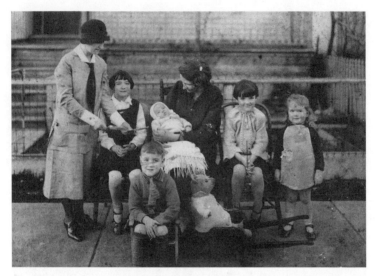

The Victorian Order of Nurses staff wore uniforms that were distinctive yet modern. This nurse, wearing a drop-waisted dress, tie, and cloche hat, was photographed during a postnatal visit in British Columbia, *circa* 1930 (BCARS/HP 78688).

SOURCE: Victorian Order of Nurses, British Columbia (PABC).

and regulations was risky. Not only might a student be dismissed for 'insubordination', but because hospital superintendents communicated with one another, once dismissed, students could not easily transfer to another institution. For this reason, much of the commentary on hospital rules and discipline was presented in humorous form. Alluding to the debate over hair length, a 1928 yearbook instalment of 'Want Ads' included 'Mary Lang—Wants nerve to bob her hair.'[20] A poem entitled 'Don't!!!' gave advice to junior nurses: 'Don't wear your uniforms up to your knees/—If you do, you are bound to feel more than a breeze!. . ./Don't stand in the hall with Tom, Dick or Harry, But send them right home and do not tarry . . ./Don't flirt with Joseph, Rezzie or Lou,/Or you will find your training days through.'[21] The Vancouver General Hospital's 1939 *Nurses' Annual* included a cartoon depicting morning roll call.[22] Nurses' popular culture also subverted the sexual sanctity of the uniform by linking nurses' ability to make heterosexual conquests to their work and dress. For instance, the 1928 poem 'The Nurse's Chance' was cheeky in its vampishness.

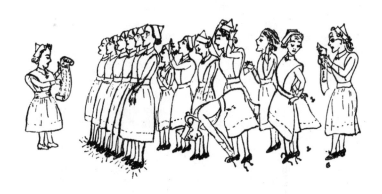

Roll Call — and so on "Behind Scenes"

SOURCE: Vancouver General Hospital, *Nurses' Annual*, 1939.

It seems to me a nurse has got
A most delightful life
Since she has many chances
To become a rich man's wife
for men will eat and men will drink
And men will raise the deuce
Until they clog their tummies up
And stop their gastric juice

When on their beds of pain they toss
With diverse groans and howls
Nurse smoothes their pillows, holds their hand
And wrings out cold wet towels
She takes a mean advantage of
A fellow when he's sick
By dressing in a uniform
That makes her look so slick

When men are getting well
They are a mighty mushy lot
And that is when the wise nurse doth
Strike while the iron is hot

> For men assume the wife will be
> Just like the nurse who cooled
> Their fevered brow so patiently
> But oh! how men are fooled[23]

The 'mean advantage' that the 'slick' uniform and bedside attendance provided permitted the nurse to improve her class position by becoming 'a rich man's wife' and to subvert conventional gender relations within marriage, for 'But oh! how men are fooled'. A 1926 cartoon from the Vancouver General *Nurses' Annual* played on the flirtatious flattery that some patients bestowed upon their nurses. While the nurse received accolades, the friend/wife bore the brunt of the patient's ill humour.[24]

This celebration of bedside flirting resonated with many of the more direct contraventions of rules that became part of the lore of nursing training. Oral testimony corroborates evidence found in nursing administrators' records that breaking the rules was part and parcel of student life. For instance, some hospital staff continued to pursue relations with male patients and staff. In the early 1920s at Halifax's Victoria General, Edna Kelly was brought up 'on the carpet' for having her 'name coupled with that of a patient . . . when on night duty.' The patient himself had reported Kelly, but the nurse had her

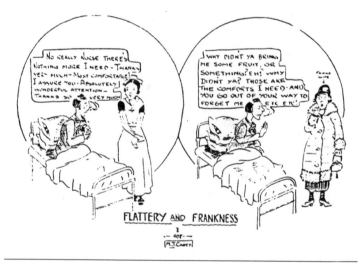

FLATTERY AND FRANKNESS

SOURCE: Vancouver General Hospital, *Nurses' Annual*, 1926.

explanation of the incident accepted and was 'given another trial', though transferred off that ward. Kelly was but one Victoria General student 'inclined to pose'. Annie Simmons was also 'constantly being reprimanded for posing and talking with male nurses and patients.' She was advised to leave the school, which she did. Doreen McMillan was disciplined for similar breach of etiquette. McMillan 'had been out two nights in succession' with a male nurse 'with whom she had no opportunity to get acquainted.' The superintendent of nurses discharged McMillan, but the sentence was commuted to a suspension 'by order of *one* of the commissioners [original emphasis].' Sally Penner did not have friends in high places. She, too, had been out 'two nights in succession', but her date was an ex-patient. The second night she arrived at the nurses' residence 'a little too late to come in by the door' and instead 'came in through a junior nurses window'.[25] Unfortunately, the matron of the residence was wise to that trick and Penner was discovered and dismissed. Such direct contravention of regulations posed the risk of discipline and punishment, but many others did not get caught.

Direct defiance of hospital etiquette could go further. In 1932 one Vancouver nurse went so far as to engage legal assistance to confront institutional power. The graduate nurse had been suspended and then 'requested to leave the Hospital on account of some social entanglement'. Unemployed, the nurse decided to apply to the Essondale Mental Hospital to pursue postgraduate work in psychiatric nursing. Essondale authorities asked Vancouver General Director of Nursing Grace Fairley for a 'confidential report on the nurse's work and character'. Fairley replied that the nurse had been 'relieved for social reasons', and the nurse was not accepted at Essondale. Likely realizing that the Vancouver General conflict would continue to limit her opportunities, the nurse hired a lawyer who demanded on her behalf one month's pay and 'a retraction of the alleged defamation of character'.[26]

Negotiating Bedside Relations and Accommodating to Conventions

Given the number and variety of women who entered nursing training programs annually, finding examples of students who resented conforming to the formal code of etiquette is not surprising. What is more intriguing is the degree to which rank-and-file nurses accommodated themselves to the prescribed feminine image. Perhaps accommodation is too strong a term. It is more accurate to say that nursing students and graduates embraced features of the élite vision and turned them to their own end. However frustrating individual nurses found the constraints of feminine deportment demanded by their educational institutions, the asexual femininity offered several positive elements that served working nurses well and account for the apparent internalization by ordinary nurses of the conventional occupational image.

One such element pertained to the internal structure of nursing. Nurses could look forward to increased personal autonomy upon graduation and thus accommodation to the strict rules and regulations reflected students' recognition that training school was a finite period. The Misericordia General Hospital graduating class of 1927 wrote a parody of the ten commandments that laid out the rules governing life in the school. The commandments began with: 'Thou shalt in no wise alter the uniform of the school if thou would'st live long and happily in the Misericordia Nurses' Home.' Other commandments referred to getting sufficient rest, not being late for morning prayers, not taking visitors to residence rooms because 'they are not of the chosen ones', and not coming in past 10 p.m. except on Wednesday, when 'thou mayst stay out until 11:30 pm and make merry, for thou hast surely earned it.' The litany concluded with the tenth commandment: 'Thou shalt obey all the commandments of the school and thy Superintendent if thou would'st graduate and obtain an eternal freedom.'[27]

While waiting for 'eternal freedom', students also used popular culture to celebrate the coming-of-age process that apprenticeship entailed. In the 1933 Winnipeg General yearbook, the beginning of each section was introduced by a cartoon representing the four phases of student life. The first phase was that of probationer. This cartoon depicted a tall, gangly, unsophisticated girl with unkempt hair and wide eyes. The absence of the hat signified her lowly probationer status, as did the scrub brush dropping from her hand. Her apparent alarm, signified by the probie's hand at her mouth, stemmed from the summons to the 'TSO' (Training School Office), which could only mean that some rule had been transgressed and discipline was pending.

The junior nurse had survived the probationary period and now sported a cap. But the cartoon for 'Juniors' indicated inexperience of a different sort. In that cartoon, the slim and attractive junior nurse once again had her hand to her mouth, embarrassed at having been caught sitting in the lap of an old man. The man had one hand out, as if in appeal and as if he had just removed the hand from the nurse's backside. The look on his face was a combination of a leer and a snarl. The matronly graduate nurse returned a look of equal force

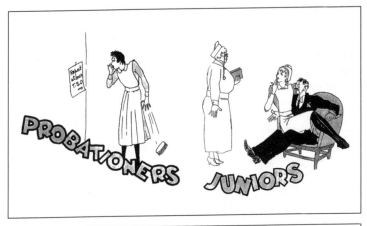

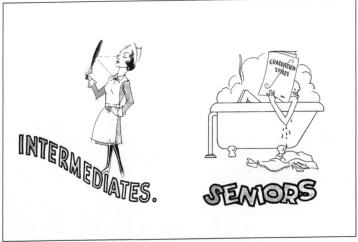

SOURCE: Winnipeg General Hospital, *Blue and White*, 1933.

with a stern glare and a thrust out chin and bottom lip. The young nurse's interest in men contrasted starkly with the portrayal of the intermediate and senior nurses. The intermediate was not interested in romance but in her new-found status. Looking in a hand-held mirror she saw the pin she has received for advancing to intermediate nurse status. The intermediate was also well-groomed and attractive, but her confidence came not from masculine attentions but from professional achievement. For 'Seniors' some of the excitement of status had worn off. The final figure in the series wore no uniform at all, but rather had shed her working clothes and was soaking in a hot bath, perusing the latest fashion for graduate nurses. Happy to be out of hospital garb, the lithe figure looked neither like her subordinate students nor like the matronly supervisor.

These images capture several elements of nurses' coming-of-age process. Firstly, they suggest that nurses' sexual identity was formed during the apprenticeship years and represented a combination of leaders' visions and nurses' own. In the final frame, the senior nurse graduated to an ambiguous sexual status, still interested in fashion and possibilities of sexual appeal, but not yet decided what direction her life will take. Because nurses were expected to retire from formal practice when they married, the 'uniform' selected would either lead to a life with a man, through marriage, or one without, through a nursing career. In either case, nursing promised the transformation from a gangly, unattractive probationer, through a phase with men, into autonomous status. These images suggested that nursing actually produced a better version of female sexuality than that offered to all women.[28]

Secondly, while the supervising nurse was overweight and overbearing, her image was not unappealing. She had small feet, petite ankles, well-manicured hair, and an ample bosom. Her authority was clear and it was an authority powerful enough to confront a well-dressed gentleman, perhaps a senior medical consultant or a member of the hospital board of governors. On a third and related point, within this cartoon the sexuality of the older man was posed as a problem. The junior nurse seemed to be enjoying her session on his lap, but the man was depicted as a lecher, and not a very attractive one at that, who was taking advantage of the young nurse and also of his power. Thus, if adhering to conventional femininity helped nurses mature, such social norms could also be used to demand a certain level of respect and dignity in workplace contexts, most of which located nurses near the bottom of the power structure.

The benefits of the conventional asexual image were made clear for graduate nurses in the workplace who daily had to negotiate working and personal relations with powerful male superiors. Given the importance of doctors' and other powerful men's recommendations and connections to secure jobs, nurses had to walk a fine line of being friendly without being too much so. Feminist author Ellen Knox addressed this issue in *The Girl of the New Day*. On the question of 'purity' Knox acknowledged to her graduate nurse readers:

'You and your classmates determined when you were set free on your own resources that "things of night at your glance should take fright"' but also recognized the perils to purity that bedside care presented. She queried: '. . . what are you to do if your patient is idle, and whenever you are off your guard, flatters you or says low, common things, better left unsaid.'[29] But as Florence Maitland of Salmon Arm Hospital discovered, patients' advances might be more subtle and more complicated. In 1940 Maitland returned to British Columbia and sought letters of recommendation from her old patient, now deputy provincial secretary, Mr P. Walker. Walker's responses to Maitland's requests were more than enthusiastic. He informed her that he had been in Kamloops recently and, had he known that the nurse was in Salmon Arm, 'would have run across to see you'. Walker expressed regrets that Maitland had not returned to BC sooner. He had been back in hospital recently and claimed he would have hired her as a special nurse again. Alluding to Maitland's nursing care during his previous hospital stay, Walker lamented that their interactions had remained within the bounds of respectability: 'I have such pleasant recollections of your attentions, unfortunately quite proper ones, when you were at the hospital here years ago.'[30] Innocent flirtations between citizens with such unequal social power could prove difficult to manage without the aid of clearly delineated rules of personal and sexual propriety.

Insisting on gentlemanly behaviour also protected working nurses from allegations that sexual favours were the basis of professional appointments. For example, in January 1936, Dr A.D. Lapp, superintendent of the Tranquille Sanatorium, took action to end the controversy surrounding his dismissal of one superintendent of nursing, Miss Sherriff, and the subsequent appointment of another, Miss Allan. 'Interested parties', claimed Lapp, were spreading 'extravagant, ridiculous and impossible' stories regarding his selection of Allan as matron. Lapp insisted: 'So far as me being friendly with Miss [Allan] I am and shall continue to be until I see some good reason why I should not. My wife is also friendly to her and she is a frequent visitor at our house.'[31] For working women dependent on the patronage of male physicians and administrators, maintaining a nonsexual status in the work-force was necessary not only for defending nurses against unwanted sexual advances but also for defending them against allegations of professional advancement through sexual relations.

Demanding genteel behaviour informed nurses' relationships with doctors in further ways, as exemplified by a 1929 conflict at

Vancouver General. That year a committee was appointed to investigate complaints lodged against one of the surgeons for alleged use of foul language. The surgeon had been so abusive that two graduate nurses resigned. The nurses' complaint was framed around the surgeon's ungentlemanly behaviour. He had used foul language ('hold up that bloody leg'), hurled ethnic insults ('nothing but your damned Scotch stubbornness'), made racist remarks ('any nigger wench on Hastings Street could wring out platers better than you'), inferred professional incompetence ('You let patients die on the table before they even get out of the OR'), and questioned the respectability of the students ('All you nurses stay in the Hospital for is to keep out of the penitentiary'). One of the nurses reminded the inquiry that she had extensive nursing experience, 'having worked with some of the outstanding Orthopedic surgeons in the East', but that the Vancouver General operating room conditions were by far the worst: although 'the surgeons generally proved to be gentlemen', the surgeon in question was not.[32] The nurses claimed that his abusive behaviour terrorized student nurses who had to work with him. While the graduate nurses could find work at another hospital, student nurses could not resign without imperilling their chances of having a nursing career at all. Therefore, demanding gentlemanly behaviour from the medical staff was particularly important for the student nurses, who held little authority while working side by side with the city's leading doctors.

Relations with patients could prove equally challenging to negotiate. At the same time that some popular culture celebrated the sexual and marital possibilities nursing presented, it was none the less recognized that transgressing clearly delineated boundaries might result in allegations of improper behaviour and dismissal. The following poem appeared in several nursing yearbooks of the inter-war decades, including the Winnipeg General's *Blue and White* and the Vancouver General's *Nurses' Annual*.

> Some people think that nurses
> Fall in love the very day
> They come to count a sick man's pulse
> Or bring his dinner tray.
> They think the tender passion
> Delightful as perfume
> Surrounds a sniffy patient
> Or the cleaning of his room.

There's nothing much alluring
About a stricken male
Who has a growth of stubble
Upon a cheek that's pale
Nor does fair romance linger
Within the tousled hair
Of a man without a collar
Who's as cranky as a bear.

So cheer up, wives and sweethearts,
Because it is not true
That artful vampires in white caps
Would wish to steal from you
To tell the truth, before a week
The poor nurse is a wreck:
The love for your man is only this—
The love to wring his neck.[33]

Despite the poem's humorous conclusion, the reality of private practice necessitated that nurses distance themselves from the dangerous image of nurse as sexual predator, for any threat to domestic and marital relations might cost private-duty nurses their jobs.

Asserting an asexual persona was particularly important for graduate nurses working in public health and private duty, where they would often find themselves alone in rough neighbourhoods in the middle of the night, travelling unchaperoned with a male doctor, or accepting rides from strangers. Nurses working for Winnipeg's Margaret Scott Nursing Mission, for example, often received offers of assistance from their logical allies in social service, members of the fire-fighting and police forces. MSNM staff were appreciative of offers for police escorts, but were proud to report: 'I am not afraid to go anywhere at any time in my uniform as all our friends and patients know us.'[34] Men from all classes could be counted on to treat MSNM staff with respect. Riding home on the streetcar 'tired, wornout workmen . . . offer us their seats if we are in uniform.' Streetcar and bus drivers would hold their vehicles to wait for a nurse hustling to catch her ride. When the nurses were walking to cases in outlying districts, 'truck drivers . . . private cars, the doctors and anyone going in our direction' would stop and give the MSNM nurses a lift. For these nurses, then, conforming to the behavioural and dress restrictions of the nursing establishment held tangible rewards. The asexual persona promoted by nursing leaders served to neutralize even the most sexually dangerous men, turning working-class and bourgeois males alike into gentlemen.

The story told by Mary Shepherd of her experiences working as a student at the Margaret Scott Mission provides a humorous insight into the symbolic meaning nurses vested in their uniform. During her rotation at the Margaret Scott Mission, Mary Shepherd was called one night to assist a local doctor in delivering twins at a North End home. 'The doctor asked me if I'd like him to wait for me and I said "no we weren't too far from Main Street", so I proceeded about 3:30 in the morning all by myself down there.' As Shepherd started her long walk to Main Street and its streetcar, a man appeared on the sidewalk beside her. He accompanied her all the way to Main Street, saying 'unrepeatable' things. Shepherd managed to make it safely to the streetcar and flagged down a policeman to escort her up George Street to the Mission. Upon her arrival there she 'just fell in the door and howled my head off'. While Shepherd did not report the incident to MSNM authorities, and while her nursing supervisors at Winnipeg General only learned of the incident when it was referred to in the annual yearbook, her story spread quickly among the students and remains a standard in Winnipeg General nursing mythology. While the story served as an important reminder of the many adventures encountered, and of the fact that nurses were breaking new ground as independent women, Shepherd's response to her harasser evoked the symbolic strength of identity nurses invested in their uniform. As the man talked to her on what seemed like her endless journey to Main Street, Shepherd simply replied, 'No thank you', and later explained, 'I wasn't getting into any fights because I was a nervous wreck.' However, as she boarded the streetcar and escaped her harasser, Shepherd flung a comment back to the offending man—what she still considers a 'noble' response: 'If you don't respect me, you might have respected the uniform.'[35]

Same-Sex Relationships

Within male-female workplaces, constrained sexuality and an asexual persona served as necessary defences against unwanted heterosexual advances, and also served to create and legitimize distinctive all-female, homosocial space. Because married women were supposed to give up their practices, most working nurses relied on other women to provide social and personal support structures. Graduates travelled far and wide, often accompanying each other on their continental and international ventures. Other practitioners stayed closer to home, establishing households shared with class-mates and colleagues.

These relationships often began in residence, where students shared meals, facilities, duties, discipline, and extracurricular activi-ties. There, students humanized the otherwise formal and impersonal institutional program of work and study by devising elaborate sets of nicknames for one another. On the wards, nurses were referred to by the formal title 'Miss' and their last name. In the residences, they were called by their first names, by their last names only, or by their nicknames. A few nurses were identified by feminine monikers, such as 'Bunny', which they may have been called by their families. Most nicknames were truncated versions of family names, and given the Anglo-Celtic patrinomial system, these versions of their family names usually became masculine nicknames. Thompson became 'Tommy', Macfarland became 'Mac', Andrews became 'Andy'. Other abbreviated family names translated into gender-neutral monikers: Shuttleworth was known as 'Shuttie', Blackwell became 'Blackie'. Occasionally, a more inventive or literary reference influ-enced students' nicknames. For instance, Anne Sawyer was known as 'Tom'. Where 'Torchy' Adamson acquired her nickname was never made clear.[36]

The result of the naming system was that large numbers of stu-dent nurses were known by non-female appellations. Within hospital residences this promoted a certain amount of gender-bending where non-feminine attributes were celebrated. For instance, many school yearbooks included a 'horoscope' wherein the aspirations and aver-sions of graduating nurses were identified or parodied. One column in the horoscope listed 'appearance'. The adjectives ranged from 'pert' or 'blonde' or 'demure' to 'boyish' and 'masculine'. In the 'ambition' category graduates were credited with seeking out post-graduate employment, with travel, with pursuing heterosexual rela-tionships, and with maintaining friendships developed during their training.

There are some allusions to intense or special friendships between two students and occasional indications that some of these couplings were oriented along a masculine-feminine dyad, a less extreme ver-sion of the butch-femme sexual personae that developed within les-bian communities in the 1950s. Overall, however, there is no evidence that the women identified as part of a couple pursued same-sex rela-tions in their postgraduate careers, nor that women who were identi-fied otherwise did not. Among other things, it is impossible to know to what degree the authors of the horoscope or other instalments in nurses' popular culture were accurately commenting on their classmates' behaviour, were alluding to 'in' jokes, were purposefully suggesting the opposite of a classmate's personality, or were just concocting information about classmates about whom the editors knew very little. Rather, this evidence is testimony to the range of personal characteristics that students were permitted to display during their off-duty hours and of the unself-conscious expressions of affection and fun that did not, in the same-sex environment of school and residence, have to conform to conventions of femininity. Nurses, either as students or graduates, were single women permitted and encouraged to pursue close relationships with other women, and those relationships took a range of forms.

For instance, one oral history informant who trained in the 1920s recalled a nocturnal skinny-dip in the Winnipeg General pool one winter night. As she and her classmate were paddling around the pool, they heard the tell-tale footsteps of the night supervisor. The two nude women hovered below water clinging to the poolside, out of sight of the senior staff member, and managed to escape detection. The retired nurse laughed at the incident, wondering if the supervisor had chosen to ignore the obvious presence of the students. Regardless, such tales serve as reminders of the intense physical and perhaps sexual encounters that were possible in the female-only milieu of hospital apprenticeship programs.[37]

This pattern whereby nurses formed intimate friendships extended well beyond hospital training. Evidence of same-sex erotic relations can only be gleaned from fragmentary documentary evidence. Yet these slight glimpses suggest the significance of the homosocial possibilities that adherence to Victorian asexuality permitted. A series of letters between a Vancouver General social service nurse, Miss Patterson, and Superintendent of Nursing Kathleen Ellis, written during Patterson's convalescence from tuberculosis, described various socializing with other women. Special affection was reserved for a nursing colleague, with whom Patterson was in regular contact. As Patterson informed Ellis: 'Am missing Miss ___ so much, but expect that she is having a wonderful time.'[38] That the senior administrative nurse at Patterson's place of employment would understand the latter's emotional attachment to another graduate nurse indicated the social acceptability of this kind of same-sex 'coupling'.

The experience of one BC nurse sheds light on this little explored part of nursing's past. In the late 1930s, Eleanor Patrick accepted a position as sole nurse in charge of the Gough Memorial Hospital, the Red Cross outpost hospital in Cecil Lake, BC. Patrick arrived in the small community north of Fort St John with an impressive record of public health work in England and Canada. She was accompanied to Cecil Lake by her partner, Rosemary Webster, who was with Patrick in March 1937 when disaster struck. Patrick contracted influenza, which had been causing havoc in the district, and by the time she received proper medical attention it was too late and she died.

Rosemary Webster was heartbroken. In a letter to Mrs Gordon, a Red Cross volunteer from Victoria who had sent gifts and money to the Cecil Lake staff, Webster wrote: 'it is very hard to realize that Miss [Patrick] has "Gone on". She was so often away from here that I think she is away now and it always comes as a shock when the fact is brought home to me that she is not returning any more. . . . I find it very difficult to be here just now for everything "speaks" of her, and if I do not keep very busy I get miserable.' Still, Webster hoped that the Red Cross would allow her to continue the Cecil Lake work. She explained: 'I love this place and the people, I also loved Miss [Patrick] and although I cannot hope to do all that she did, I can at least do my little bit.'[39]

If Webster's letter revealed the depth of her sorrow, her correspondence with Gordon also indicated that within the world of Red Cross women Webster was considered Patrick's life partner. Gordon clearly knew that the two women were living together—even though Webster did not have any apparent occupation in Cecil Lake—and had in the past sent 'care' parcels to the two women. Upon Patrick's death, Gordon wrote Webster a 'kind letter' of condolence. Sadly, although Webster's relationship with Patrick was acknowledged within the nursing world, it was denied by society at large. Here the limits of nurses' relationships were made clear, as Patrick's obituary revealed. While Webster was writing her poignant letter to Gordon requesting to stay in Cecil Lake, the newspaper obituaries announced that Patrick was survived only by her parents and brother.[40]

That single women like Webster, Patrick, and Patterson would establish companionate relations with other women was not unusual. In the nineteenth and early twentieth centuries, when industrial economies began offering women educational and employment options outside the domestic sphere, women who chose work over marriage often forged close emotional and social bonds with other women. Whether those bonds had a physical dimension is the subject of substantial historical debate. Some historians of sexuality have argued that, for many women, emotional intimacy extended into sexual intimacy as well. Other scholars have cautioned against imposing late twentieth-century sexual categories, such as lesbian, onto previous eras when verbal expressions of love and passion were not necessarily accompanied by physical ones.[41] In her biography of the American nurse and reformer, Lillian Wald, Doris Daniels articulated the 'troubling questions' the debate around same-sex relations has posed for historians and feminists: 'Do all intimate relationships between women have a sexual component and should such relations be called lesbian if that erotic dimension is absent or unprovable?'[42] For nursing historians these questions are particularly meaningful. The intense experience of apprenticeship training and residence life, combined with the social imperative that nurses maintain safe distances from male co-workers or patients, made relations with other women the logical choice for many nurses. Nursing's occupational structure thus fostered women's friendships, some of which evolved into permanent companionate relationships that were acknowledged in and around nursing circles, if not by all elements of society. The degree to which women's companionate relations were also sexual ones awaits further research.[43] The evidence presented here does not indicate the sexual preference or activity of women like Patrick and Webster, but does underscore the fact that the love and support women offered each other was an important, if understudied, element of nursing's past.[44]

For Canada's third generation of trained nurses, the occupation's conventional asexual feminine persona created a social space that permitted women to forge intense and important same-sex relations, provided a social distance from sexual danger on the job, and at the same time enhanced nurses' claim to social respectability. But nursing leaders and working nurses did not always agree on where the boundaries of respectability should be placed. In hospitals, administrators held the balance of power; thus, if nurses wanted to challenge the conventions established by their superiors, such resistance had to be undertaken with caution. Being suspended from training or losing favour with local health authorities, in an era when alternative occupational options were few, held serious fiscal repercussions for working nurses who were already struggling with underemployment. Still, however much working nurses chafed under the regulatory regime imposed by their superiors, they could use that feminine and sexual persona to their advantage. This equilibrium between the vision of occupational leaders and rank-and-file practitioners strengthened the bonds of gender among nurses. On the other hand, heterosexual or lesbian women wishing to transgress openly the sexual mores of the day were not empowered by the restrictive sexuality inherent in nursing's conventional feminine image.

Transforming the Ideal: 1942–1968

The economic and social upheavals that accompanied and followed World War II shattered this equilibrium and forced nursing leaders to abandon their long-held Victorian ideal of femininity. In the first few years of the war, the surplus of nurses from the depression decade, like the surplus of Canadian workers more generally, had been reabsorbed into the wartime economy. By 1942, the Canadian military, industry, and government began actively to recruit women into sectors of employment previously dominated by men. So, too, the health-care sector began, for the first time in several decades, to experience shortages of personnel. As hospitals and private patients sought to recruit greater numbers of students and nurses, they found out that new graduates and long-serving staff alike were taking advantage of their improved employment options by signing up for military duty, quitting to take better-paying health-care jobs, or abandoning nursing altogether. In another era, hospitals would have adapted to these shifts by reducing patient size, but the increasing patient demand on institutional services combined with improved federal funding for hospitals made earlier strategies for balancing the patient-staff ratio unrealistic. Facing sufficient funding bases for the first time, hospital administrators looked instead to find new ways to increase radically the available pool of student and trained nurses.

These new economic and social conditions for hospitals proved to be more than just wartime ones. During the 1950s and 1960s the private-duty market shrivelled and hospitals emerged as the dominant site for health services. At the same time, high turnover in the nursing work-force continued. Despite the eradication of barriers to married women and women of colour, nursing administrators struggled to maintain a sufficient supply of trained nurses because of relatively improved occupational options for women and because many women left paid employment upon pregnancy. Confronted with this new set of demands, nursing leaders and educators moved to make nursing an attractive occupational option. Given different circumstances and traditions, they might have accomplished this goal by degendering the job to attract more male nurses. Instead, they modernized nursing's sexual and social feminine image, thereby ensuring that the occupation would remain, in this era, women's work.[45]

Changes in nurses' uniforms served as the most telling evidence of the new feminine ideal being promoted. During World War II nursing schools moved to bring nurses' official dress into line with that of other uniformed women, though not domestic servants this time. Rather, nurses' uniforms began to resemble those designed for women in the military. In *They're Still Women After All*, Ruth Pierson demonstrated that the wartime propaganda campaign to recruit women into military and civilian production hinged on the depiction of women in uniform—be it a CWAC dress or a welder's suit—as uncompromisingly heterosexual and feminine.[46] Nursing leaders followed suit. While it is unclear whether this was a self-conscious manoeuvre to capitalize on the positive image of women in the military or simply part of the larger fashion trend of the day, nursing schools raised the hemlines, tailored their skirts, shortened the sleeves, relaxed the collar, and, eventually, removed the apron.[47] By the 1950s, further modifications occurred as many hospitals introduced uniforms with full, soft skirts, a design that conformed to what historian of fashion Maureen Turim has termed the 'sweetheart line' of female dress design. With respect to Hollywood movie uses of the sweetheart line, Turim argues that this shape was able to 'annex the connotations of princess, debutante, or bride that became attached to this exaggerated feminine' appearance and that it contrasted with the 'slinkier tight skirt . . . [that represented] women as sexual warriors and golddiggers.'[48]

There was, of course, an economic consideration in modifications to institutional dress. For instance, the Toronto General Hospital discovered in 1943 that the English-made material used for the traditional uniform was in short supply. Initially, the hospital economized by shortening the uniform sleeves and removing cuffs and then by using Canadian-made white fabric. At war's end, rather than return to the original fabric and design, 'it became evident that the whole question of style, material and other details . . . should be reviewed.' A committee of hospital staff, students, and alumnae members along with representatives from the uniform industry were empowered to recommend a new outfit for Toronto General nurses. The committee even consulted an 'internationally known designer who has definite ideas concerning the uniforms'. The designer's advice that 'a charming appearance in every field of activity is a helpful tonic and especially so in nursing' obviously struck a chord in the health-care world because when the all-white uniform was introduced the *Canadian Hospital Magazine* reported its debut in terms that inferred a model's runway and fashion show.

This Class wore smart white uniforms with short sleeves and deep inset side pockets, thus doing away with starched cuffs, collars, bibs and aprons. The all-white uniform is a departure which will establish a precedent at the Hospital. Not only is it attractive in appearance but it is practical and should prove very popular.

This assessment of the new dress was proudly reported in the TGH alumnae newsletter by none other than Toronto General Superintendent of Nursing Mary Macfarland.[49]

At the same time that nurses' public image was modernized to conform with wartime and post-war fashion trends, the image of nursing was reconstructed to highlight that nurses enjoyed the same opportunities for social and leisure pursuits as did all 'modern women'. That nursing recognized young women's needs for leisure time and social lives was a message carried into the public education system by nursing school recruiters commissioned to promote their occupational option to graduating high school students. For example, in May 1943 Julia Walters, clinical instructor at Vancouver General Hospital, arranged daily tours of her hospital for high school girls. Walters responded to the prospective applicants' many questions about 'conditions, living arrangements and hours of work' with assurances that life in the nurses' home involved many leisure activities, including 'parties, dances, glee club, ping-pong and a good library of up-to-date fiction.'[50] A CNA recruiting pamphlet reiterated that message. Emphasizing that 'reasonable hours of duty, recreation and social contacts are now recognized as essentials in the life of the student nurse', the pamphlet promised young women that the occupation was 'studded with opportunities and adventure'.[51]

In these new circumstances, student nurses enjoyed slightly relaxed rules of residence life. Institutions like Winnipeg General established a 'smoker' wherein nurses could enjoy cigarettes without having to sneak onto the roof or into a nearby café as they had done in the previous generation. Marjorie McLeod recalled that until she enrolled at Winnipeg General, 'I don't think I'd ever seen a woman smoke.' But because 'the smoking room was where all the fun was . . . all the student nurses went in that room, usually after every shift, that's where the people got rid of their tensions, and told all the jokes', McLeod realized that if she wanted to be part of the after-hours socializing she had to 'smoke in self-defence'.[52] In this more relaxed climate, nurses' popular culture contained more explicit references to sexual activity. The 1949 Calgary General Hospital yearbook included a cartoon of a student dreaming in her bed. The student had dropped her gynaecology text and drifted off to her romantic fantasies.

Cartoons such as this highlighted the new occupational identity being promoted within nursing's popular culture. In contrast to the previous generation, which had used science to differentiate nurses from other women, nurses in the post-war era celebrated the ways that scientific knowledge enhanced their heterosexual desire. An item in the Vancouver General *Annual* of 1957 recited the 'Ten Commandments

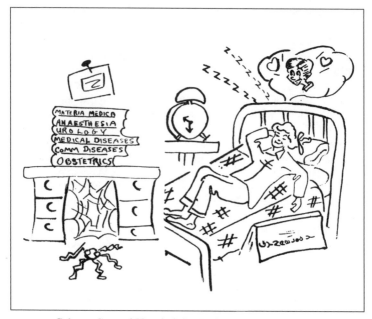

SOURCE: Calgary General Hospital, *In Uniform and Cap*, 1949.

of Nursing', including sanctions against parking in a darkened car in front of the residence, flirting with 'any handsome young intern', and arriving home past the midnight curfew.[53] References to students borrowing each other's clothes to go out on dates highlighted the romantic encounters apprentices enjoyed. Such encounters were celebrated at class formals and seasonal dances, sometimes organized in conjunction with engineering students at the local university. A 1958 Vancouver General yearbook photograph of a young woman, decked out in a full-length, sleeveless 'sweetheart' gown, walking down steps of the nurses' residence holding the hand of a dapper young man wearing a tuxedo, reminded nursing and non-nursing readers that apprenticeship training did not insulate nurses from the broader heterosexual culture of the day.[54]

As part of this rearticulation of nurses' femininity, nursing was no longer portrayed as an occupation women pursued until marriage or in place of marriage, but was recast as an occupation that prepared women for, and could be pursued after, matrimony. Nursing leaders campaigned to resolve the dichotomies between heterosexual

pursuits and paid work by emphasizing that any woman could use-
fully train as a nurse and that training would enhance not only a
woman's marital prospects but also her skills at making a marriage
successful. A *Vancouver Daily Province* article of July 1944 captured
the romance of adventure and matrimony that nursing leaders were
trying to promote. The article began:

> She is everywhere. On the battle field. . . . On the high seas. . . . In
> the hospitals and the homes and crowded tenements and the lonely
> prairie farms, where Canadian babies are being born. In the far
> reaches of the north and isolated places of the Dominion. . . .
> Tramping the streets of the big cities, her bag in her hand, calling
> at the little houses and the big houses, checking on the old and the
> young and the weak. In industrial plants and sanatoriums and
> schools. Perhaps she is not always in her traditional starched
> white. She may change that for a serviceable dark suit, or heavy
> weather togs, or even battle dress. And there are too few of her.
> The burdens she carries are too heavy, the hours—often—too long.

As it focused on the daily life of one aspiring practitioner, Miss
Leone Elliott, president of the Vancouver General student council, the
article made clear that there was 'no better training for motherhood
anywhere than working in the children's ward of a hospital'. About
nurses' training in nutrition, the article declared: 'That's another science the nurse studies which comes in handy for the housewife—it's
not surprising that the matrimonial rate among nurses is higher than
in any other profession.'[55] Thus, the renovation of the occupational
dress did not only serve to expose more leg and accentuate more
curves, it also served as a powerful symbol of the fundamentally heterosexual status of nurses and represented nursing leaders' broader
campaign to bring their occupational image more in line with that of
all 'modern' women.[56]

This did not mean that working nurses or nurse administrators
abandoned the older image of asexual saint, a persona that continued
to help nurses negotiate relations at the bedside. Throughout the war
years, especially, some images continued to celebrate nurses' devo-
tional calling and public duty. The front cover of the October 1940
Canadian Home Journal, for example, presented a Rex Woods drawing (*à la* Rockwellian realism) of an army nurse. The background
was white with a red cross in front of which stood an army nursing
sister dressed in blue double-breasted tunic, white square-cut apron,
and white nun-like head dress. The nurse's arms were at her sides,
and because the picture showed her from only the waist up, the

viewer could not see her hands. The figure's power clearly came not from her ability to 'do' but from the moral strength that her quasi-religious status—reinforced by the cross behind her head and the nun's cap—provided her.[57] Similar images were generated to advertise Red Cross blood drives. When advertisers wanted to applaud participants in wartime, community-duty nurses were frequently included among the characters presented.[58]

The proliferation of nursing imagery, especially sexualized imagery, in the media resulted from changes occurring in the occupation's structure. As hospitals emerged as the primary location of employment, nurses were less reliant on the patronage of male physicians or community members. Nurses were less frequently called to individual homes where doctors, family members, or men on the street might harass them or misinterpret their behaviour. Instead, practitioners applied for jobs through hospital personnel offices and answered to hospital administration. This did not mean that harassment and assault disappeared as social problems. Rather, it meant that nurses' employment options were not dependent on or prey to the whims or dangers of individual community members. In this context, media images that emphasized nurses' heterosexuality and femininity were less threatening to the occupation and highly appealing to advertisers. Whereas in earlier decades nursing leaders resisted corporate efforts to use the nurse's uniform for 'commercial purposes', the frequent use of this type of nurse-figure now supported the larger efforts to celebrate nursing in the public sphere.

Advertisements in CN, for example, began to parallel those of commercial publications, emphasizing the feminine goals of beauty that nurses pursued in their off-duty hours. Noxzema ads reminded CN readers that 'Nurses Have Private Lives, too!. . . But you can't look forward to much fun on your time off if your feet burn, or if your hands are red, rough and sore!'[59] Another began 'How to be a prettier nurse'.[60] An ad for Mum deodorant depicted a male physician at the bedside of a male patient. As the doctor picked up the telephone to call for a private-duty nurse, the patient requested, 'for heaven's sake don't send for Miss H. . . . again!. . . she's a good nurse all right . . . I could overlook perspiration odor in a truck driver. But in a nurse—it's unforgivable!'[61] As the latter advertisement indicated, maintaining standards of attractiveness were prerequisites for positive work experiences and heterosexual attentions. A Noxzema ad that began with the statement/question 'Best Medicine A Man Ever Had . . .?' included a sketch of an attractive nurse casting her eyes demurely backwards in the direction of two male patients who

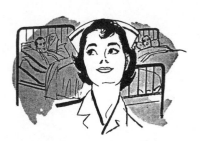

"Best Medicine
A Man
Ever Had...?"

SOURCE: *Canadian Nurse*, 1958.

were watching her appreciatively.[62] Promotions for a menopausal estrogen therapy conveyed a similar message. An attractive nurse held the wrist of a male patient as she looked at her watch to monitor his pulse. The heading 'still serving a good cause' referred explicitly to the drug being promoted, but also alluded to the social 'causes' served when nurses attended patients and when attractive women retained the attentions of men around them.[63]

Nursing commentators were aware of the necessity and, in fact, inevitability of their occupation receiving such attention from purveyors of commercial and popular culture. Not only did the national nursing journal need the advertising revenues of corporate sponsors, *CN* authors realized that in the post-war economy of state-funded medical care nursing was open to substantially greater amounts of external comment. *CN* editor Ethel Johns informed her readers of her recent correspondence with a member of the public who 'told us right out . . . that she thinks nurses are the last vestigial remnants of the Victorian Era. . . . Her general idea seemed to be that it is high time for us to take a good square look at this strange new world we are living in . . . and then go out and do something courageous and constructive on our own behalf. . . .' Johns agreed that her occupation could no longer shape itself with only internal priorities in mind: '. . . we are in for a reconsideration of nursing values . . . and we are not going to be allowed to make the appraisal all by ourselves. . . . The community is going to take a hand this time. . . .'[64]

Indeed, it was non-nurse commentators who popularized this new definition of nursing's heterosexual complementariness, and among the non-nurse commentators, no one did it better than Harlequin

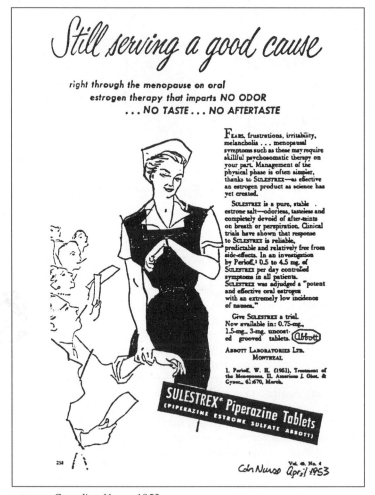

SOURCE: *Canadian Nurse*, 1953.

romances. One of Canada's largest multinationals, the Winnipeg-based company soon discovered that a significant international market existed for romance novels. Throughout the 1950s and 1960s, Harlequin began to corner the market in this genre by re-publishing the English serials by Boon and Mills. In the early years of the Harlequin business, nurses were standard characters around which the plots of love, disagreement, misunderstanding, and resolution revolved. Like the teachers and governesses who also served as Harlequin heroines, the nurse-protagonists were of humble origin, orphans (or far from family support networks), independent and proud, principled sometimes to the point of stubbornness, attractive (more from internal radiance than from physical beauty), and chaste. They also loved their work.

A number of scholarly analyses of Harlequin romances have been published, among them Margaret Ann Jensen's Love's Sweet Return: The Harlequin Story, but several additional nurse-specific points require emphasis.[65] Firstly, nursing provided this genre with the perfect occupational setting in which to reveal the characters' sterling qualities. The hierarchical structure of the occupation ensured that the heroine would have to demonstrate strict internal discipline and a willingness to be subordinate. The heroine was never a supervisor or senior administrator, always a plucky student, private-duty, or staff nurse on the brink of becoming an excellent practitioner. Her subservience to the male lead therefore was explained not in patriarchal or personal terms—our heroine was no snivelling coward—but in terms of her own acceptance of the importance of hierarchy in ensuring patient health.

If nursing served Harlequin authors well, so, too, did Harlequin authors reinforce the modern image of nursing that leaders were trying to inculcate. Perhaps recognizing that many readers might be working women, the novels did not pose a contradiction between paid nursing work and unpaid domestic marital duties until the end of the stories, if at all. Rarely did the nurse heroines quit work to be married. Rather, they resigned for other reasons and marriage then fit into their plans. For example, in a 1963 publication, Nurse of My Heart, heroine Sally Gaskell resigned from her hospital to return home and nurse her invalid sister.[66] In Nurse in Training Christy abandoned her training to be married, but only because once married she planned to go to medical school, a plan that her true love, once they were reunited, endorsed wholeheartedly.[67] In Nurse Wayne in the Tropics, English nurse Triss Wayne, working on a plantation on the Gold Coast of Africa, finally assented to marry the man of her dreams, but they agreed that Triss must first return to England to complete her contract with her clinic there. Upon her return to Africa, Triss would assist her husband in establishing a local hospital for colonists and Africans.[68]

As the above examples illustrate, Harlequin romances were rarely set in Canada, but in unspecified villages in England or in 'exotic' colonial settings. Jensen has observed that persisting racist stereotypes were used to create 'exotic' settings for the novels, but depictions of native and non-Western peoples did more than just that.[69] The adventures around the world that Harlequin presented offered Canadian nurses a universal image that united practitioners from different Western nations under the single identity of White European female. This message was particularly important to Canadian nurses, who in the post-war years were experiencing a significant ethnic and racial diversification of their occupation. As formal barriers to Afro-Canadian, Asian-Canadian, and First Nations women pursuing nursing credentials eroded, popular culture reinforced the privileged position of White women in the occupation.

Central to the Harlequin message of European or, more specifically, English superiority was the sexual representation of non-White and non-English speaking women. Depicted as the mothers of many children, the 'exotic' women demonstrated limited abilities to care for their offspring. In *Nurse of My Heart*, Sally Gaskell encountered a young 'Gipsy' woman who had entered a store to buy baby necessities. Unlike most of the village women, Sally did not condemn this outsider who 'had the magnificent profile one might find on a Grecian coin—a beauty as old as Time, delicately chiseled', although Sally noted that 'her hair was lank and greasy, her fingers stained with nicotine. The stub of a cigarette clung to the splendidly-moulded lips. . . .'[70] When news reached Sally that the young woman had died and the baby was in jeopardy, she rushed to the rescue, providing modern medical care and superior maternal attendance to that of the 'Gipsy' woman.[71] Like other Harlequin heroines, Sally was distinguished not by procreative heterosexuality *per se* but by the superior mothering skills that nurses like Sally had, even if they were themselves as yet childless.

Nurse Wayne's experiences in the tropics emphasized the same conclusion. En route to the Gold Coast, Triss's ship docked at 'Las Palmas, that fairyland satellite of Spain', where she spent the day with the soon-to-be object of her affections, Stephen Graham. There Triss observed 'the dark-eyed, luscious-lipped Spanish women with their inevitable ear-rings and brown babies.' The procreative sexuality of the local women was implicitly explained by the presence of the 'idle, good-looking men who lounged everywhere'. One of the 'husky loungers' touched 'Triss' soft cheek' and spoke to Stephen in Spanish. Stephen translated: 'He compliments me on my pretty wife with the roses in her cheeks, and hopes we will become blessed with ten ninos!' Once again Triss's temporary childlessness did not divide her from other women, for her potential was obvious. Instead, as the plot developed, it became clear that Triss and other White women like her were superior to the local women because they retained control over their sexuality and over childbirth more generally. When Triss provided emergency obstetrical care for an African woman, she also gained a reputation as a skilled midwife and healer who could manage childbirth in a manner superior to the community wise women, such as 'one old granny' who refused to heat water for Triss and insisted that the 'child would probably be drowned in the process. Defeated finally by a majority vote, the granny refused to take further part in the proceedings, and sat muttering by the fire while Triss delivered a beautiful, female child.'[72]

It is equally significant that throughout the novels the young heroines retained their heterosexual femininity. Same-sex sociability was rarely applauded. The heroines had few female friends and the women around them were portrayed as weak and, indeed, often had to undergo a radical transformation to heterosexual complementariness themselves. In relations with men, the Harlequin heroine set the standard of heterosexual femininity. She was chaste and loyal, and recognized her own true love at first sight. Proximity to male patients' bodies did not liberate her heterosexual desires, but rather confirmed the heroine's monogamy. When in *Nurse of My Heart* Sally's brother-in-law, Chris, on whom she had had an adolescent crush, made a pass at her, she was disgusted. Although Sally had not yet identified the object of her true and endearing passion, Sally knew that Chris was definitely not her man.

If their heterosexual monogamy was firmly in place, it was threatened by the possibility of never marrying. Nurse novels regularly included one senior nurse who was so committed to her work, and so unable to combine work and love, that she became 'hard'. Even Christy momentarily ran the risk of losing her femininity. During the brief moments in *Nurse in Training* when Christy had broken off with both of her male marital possibilities, she decided, 'That was that, then. She was done with men, oh, thank goodness she was done with them!' But then the reader learned: 'Her face took on a harder outline and her red mouth became a grim straight line as she went about her afternoon duties. . . .' Fortunately, Christy's curves returned in time to resolve her affair with Brent. These images of the non-heterosexual nurse are stock in trade of Harlequins, designed to identify the danger inherent in life without men.

Other sources of popular culture also addressed nurses' heterosexual complementariness, but unlike the Harlequin novels, they did not necessarily rely on positive images of nurses to sell their goods. As nurses became popular figures in mass circulation magazines and newspapers, so, too, the question of nurses' sexuality became re-examined in a less flattering way and the image, with which we are now familiar, of the sexually knowledgeable nurse began to appear. For example, a 1945 cartoon from the *Halifax Herald* depicted two nurses at the bedside of a young male patient. As the patient, not ter-rifically attractive himself, sucked on a thermometer, his eyes bugged out at the young, voluptuous nurse. The second, older, grey-haired, bespectacled nurse requested her colleague to leave the bedside because she was causing the patient's temperature to rise unnaturally high. Scientific medicine was being interrupted by female sexuality.

At the same time, the fact that the patient was a young man who was clearly more responsive to the ministrations of the curvacious young nurse suggested that sexuality and science could be combined in powerful ways. According to some popular commentators, nurses' technical knowledge and scientific skills were made more potent when combined with sexual appeal. For instance, the 10 November 1950 edition of the University of Manitoba students' union newspaper, *The Manitoban*, announced that the Red Cross would be on campus that week. The announcement began with the statement: 'Roll up your sleeve and smile for the cute little blonde nurse, boys—she wants some of your blood for her collection.'[73] The nurse's professional man-date to administer a blood bank was recast *à la* Dracula, as if it were her collection and her sexual appeal that lured potential victims.

A 1962 issue of *Hospital Guardian*, the official voice of British Columbia's Hospital Employees Association, also suggested a con-nection between sexuality and science. The cartoon was intended as a critique of mechanization of health care; the foolishness of need-ing a machine to change a diaper on a baby was self-evident. The joke, however, was premised on a particular relationship of sexual-ity, femininity, and work. The machine-tender was an older nurse whose lack of physical appeal was accentuated by the out-of-date fashion she wore. Flat-chested, with unkempt hair, in need of glasses, and wearing a long uniform and 'granny boots', she blithely fed the happy babies head first through the diaper-changer, until a younger nurse rushed over to correct the obvious error. Youth was not this practitioner's only attribute. She boasted a curvacious figure (including a well-developed bust), slim legs, long hair fram-ing a pretty face with wide eyes, a short uniform, and modern shoes. The humour, therefore, lay not only in the uselessness of the machine, but also in the older nurse whose experience in the work-place undermined even the most basic elements of femininity, such as knowing which end of a baby was up. By contrast, the younger nurse, while having less professional experience, none the less was

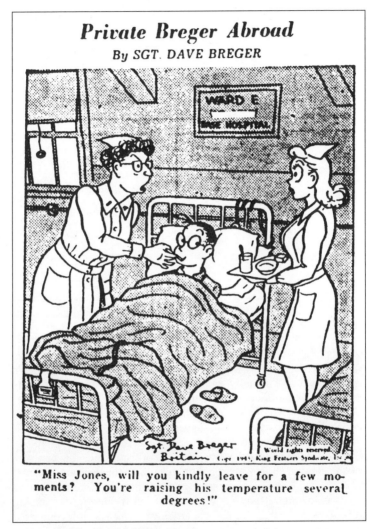

Private Breger Abroad
By SGT. DAVE BREGER

"Miss Jones, will you kindly leave for a few moments? You're raising his temperature several degrees!"

SOURCE: *Halifax Herald*, 1945.

interpreted as a better practitioner because she had not lost touch with her femininity.

By the late 1960s and early 1970s, the sexualized image of the nurse would be carried one step further. Within American popular culture, such characters as *MASH*'s 'Hot Lips' Hoolihan and Ken

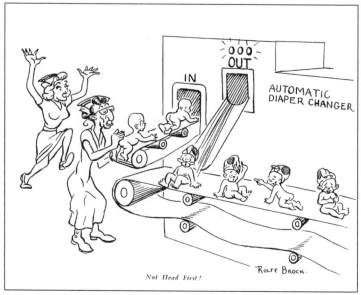

Not Head First!

ROLFE BROCK.

SOURCE: British Columbia Hospital Employees Association, *Hospital Guardian* (Oct. 1962), p. 7.

Kesey's 'Big Nurse', nurse Ratched in *One Flew Over the Cuckoo's Nest*, were depicted by left-liberal writers as symbolic of women's heterosexual and socially damaging power. At a more grassroots level, popular culture positioned nurses as more sexually knowledge-able than other women, as nurse-characters' frequent appearances in pornographic films and novels suggested.[74]

Working nurses were not necessarily liberated by this vigorously heterosexual femininity that was expected of them. True, this new sex-ual-social occupational paradigm did legitimate the decision made by many women in the post-war era to combine nursing careers with mar-riage, as the significant numbers of married women in the nursing work-force indicated. But the unmarried women, who still comprised the majority of young women entering the occupation, confronted a definition of femininity in which sexual space was in some ways even more difficult to negotiate than it had been before. Heterosexual women were on the one hand encouraged to participate in the youth culture of heterosexual and male-female activities, but at the same time they had to avoid crossing the line into promiscuity. The conflict that brewed at Vancouver General Hospital highlighted this contradiction.

'The Case of the Kissing Nurse'

On a lazy Sunday afternoon in January of 1959 Mrs Bew and Mrs Sulman discovered they had a problem. Right in front of their office window sat a parked car in which a young couple were engaged in passionate kissing. As matrons of the Vancouver General nurses' residence, Bew and Sulman were responsible for ensuring that more than 500 student nurses adhered to the institution's residence rules and thereby helped to maintain a sterling reputation for their school and hospital. Here lay the dilemma. Owing to the nature of the activity in the car, the matrons could not see the woman's face. If she was a student, the school representatives could interrupt the couple and insist that the woman return to her residence. After all, not only was her behaviour unseemly, but it was past 2:30 p.m. and all student nurses were expected to be back in the hospital a half-hour before their 3 p.m. shift began. If she was not a Vancouver General student, could the matrons rightfully request the couple to move to another location? Unsure as to their jurisdiction, the matrons telephoned various administrative offices until they finally reached someone in the Department of Nursing office who assured the matrons of their authority over the matter. Just as the diligent overseers were about to take action, the car door slammed and the young woman—a senior student at Vancouver General—sauntered towards the residence. The matrons intercepted the student, reported her to the school authorities, and the student was suspended for two weeks.

To be sent home for two weeks was a stern penalty, though not unusually so. Suspension was more serious than the frequently invoked punishments of having time added to the three-year training period or having late leaves revoked, but it was also less extreme than the other possibility, outright dismissal. Yet the penalty of having to return home to explain to her parents why she had been reprimanded was severe enough to prompt immediate sympathy from her colleagues in the nursing school. Protesting what they considered harsh and inconsistent punishment, the student nurses threatened to strike if the errant nurse was not reinstated. News of the conflict leaked to the press and by the end of the week it was receiving not only local but national coverage. Faced with public humiliation and the potential loss of 500 bedside attendants, the hospital administration met, first with the vigilant matrons to sort out the details of the case and then with the student council to pre-empt the strike and to negotiate the rules governing residence life and nurses' leisure time.[75] Meanwhile, newspapers, radio stations, and television networks debated 'the case of the kissing nurse' to understand why, as the *Toronto Daily Star* put it, 'are certain women's professions discriminated against in romance?'[76]

Like other labour disputes between hospitals and their employees in the pre-Medicare era, the conflict was resolved through a combination of negotiation, paternalism, and threats. But events at Vancouver General in 1959 revealed long-standing tensions involving health-care administrators, working nurses, and the public over how nurses' sexuality, femininity, and respectability would be defined and the importance of those definitions in situating nurses in the world of work. When Matrons Bew and Sulman met with hospital administrators such as the chairman of the board of directors, Mr Banfield, the discussion centred not on whether the kissing had occurred, but whether it had gone on for too long. One matron proclaimed, 'I'm not a prude but 25 minutes is too long.' Another administrator asked, 'Who initiated the contact?' And another queried, 'Were his hands in evidence at all times?'

In the midst of these mixed messages and ambiguous limits, nurses' claims to respectable femininity hinged on their ability to negotiate the messages and limits they encountered. Not surprisingly, then, the essence of the students' complaints was not about rules regarding deportment *per se*, but rather the inconsistency with which those rules were applied. This point was not lost on all observers. Mr McNaughton, second vice-chairman of the hospital board, observed that at 10:30 at night he had often seen seven cars lined up outside the residence as students said good-bye to their boyfriends, and asked, 'was it a crime to kiss your boyfriend at 2:30 in the afternoon but not one at 10:30 at night?' Here McNaughton captured the crux of the problem, for heterosexual desire was to be applauded and encouraged in daylight but practised only after dark, preferably with a man who would become the young woman's husband.

If these expectations were difficult to meet within a heterosexual context, so, too, was the space for all-female social and sexual relations narrowed in this era. While nursing residences continued to serve as fertile ground for intimate friendships among women, the homosocial possibilities of nursing became an embarrassment to the occupation. For single working women, same-sex friendships lost their social legitimation and, with it, the space for occupationally accepted homoerotic relationships vanished. Nursing's refusal to recognize any female friendships save those pursued by heterosexually active women was fuelled by the post-war climate of homosexual repression and regulation, what Gary Kinsman has termed the era of heterosexual hegemony.[77]

In a recent study of American sexual deviance in the post-World War II years, Donna Penn has suggested that rather than female sex roles being understood as 'a kind of duality or polarity with deviant and normal bolstering up either side of the line that divides them from one another', a 'circular metaphor' better captures the shape of female sexuality. Penn argues:

> Proper female sexuality, heterosexual in orientation and reserved for the home and within marriage, was, in the postwar framework, surrounded by uncontained, rather public expressions of illicit sexual behaviors. These behaviors were constituted in the form of the prostitute, the lesbian, and the prostitute as lesbian.[78]

As Canadian nursing élites emphasized the heterosexual complementariness of their occupation, they had to come to terms with the possibility of open displays of heterosexual activity—whether in front of the nursing residence or in popular representations of nurses—and with the tradition of same-sex social relationships, some of which may have been constructed as private homoerotic ones. As 'the case of the kissing nurse' revealed, containing female heterosexuality within monogamous, matrimonial relations with men created a very narrow set of sexual options for working nurses.

Conclusion

It is now considered a truism to state that nursing is women's work, but the particular attributes that comprised femininity were neither natural nor uncontested. This is especially clear when the question of female sexuality is considered. Over the course of the twentieth century, the sexual image of nurses has changed significantly, sometimes reinforcing the broader social representation of female sexuality and other times deviating from that social norm. Nursing leaders and educators advocated particular sets of appropriate sexual and social behaviour according to the political economy of their occupation. Second- and third-generation nursing leaders used their positions in hospital training schools to instil an exaggerated version of Victorian femininity. This asexual workplace persona was necessary to enhance nursing's reputation of respectability and at the same time to convince young women to dispense personal and physical care to the bodies of strangers. When, in the 1940s and 1950s, the occupation's leaders needed to increase dramatically the size of the nursing workforce, they reconstructed nursing's image to emphasize the fundamentally heterosexual nature of nursing, that nursing and marriage were mutually reinforcing occupations for women.

Nursing students and graduate nurses did not always endorse the occupational image promoted by leaders and educators. In the pre-World War II years many resisted the restraints placed on sexual and social behaviour. In the post-World War II era many continued, as they had done in previous generations, to pursue careers as single working women and others rejected the compulsory heterosexuality of nursing's new sexualized persona. Throughout the twentieth century, the Victorian image of the asexual nurse continued to help working nurses negotiate power relations at the bedside, although the utility of that image diminished as hospital employment supplanted private-duty work as the dominant mode of employment.

The reconstruction of nurses' image along heterosexually complementary lines did bring nurses into line with other women, and, in fact, nursing emerged in the post-war era as an occupation signified by the sexuality of its members. This did not constitute sexual liberation, any more than did the asexual persona of the earlier generations. Heterosexually active fourth-generation Canadian nurses found that they had to walk the fine line of pursuing 'healthy' sexual relations with men without slipping into promiscuity. Same-sex-oriented nurses found that companionate relations between women were no longer easily accepted.

The power of popular imagery was perhaps most dramatically demonstrated when, in the 1960s and 1970s, the feminist movement developed its critique of sexuality and femininity. Insisting that women could and should express their sexuality as freely as men and questioning whether equality could be attained in heterosexual relations, feminists constructed a vision of liberation that criticized heterosexual complementariness. Nursing, with its celebration of heterosexuality and deference to male doctors, thus appeared to feminists as a model of unliberated sexuality.[79] In spite of the facts that working nurses had struggled to resist exploitive sexual relations in the workplace, that nursing was one of the first occupations to accommodate working mothers, and that many of the more exploitive sexual images came from non-nurse commentators, common ground between nurses and feminists was quickly eroded. Tensions between the two groups appear even more unfortunate when placed in contrast with the mutual support that nurses and feminists provided each other in the early twentieth-century drive for suffrage.[80] In recent years, this rupture has begun to heal, but nurses and feminists alike have yet to appreciate fully the particular contradictions that femininity and sexuality have posed for the modern trained nurse.

6

Contradictions and Continuities: The Fourth Generation of Canadian Nurses, 1942–1968

When nursing leaders and historians reflect back on the period from 1942 to 1968, they frequently characterize that era as one of resolution and progress, in which the problems of institutional reliance on student labour, the uncertainty of private-duty work, and the lack of professional recognition were solved.[1] In these years, nursing education was released somewhat from its subordination to hospital staffing needs and as a result, permanent hospital employment became the dominant subsector of nursing work. Professional advancement of this kind was not the only force shaping nursing in the post-war era. A contradictory impulse of proletarianization was also in effect, as hospital staff confronted the realities of working regular shifts for a large third-party employer and of a two-tier system of nurse-managers and nurse-workers on hospital wards. Several recent studies have argued that this process of proletarianization proceeded alongside professional achievements, creating a particular pattern of 'occupational struggle' and an ambiguous class status for nursing.[2] Although such studies have constituted an important corrective to the portrait of progress presented by earlier generations of nursing scholars, they have rarely calculated gender into their historical formulations. The ambiguous occupational identity of the post-World War II era was also influenced by the continuities from and commonalities with older patterns structuring nurses' work that kept nursing the preserve of White women. Ongoing pressures for nursing staff to complete a multiplicity of overlapping functions and to perform whatever duties patient health required, in conjunction with the persistence of a powerful gender division of labour and authority, reinforced common bonds between nurse leaders and rank-and-file practitioners.

Rather than interpret the post-war era as one of professional development or of proletarianization and declining class status, this chapter explores the contradictions and continuities of gender and class, as well as ethnicity, that combined in this fourth generation to create new tensions at the bedside and within nursing organizations. Because the hospital sector employed the majority of graduate nurses and provided most medical and surgical treatment, the focus of this chapter is on institutional work. The paradox faced by hospital and non-institutional nurses alike was that at the very moment when a more conservative, heterosexualized image of the occupation was being promoted in popular culture, nurses at the workplace were experiencing enhanced social authority, but also greater alienation and militancy as they sought new modes of coping with the gendered structure of health-care work.

Redefining the Boundaries of Occupational Membership

As post-war popular culture was redefining nursing as a quintessentially heterosexual and feminine pursuit, events at the workplace underscored nursing's traditional link with femaleness. After two decades of unstable employment for third-generation nurses, in the years after 1942 the job market inverted as dramatic hospital growth demanded substantial increases in institutional nursing staffs. Nursing leaders and administrators responded to the undersupply by increasing the size of the nursing work-force. The occupational boundaries were stretched to include more men and more recruits from diverse ethnic and national backgrounds, but the greatest point of expansion was the welcoming of married nurses back into paid labour. These strategies resulted in labour force growth, but they lagged behind the demand for nursing personnel. Indeed, observers of the inter-war employment crisis could not have predicted that in a few short years the supply/demand ratio would change so quickly or so thoroughly.

The outbreak of war in 1939 did not immediately reverse the oversupply and underemployment that had plagued nursing in the inter-war decades. For the first few years of World War II, opportunities for work in the three traditional subsectors of nursing stabilized, while a modest number of new positions were created in the military and in civilian sectors such as transportation. The career of Ottawa Civic graduate Elsie Dunnet illustrates the meaning of these opportunities. Dunnet resigned from the staff of the Gravenhurst Tuberculosis Sanatorium in 1939 to take a job as hostess with Trans-Canada Airlines

(TCA). Like other companies, TCA hoped that hiring graduate nurses as flight attendants would convince customers that air travel was safe. Dunnet flew the western Canada circuit until 1942, when she again changed jobs, this time signing up with the Canadian Army.[3] Dunnet, along with many other registered nurses, had been applying to the armed services for several years, but nursing opportunities in the RCAMC did not open up until 1941–2, when 300 Canadian nurses were sent to South Africa and when, in the wake of Dieppe, Canadian nurses were needed for service in British military hospitals and European field stations. By the end of the war, close to 4,000 Canadian nurses had served in the military.[4]

Thus, not until midway through the war did the demand for nurses, as well as other working women, accelerate in the civilian as well as military sectors.[5] By 1942, when Fraudina Eaton, author of the 1938 report on labour conditions in British Columbia hospitals, took charge of the newly created National Selective Service Women's Division, shortages of nurses were being reported in most areas of employment. Nursing leaders and administrators worried over how to recruit more students into hospital programs and more graduates onto their staffs. In 1942, Vancouver General Hospital's director of nursing, Grace Fairley, reported that the shortage of nurses had become so serious that at one point in the year two wards were closed due to lack of nurses.[6] By 1944, hospitals across the nation were reporting 'extreme instability of the graduate nursing staff'. That year, Vancouver General faced 249 resignations, a more than tenfold increase over rates in 'normal' times. At Winnipeg General Hospital more than half of the graduate nursing staff in 1944 were new appointments hired to replace the 40 nurses who had resigned in the previous 12 months. Ten of those resignations were attributed to nurses who joined the army or allied services, five were for marriage, seven returned home, and 19 were for 'miscellaneous reasons'.[7] By the war's end, the Manitoba Association of Registered Nurses executive was devoting entire meetings to the issue of nursing shortages, but admitted 'to date there has been no remedy'.[8]

When hostilities ceased, it became apparent that the shortage of nurses had more systemic origins than just military emergency. In 1947, Calgary physician Dr E.P. Scarlett concluded that 'the serious shortage of nurses at the present time, and changes in our society have brought the whole organization of the nursing profession under scrutiny.'[9] As predicted, nursing issues did receive regular scrutiny in publications like Winnipeg General's *Accounts and Reports*, which almost every year from 1942 to 1966 identified the lack of graduate nurses as a major brake on expanding hospital services.[10] Nursing leaders responded to the crisis by conducting surveys and researching strategies designed to augment the graduate nurse work-force. A 1958 BC report claimed that between 21 and 35 positions for general staff nurses were vacant in the spring of 1958, and 13–17 positions 'above General Staff' were open. A further 28 public health nurses were required.[11] The Association of Registered Nurses in the Province of Quebec (ARNPQ) estimated in 1962 that 26 per cent more general-duty staff were needed to prevent further reductions in the number of hospital beds.[12] A 1968 study by the Ontario Department of Health, _The Untapped Pool_, concluded that 'for every working nurse there is at least one who is not actively nursing. In fact the Untapped Pool composes 56 per cent of all nurses.'[13]

The growing demand for medical and nursing services reflected the broader reorganization of health-care financing in the post-war era. Enjoying increased wage levels in the wartime and post-war economies, ordinary Canadians could afford health-care services that in the previous decades had been beyond their budgets. This purchasing power was enhanced by hospital insurance programs developed first by private companies such as Blue Cross and then, in the late 1940s, by publicly financed hospital insurance programs instituted by four provincial governments. Meanwhile, hospitals struggled to obtain a greater degree of financial stability. Measures like the 1948 Federal Hospital Grant Programme provided institutions with direct funds for education and capital costs, but expenses continued to sky-rocket. In the 1950–5 period alone, Canadian hospitals increased their patient loads by 40 per cent, at the same time that costs per patient day grew by 75 per cent and total operating expenses grew by 260 per cent.[14] The federally administered hospitalization insurance plan of 1957 did make institutional services universally available, but in spite of the increased funding, hospitals continued to face mounting pressure for a greater number of specialized patient services.[15]

Expansion of hospital services was dependent on the increased employment of graduate nurses. In 1951, the Canadian _Census_ listed 35,138 graduate nurses as gainfully employed and by 1961 that figure had nearly doubled to 61,699.[16] Although this rate of growth surpassed that of the Canadian population, which increased by 50 per cent in the 1950s, the rapidity with which the nursing work-force grew was consistent with the more general expansion of the nation's female labour force. Reflecting that fact, nursing continued to represent approximately 3 per cent of Canada's working women.[17] What was new to the post-war era was that most nurses now worked in hospital wards, either as general-duty nurses or as supervisory staff.[18] The ARNPQ calculated that in Quebec hospitals in 1962, 62 per cent of graduate nurses worked in general duty performing direct patient care and a further 16 per cent were employed as head nurses and directors of nursing. Only 11 per cent worked in public health or industrial nursing and fewer still, 9 per cent, in private care.[19]

To secure the requisite number of practitioners, the nursing workforce was expanded in several ways. First, efforts were made to increase the number of students trained. Between 1939 and 1946, the number of graduates each year increased by 45 per cent, and between 1951 and 1961 the student population grew by another 50 per cent.[20] Large schools nearly doubled their size. At the Toronto General Hospital, for example, the annual average graduating class for the pre-1940 years was 53, whereas after 1940 it averaged 100 graduates per year and by 1952 the largest-ever class, 121 nurses, completed their education.[21] Enlarging the supply of students was no easy task, especially given wartime expansion of jobs open to women followed by the post-war retraction of women from the work-force. BC statistics showed that in 1944 nursing attracted one-quarter of women with junior matriculation, but by 1962 only one of ten such candidates chose to pursue nursing. While this reflected the growing numbers of Canadians achieving high school education, it also revealed that in an era of expanding job options for women, nursing had to work hard to attract its share of recruits.[22] To compete with other occupational options, provincial associations and hospital schools mounted recruiting campaigns that involved visiting high schools, giving talks to youth groups, gaining newspaper coverage, staging displays in public centres, and even running radio programs.[23] Among the latter was a January 1947 program, 'People Ask', in which the Viscountess Alexander spoke on 'Opportunities for Girls in Nursing'.[24] During the war, nursing leaders such as Brandon General Hospital's Christina Macleod had recommended, to little avail, that hospitals appeal to the federal government 'to direct some [nurses] who are educationally qualified, to hospital service instead of military duty'.[25] Nurses had more success convincing the federal government to establish a grant for hospital schools, the bulk of which was devoted to recruiting students.[26]

One ready supply of new recruits lay in the countryside, where, as was the case for previous generations, rural economies offered young women limited occupational options. Data for Halifax's Victoria General Hospital in 1944–6, 1949, 1951–3, and 1955 reveal that urban-born women represented only a small percentage of nurses trained there. In those years, only 36 graduates hailed from Halifax and Dartmouth, as compared to 255 from the rest of the province.[27] At Winnipeg's Misericordia General Hospital, the classes of 1948 and 1953 together included 11 women from Winnipeg and St Boniface, 24 women from rural Manitoba, 20 from rural Saskatchewan and Alberta, along with 6 others.[28] On the west coast, the rural-urban ratio was more balanced, with Vancouver General graduates evenly divided between urban home towns in BC or the prairie provinces and those with addresses from rural parts of the four western provinces, but even at 50 per cent, rural women remained a significant supplement to the available labour pool of recruits.[29]

Included in this expansion of the student work-force was a renewed interest on the part of nursing educators in recruiting men into training programs. In 1951, only 42 male students were enrolled in hospital schools, but by 1961 there were 326 male apprentices. Although their presence signalled the existence of new possibilities within the occupation, which men would take greater advantage of in future generations, in the fourth generation of apprenticing nurses men remained a small minority. Hospitals like Halifax's Victoria General attracted slightly greater numbers of male students in the early years of the war, but after 1943 usually no more than two, if any, enrolled,[30] while in Quebec, the provincial nursing act specifically excluded male practitioners.[31] For these reasons, male nurses constituted only 0.3 and 1.4 per cent of the total student work-forces in 1951 and 1961.

The existence of better-paying jobs in industry discouraged most men from pursuing a career in nursing.[32] Those who did found that some co-workers resented male incursions into otherwise female-dominated territory. A 1964 letter to CN from Mrs Eileen De Witt, claiming that 'this business of employing male nurses to care for female patients is disgusting and ridiculous' and that obstetrical training for male nurses 'is really inane', prompted heated replies from two male colleagues. Defending the right of male nurses to attend female patients and obstetrical cases, Albert Wedgery, RN, called De Witt's attitudes 'Victorian' and 'outmoded'. RN Richard Palmer pointed to the double standard underlying De Witt's opinions—after all, female nurses provided care to male patients—and agreed with Wedgery that 'education' of female nurses was necessary to remind them that 'the function of a nurse is caring for the sick—irrespective of race, color, creed or sex [italics in original].'[33]

Palmer's critique of discrimination in nursing was timely, for the post-war shortage of nurses was also accelerating the erosion of racial and ethnic barriers. Formal exclusion of African-Canadian and First

Nations women from nursing training programs ended during and after World War II. Chinese- and Japanese-Canadian women, who had been represented in small numbers in BC schools since the 1930s, made their way into programs elsewhere in Canada. In 1951, 15 'Indian and Eskimo' and 87 'Asiatic' women were listed as students in the *Census* and in 1961 those figures had grown to 38 and 117. Many students of non-European descent were Canadian-born, but a small number were immigrants. Of the Asian women enrolled as student nurses in 1951 and 1961, 16 and 32 were born in Asia. Ethnic diversity was also enhanced in this era by the growing presence (16 per cent in 1961) of women of European ancestry who were neither British nor French.

Eradicating racial and ethnic barriers was not an easy task. In the 1930s and 1940s, nursing administrators in British Columbia had advocated nursing training for Japanese- and Chinese-Canadian women on the grounds that 'it is necessary to give to them health teachers of their own nationality.' Adhering to the racist belief that 'the Oriental . . . is a fatalist and still has many of the characteristics of the Dark Ages', these administrators expected Japanese- and Chinese-Canadian nurses to be 'instruments of reform' who would 'break down these native inhibitions' to Western public health programs.[34] In the years after World War II, official rhetoric changed as nursing leaders, playing on the post-war theme of international equality, condemned discrimination in more democratic terms. A resolution passed at the 1944 Canadian Nurses' Association general meeting 'reaffirm[ed] its policy to support the principle that there be no discrimination in the selection of students for enrollment into schools of nursing.'[35] Yet contrary to the national body's official and supposedly well-established position, nursing programs and provincial associations were slow to open their doors to non-White women. In 1943, the Registered Nurses' Association of Nova Scotia reminded nursing's national office that only White Canadian nurses were eligible for postgraduate training in the United States, since there were no programs for training 'coloured girls' in Canada.[36] The following year Ontario's Council of Nurse Education informed a young woman from Owen Sound that she would have to apply to Detroit or New York, since training in Ontario was not available to Black Canadians.[37] In 1947, the CNA was forced to restate its egalitarian position when a YWCA survey alerted the press to persisting racial discrimination in nursing schools.[38]

Meanwhile, racial barriers were being attacked by local activists such as Halifax's Pearline Oliver. A founder of the Nova Scotia

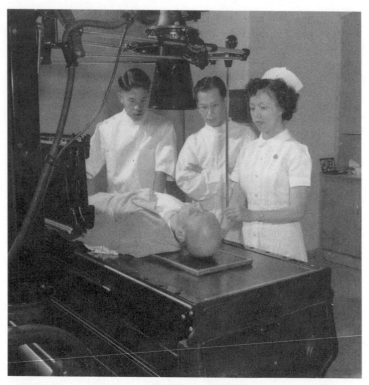

After World War II, the formal barriers to non-White nurses were lifted in Canada. None the less, an expectation remained that those women would serve 'their' ethnic communities, as this nurse at Vancouver's St Joseph Oriental Hospital did (National Archives of Canada PA 112794).

Association for the Advancement of Coloured People, Oliver successfully campaigned in the late 1940s to make local hospitals accept African-Nova Scotian students into their training programs.[39] Efforts by individual Black women in Ontario to gain access to nursing education finally paid off when, with the help of a local priest, Marisse Scott was accepted into Guelph's St Joseph's Hospital school. Resistance to admitting women of African descent persisted in Quebec until the 1960s.[40]

The eradication of racial and ethnic barriers represented an important moment in nursing history, but for non-White women, getting accepted into a training program was only the first step. Their small

numbers and the ongoing prejudice they faced made surviving nursing training a painful process for many visible minority nurses.
Recalling her first day at the Brandon General Hospital School of
Nursing, Irene Desjarlais said, 'I was so scared I felt like turning
around and running down the steps and home. This was the first time
away from my people. I heard someone say that I'd be just like the
rest of the Indians and quit, wasting the government's money.'[41] Similarly, racism within a hospital training school in western Ontario
prompted Wilma Major, a woman of Ojibway-European descent, to
transfer to Chicago's Cook County School. There she 'was just
another minority. Some people even thought I was Jewish.'[42]

Once graduated, minority nurses were joined in the work-force by
foreign-trained practitioners. Like other immigrants, their contribution to the economy and the nation received greater public endorsement than in previous decades. Between 1962 and 1968 alone, nearly
20,000 graduate nurses immigrated to Canada, an average of 2,800
per year, though at its peak in 1967 immigration of graduate nurses
reached 4,262.[43] Among female nurses, the percentage of immigrants
rose from 12 per cent in 1941 to 17 per cent in 1961, while among
male nurses, foreign-trained practitioners reached 32 per cent in the
early 1960s. Like the immigrant work-force more generally, more
than two-thirds of male and female immigrant nurses had arrived
after 1946.[44]

Negotiating the immigration process could be difficult, especially
for nurses from non-European nations. While Canadian authorities
and nursing leaders agreed that some system of evaluating European
nursing training programs was needed and that graduates of those
programs 'have had professional education and we should not fail to
make use of trained minds and hands',[45] when assessing the 'trained
minds and hands' from non-European nations, immigration officials
and nursing leaders were less ready to value immigrant nurses' credentials. It took Beatrice Adassa Massop from October 1952 until
December 1953 to convince Canadian immigration authorities that
she was a case of 'exceptional merit' and should be allowed to emi-
grate from Jamaica to Toronto. During those 14 months, with the help
of Canadian activist Donald Moore and the Negro Citizenship Association, Massop had her nursing qualifications approved by the Registered Nurses' Association of Ontario, secured a job at the Mount
Sinai Hospital, was denied entry by the Immigration Department,
and, upon appeal, was finally granted entry into Canada. In the years
following, numerous other African-Caribbean women immigrated as
nurses.[46] Between 1954 and 1965, 982 trained or graduate nurses and

286 nursing assistants from Caribbean countries gained landed-immigrant status in Canada, all having been obliged by law to inform their prospective employers that they were 'coloured'.[47] For some, like Massop, who boasted 21 years' experience as a nurse and midwife, having RN credentials approved by Canadian nursing organizations was a straightforward process. But as Agnes Calliste's research has demonstrated, many Caribbean-trained practitioners were required to 'upgrade' their skills to be eligible for RN status and therefore entered Canada as assistants who worked in hospitals while completing a three-month obstetrical course. Many of those women did complete their extra training and obtained RN status, but it was not always possible to gain immediate access to the upgrading courses. As a result, some immigrants remained as highly qualified nursing assistants, joining the other minority women who constituted an important addition to the pool of aides and assistants.[48]

Formal eradication of colour bars notwithstanding, immigration and entrance restrictions ensured that the fourth generation of Canadian nurses continued to be comprised of predominantly White Canadians.[49] Nursing also remained the domain of women. By 1961, only 2,354 male nurses were gainfully occupied in Canada as compared to nearly 60,000 female practitioners. Since the small numbers of Anglo-Canadian men or practitioners of European, Asian, African, and First Nations descent could not begin to provide the volume of nursing services required in the post-war era, a revolutionary policy was introduced: the employment of married women. As in other fields of employment, marital status had never been a factor with male nurses. In 1951, 70.5 per cent of male nurses were married, as compared to 25 per cent of female practitioners. By 1961, however, 47 per cent of female nurses were married women, while a further 6 per cent were widowed or divorced.[50]

Recognizing the potential of the pool of 'inactive' married nurses, occupational leaders and institutional administrators took steps to encourage the return to the work-force of women who had left for marriage and motherhood. In 1942, CN explained to readers that the wartime income tax provisions allowed wives to work without jeopardizing their husbands' rights and that 'there is nothing . . . that should cause any hesitation on the part of married nurses to resume whole or part-time practice on a remunerative basis.'[51] Five years later the CNA publicly criticized employers who discriminated against married women.[52] Published testimonials from retired nurses who had re-entered the work-force sought to assure older practitioners that they could make the transition back into active service. Mrs A. Chisholm provided *CN* in 1944 with an account of her first day back at work. As she articulated her experiences with 'sinapism BID', new medicines, intravenous (IV), surgery, and obstetrical care, Chisholm made light of her initial fears, claiming that doctors, patients, and other nurses were all supportive and co-operative, despite her many fumbles. While assisting with surgery she thought, 'Wonder if anyone notices how jumpy I am. . . . No one is paying the slightest bit of attention.' After frantically trying to ready a parturient woman for labour, Chisholm learned that the labour was false, and concluded, 'Next time I won't rush things so much.' The RN survived her first day, but realized, when watching over a postoperative patient, that she had to 'stop being so jittery or [I'll] scare the poor man into a haemorrhage.'⁵³

Chisholm's self-effacing account gently pointed to the challenge facing graduates who returned to duty. While a small percentage of practitioners had always been married women who, for reasons of divorce, widowhood, or spousal disability, returned to active duty, in the post-war years the resumption of duties entailed learning new sets of rapidly changing procedures and techniques. Jo Mann left active practice upon her marriage in 1939, but her husband's ill health necessitated Mann's resumption of paid work nine years later. Mann recalled: 'It was quite a change because you see I'd been away from hospital work for quite awhile and I had to really study it and go over everything.' None the less, the nursing shortage ensured that she was welcomed by the local hospital: 'The minute I applied they wanted me to start right that day.'⁵⁴ When Violet McMillan's husband died in 1959, leaving her with three children to support, she returned to work at the Winnipeg General maternity pavilion. Thinking that 'maybe babies were still coming from the same place [and] I'd know something', McMillan first requested to be placed in the nursery and then later transferred to the postnatal ward. Having raised three children of her own, McMillan was comfortable feeding and caring for newborns, but after an absence of 24 years from active nursing, she still relied heavily on the informal instruction she received from co-workers. One nurse in particular 'was very kind to me and helped me . . . because I really had to learn, every day, every day until I got familiar with the whole thing.'⁵⁵ Other practitioners, including Sarnia nurse Barbara Burr, combined marriage and motherhood precisely because they wanted to maintain their skills. Burr explained: 'Nursing was the only thing I knew how to do. You had to keep into it or you were lost. I always knew that if something happened [and] I had to be my own support or support the kids, that if I didn't keep it up I wouldn't have anything to fall back on.' She returned to work shortly after the birth of her second child because 'I figured by that time if I didn't go and keep it up then I was going to be lost.'[56]

Capitalizing on such motivations, hospitals nurtured married women's relearning process and facilitated their return to work. Already facing shortages of residence accommodation, institutions relented on their long-standing policy that staff must 'live in' and thus established differential pay scales for resident and non-resident staff.[57] Hospitals also created part-time categories of nurses. Of the 938 Ontario graduate nurses surveyed in 1968, 12 per cent were married women working full time and a further 20 per cent were married women working part time.

For women themselves, the opportunity to continue working after marriage represented an important possibility for supplementing, or generating, their family income. Barbara Burr graduated from the Hôtel Dieu in Windsor in the late 1950s. After three years on staff at Sarnia's St Joseph's Hospital, she married and had children. In the early 1960s, Barbara was recruited back to the staff of Sarnia General, where, for seven years, she and two other women shared night duty in the surgical ward. The three women worked out their own part-time shift rotation, and the hospital administration 'just left us alone . . . as long as the nights were covered.' This arrangement allowed Barbara to work from 11 p.m. to 7 a.m several nights a week. After those shifts she returned home and minded her children all day, grabbing a nap when they had theirs. After dinner, while her husband took care of the children and did the dishes, Barbara would sleep for several hours, rising at 10 p.m. to return to work. In spite of this gruelling schedule as a mother of two children, Barbara's work enabled her family to pay off their house, take family holidays, and purchase 'family things'. When the administration decided to end permanent night duty and to rotate all nurses through the three shifts, Barbara and another co-worker quit. Barbara remained out of paid employment for five years before resuming her work career in the early 1970s, working for 18 years at a senior's care home.[58]

The desire to contribute to their household budgets cut across class lines. The 1968 Ontario study *The Untapped Pool* discovered that 20 per cent of working nurses were married to men with professional and executive jobs, whereas 44 per cent were married to men in managerial, proprietary, clerical, and sales; a further 26 per cent were skilled, semi-skilled, and unskilled workers. Clearly, the imperative to continue working was more keenly felt by working-class women. Of the 495 inactive nurses, 48 per cent were married to men in professional and executive positions, a further 39 per cent to husbands in managerial, clerical, and sales jobs, and only 7 per cent to men in working-class occupations.[59]

Nursing leaders and working nurses recognized the persisting tensions between home and work that complicated married nurses' lives. Marital conflicts sometimes erupted when wives pursued paid work. Of the Ontario nurses surveyed in 1968, 43 per cent of inactive nurses reported that their husband objected to having a working wife, as compared to only 15 per cent of full-time practitioners and 25 per cent of part-time workers. More substantial tensions existed over parenting responsibilities. Of the 114 full-time working women included in *The Untapped Pool*, only 15 per cent were childless and 11 per cent had one child. The remaining 74 per cent had two or three children, but only 26 per cent had four or more children. The part-time group of married nurses surveyed were more likely to have more children than did the full-time contingent: 27 per cent had three children, 19 per cent had four, and 9.5 per cent had five or more. The inactive nurses tended to have even larger families. Married nurses agreed that lack of child care constituted a significant obstacle to rewarding paid work. Although the study did not go so far as to recommend making child-care facilities available, its conclusion that inactive nurses needed to be encouraged to resume employment suggested that some resolution of the parenting-nursing conflict was necessary.[60]

Nurses themselves were divided over how to resolve the parenting-nursing tensions. Marjorie McLeod recalled one incident that occurred when she was on staff at Victoria's Royal Jubilee Hospital in 1950. During coffee break, a co-worker announced that although she had children, she preferred to work and, in fact, considered it healthier for her children to spend the days with a babysitter and play with their mother in the evenings. The colleague's comments were then the subject of intense debate. As McLeod recalled: 'We had a great controversy . . . we were late getting up from coffee that morning.'[61]

Individual nurses devised various schedules to facilitate both paid labour and maternity. In a 1953 *CN* article, nurse Vera O'Dacre of the Pembroke General Hospital assured her sisters across the country that anyone claiming 'marriage and nursing career cannot be combined satisfactorily' was wrong; 'it can be done'. O'Dacre's household included her husband and three children, aged 5, 12, and 17 years, as well as a high school boarder. Identifying the three preconditions to being a working mother, 'good health, an understanding cooperative husband, and time well organized', O'Dacre explained that her home was 'equipped with many labor-saving devices' and that each household chore was assigned to a particular day of the week. Every morning, O'Dacre got her family up and out of the house and then prepared the noon meal. In the afternoon, she rested with her youngest child and then prepared supper, 'either a cold plate for supper and leave it in the frigidaire or a hot supper dish which I leave in the automatic oven' before her eldest son returned from school to drive his mother to her 4:00 p.m. shift. O'Dacre's responsibilities as a general-duty nurse on the private ward ended at midnight. Meanwhile, her eldest son provided child care for his two siblings, a chore for which he received an allowance and 'a greater sense of responsibility', until his father returned home at 5:00. Echoing the 'quality time' argument, O'Dacre took every opportunity to spend time with her children: 'I know that in later years they will not remember how hard I worked but how much I played with them and the good times we had together.' But she also believed that time away from her family was more than compensated for by her pay cheque. Nursing income was, according to O'Dacre, 'a great boon to our family budget, making it possible for me not only to offset the rising cost of living but to provide my growing family with the many extras we could not otherwise have, besides contributing to the little "nest-egg" we have provided for that "rainy day," should it ever come.'[62]

Tactics deployed by nurses such as O'Dacre ensured that married women could re-enter paid labour while maintaining their primary domestic commitments. As a result, nursing remained a solidly female occupation, only marginally more ethnically diverse than in previous generations, but it had been transformed from an occupation that proscribed against linking matrimony with work into a job that could easily accommodate large numbers of married women. The result was an occupation in which the largest group of practitioners were, like working women more generally, in the 35–54 age category. And in making room for practitioners with substantial experience, in facilitating part-time work, and in recognizing the tensions between home and work, nursing participated in the broader post-war changes in women's work patterns.[63] Testimonials like O'Dacre's must, therefore, be interpreted not only as encouragement for other mothers to return to paid work, but also as an affirmation of women's ability to pursue a career without jeopardizing their domestic happiness. These affirmations were particularly important in the post-war years, which were dominated by expert prescriptions on the importance of maternal domesticity and the social and psychological dangers presented by working mothers.[64]

For all the commonalities between nurses and other working women, it was the distinctive features of nursing that more often received comment. A *CN* discussion in 1944 entitled 'The Position of Women in the Post-War World' articulated this sense of difference, stating:

> you nurses can face the future with greater equanimity than any other group of your sex. You are trained to offer a service which the world needs in peace or war. . . . You do not need to question the value of your profession . . . we recognize that you are in a fortunate field—free from male competition. You contemplate a world in which no man wishes your job or thinks that your earnings cut him off from legitimate employment.[65]

However much individual nurses were driven by economic need or by a desire to maintain hard-earned skills, the rhetoric of service continued to dominate public discussions. As a 1954 article stated: 'Married women return to nurse because of their love of nursing or to supplement their husbands' incomes before or after their child-rearing responsibilities.'[66] Even O'Dacre, having laid out the pragmatics of combining home and work, insisted, 'I do not think there is a married nurse anywhere who has not had, at some time or other, a secret ambition to go back to nursing, at least once in a while. The cherished ideals of her youthful years cannot easily be forgotten, and the satisfaction of knowing she can help in some small measure to bring back the bloom of health to suffering humanity is an experience that brings its own reward.'[67] While other working women were struggling to justify their presence in the work-force, nurses' position was legitimated by the unique occupational service ethos and by the long tradition of female caring that the vocation represented.[68]

Contradictions: Professionalization and Proletarianization

The continued legitimation of nurses' work in terms of a tradition of female caring contrasted with the very real changes occurring in the workplace. One set of these changes appeared to elevate nursing's position within the health-care system and to signal the occupation's achievement of professional status. Simultaneously, other forces appeared to be eroding nurses' autonomy and independence, thereby fuelling a process of proletarianization. As several sociologists have shown, the contradictory effects of professionalization and proletarianization produced an uncertain class identity.[69] These contradictory forces also produced a new degree of formal stratification, as a hierarchy of female patient-care personnel placed nursing administrators at the top, followed by general-duty staff, and then various levels of

auxiliary attendants. This hierarchy created fixed relations of subordination and dominance between nurses and among hospital caregivers
that were new to an occupation that had heretofore been characterized
by an equality of practitioners.

The professionalizing impulse within nursing had several dimensions. In the years during and after World War II, the rapid proliferation of new drugs and procedures complicated medical therapeutics
and necessitated the reallocation of specific tasks from doctors to
graduate nurses. Nurses were now expected to administer and understand the principles of newly developed drugs like penicillin, streptomycin, sulphonamides, and pituitrin.[70] As a result, the frequency with
which nurses gave intramuscular injections increased and nurses'
scope of practice was expanded to include intravenous injections. The
establishment in 1945 of a team of intravenous nurses at Winnipeg
General facilitated the dramatic increase in intravenous treatments
performed there, from less than 1,000 in 1945 to nearly 24,000 in
1948.[71] As well, the new techniques for transfusing, banking, and

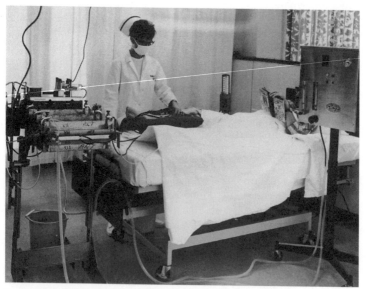

By the late 1960s, graduate nurses were responsible for a range of new
technologically based procedures, such as the renal dialysis this Winnipeg
General Hospital nurse performed in 1966 (PAM Winnipeg General Hospital Collection #224).

processing blood products all demanded the skills of nursing staffs,[72] while taking blood pressures soon became integrated into nursing therapeutics.[73] These were all 'procedures which, until recently were confined to medical personnel, and which have now devolved upon the nursing staff.'[74]

The assumption of new technical responsibilities accentuated the need for more extensive nursing education and facilitated specialization within the occupation. Institutional employers sponsored postgraduate education for staff nurses at the many certificate programs for RNs offered through universities and hospitals. Certificate courses lasted from four months to two years, in subspecialties ranging from public health nursing to instructing in nursing schools, X-ray technique, operating room technique, and obstetrical nursing.[75] To encourage staff to pursue such qualifications, and to ensure that the home institution benefited from postgraduate nursing education, hospitals made scholarships available, with the proviso that the nurse would return to the host institution or locale for at least a year.[76]

The occupation's professional standing was also enhanced by the expansion of university nursing training programs. Grants from international foundations such as Kellogg and Rockefeller, combined with funding programs by such agencies as the VON, supported students enrolled in baccalaureate programs and provided a new financial basis for the five university degree programs and two university diploma programs that were in operation at the beginning of the 1940s. By the end of the decade, five more universities had Bachelor of Nursing or Bachelor of Science in Nursing programs in place.[77] While enrolment in university nursing schools remained small—in 1962 only 148 practitioners graduated from basic baccalaureate programs as compared to more than 6,000 from three-year diploma programs[78]—the proliferation of university programs was none the less heralded as a significant professional accomplishment.

The trend towards new responsibilities and techniques necessitated new levels of education, but also exacerbated the pressure on overworked and understaffed general-duty nurses. To free graduate nurses for their recently acquired tasks and to address the persisting personnel shortage, hospitals began to employ various categories of subsidiary workers. While the precise pattern whereby 'non-professional' workers were introduced differed from institution to institution, some combination of practical nurses (later licensed practical nurses, LPNs), nursing assistants (later registered nursing assistants, RNAs), ward assistants or aides, and ward clerks was integrated into patient health services. The overall goal was to relieve graduate nurses of 'routine' personal care patient services and elementary ward administration. Auxiliaries or practical nurses were not entirely new. Manitoba and Quebec had introduced trained attendants or aides on their staffs or registries since the early 1920s.[79] But in the post-war years the number of subsidiary workers increased dramatically and became a regular feature of institutional staffing. Provincial licensing acts and hospital-based training programs, which by the early 1960s were preparing 2,000 attendants annually, validated the place of nursing assistants at the bedside.[80]

These categories of caregivers were ranked according to their skill and, to some degree, gender. The tasks retained as the prerogative of RNs included charting on permanent records, administering medications, taking blood pressure, inserting catheters, and supervising subsidiary workers. Practical nurses (PNs) or nursing assistants shared with RNs responsibility for administrative tasks, diagnostic tests, elementary nursing therapies, personal patient-care services, and preparation of equipment. In other words, PNs were empowered to perform all nursing tasks that did not involve assisting doctors with procedures or injecting/inserting anything into patients' bodies.[81] Practical nurses were considered especially useful in non-acute, convalescent, and chronic-care cases, and were expected to work under the supervision of a physician or graduate nurse. Male nursing assistants were concentrated in the mental health sector, where their physical strength was considered an asset when dealing with psychiatric patients.[82]

The responsibilities assigned to nurses' aides were limited to personal patient care and preparation of ward and supplies. This position was created initially as an emergency measure, and therefore, when possible, prospective aides were encouraged to train as practical nurses. Ward aides, on the other hand, quickly became permanent features of ward life, performing housekeeping and cleaning duties on the ward and around patients' beds, carrying and collecting trays, tidying linen and supply cupboards, and performing messenger duties. As personnel who cleaned in the vicinity of patients' beds, these workers were considered part of the nursing, not housekeeping, staffs. Because even head nurses spent 'valuable time copying timetables, requisitioning supplies, writing up reports on charts, answering the telephone and directing traffic generally', ward clerks or ward secretaries were introduced to perform basic clerical duties, including simple charting, copying reports, completing requisitions, making time sheets, checking inventory, answering telephones, taking messages, and delivering patients' mail and flowers.[83] The ranks of aides and clerks were filled predominantly by women, whereas the position of orderly remained the domain of men. As in previous decades, orderlies helped move or care for male patients and those hard-to-manoeuvre patients of either sex.

Winnipeg General provides one example of how subsidiary workers were incorporated into ward work. During World War II, the nursing shortage was met through volunteer labour comprising Voluntary Aid Detachment (VAD) members who had received rudimentary training in nursing technique. In 1943, Canadian Red Cross VADs provided Winnipeg General with over 25,000 hours of free nursing service, while the St John Ambulance VADs provided over 600 hours of nursing assistance.[84] This temporary solution gave way to more permanent arrangements in the post-war period, when a small number of practical nurses were added to the staff.[85] By the early 1950s, the 25 PNs had been augmented by over 75 other 'non-professional staff', nurses' aides, diet maids, and ward maids.[86] Then, in 1958 staffing problems and the introduction of the 40-hour work week prompted the hospital to employ 27 ward clerks and more nurses' aides, as well as to establish training programs for nurse technicians in the operating room, for orderlies, and for laboratory technicians.[87] In 1965, the hospital's intensive care unit implemented a plan whereby licensed practical nurses who had received training in ICU activities 'be permitted to carry out certain procedures which are normally restricted to graduate nurses'.

Nursing leaders and administrators applauded the introduction of subsidiary workers not only because nurses' workload was reduced but because personal care tasks, traditionally part of nurses' repertoire of skills, were being defined as inappropriate for highly trained 'professionals'. In 1950 Helen King, assistant director of nursing at Vancouver General, addressed the virtues of auxiliary nursing personnel: 'From an economic viewpoint, it seems ridiculous to use expensively trained people to carry out purely routine tasks which less skilled people can, under supervision, perform very satisfactorily.'[88] So, too, cleaning and preparing supplies, such as basins, bedpans, and instrument trays, was defined as 'non-nursing' activity.[89] The ideological and formal divestment of those tasks that had bordered on the domestic and personal constituted a crucial line of demarcation between 'professional' graduate nurses and 'non-professional' subsidiary workers.

Difference among ranks was signified not only by job description but also by educational qualifications, pay, ethnicity, and gender. While many PNs gained their positions based on their extensive experience, efforts were soon made to establish formal training programs and licensing standards for this category of worker.[90] By 1960, LPNS or RNAS received between 9 and 18 months of training. Nurses' aides were preferred to have some high school education and to be at least 18 years old when they began their three months of basic training and then six to nine months of ward experience.[91] Ward aides needed only elementary school education and had to be at least 16 years old. They received four weeks of basic training and then on-the-job training. Ward secretaries were required to be 18 years of age and high school graduates in order to qualify for a one-two week basic training program and the subsequent ward instruction. Recognizing that members of this subsidiary work-force would draw on a different pool of applicants than did diploma nursing programs, nursing leaders advertised training programs as designed 'to open the door of opportunity to those who have a desire to care for the sick but who are not equipped to enter a professional school of nursing.'[92]

In addition to these educational differences, the labour force of nursing assistants was distinguished from its graduate nurse counterpart by gender and ethnic composition. Although the number of men and women filling subsidiary patient-care positions continued to grow throughout the post-war years, the proportion and growth rate of female attendants surpassed that of male assistants. Between 1951 and 1961 alone, the work-force of male attendants nearly doubled to 13,000, while the female corps grew more than 2.5 times to nearly 50,000.[93] Health-care work remained a relatively more important sector of work for women than men, with male attendants comprising only 0.3 of the total male work-force and female assistants 3 per cent of all working women. The female nursing assistant work-force also boasted a slightly more diverse ethnic composition than did the corps of graduate nurses. Only 71 per cent of female nursing assistants working in 1961 were of British or French descent, as compared to 81 per cent of graduate nurses. Male attendants of French or English origin represented roughly the same proportion of male nursing assistants (71 per cent) and male graduate nurses (73 per cent) as were present in the total male work-force (72 per cent). Similarly, the cadre of male assistants included an equal percentage of foreign-born members (31 per cent) as did the male graduate nursing work-force (32 per cent), whereas a significantly greater number of female nursing assistants (24 per cent) were immigrants than appeared among graduate nurses (17 per cent) or female students (only 4.2 per cent).[94] Thus, divisions among female patient-care personnel were solidified by educational requirements dictating that women with fewer personal and social resources, whatever the function of their class background, immigrant status, or racial category, were concentrated in the lower levels of the nursing hierarchy. Differences of class origin, nativity, and ethnicity, manifest in differential access to training programs and jobs, reinforced the privileged position of RNs over subsidiary workers.

Wage scales reflected and entrenched distinctions among the ranks and orders of patient-care personnel. At Toronto General Hospital in 1947, wages paid to female staff ranged from the administrative and educational nursing staff, who earned between $165 and $200 per month, to head nurses, who earned $160 to $175 per month, to general-duty nurses, who earned $140–$150 per month. Salaries paid to dietitians, physiotherapists, occupational therapists, and laboratory technicians, ranging from $100 to $200 per month, approximated those of graduate nursing staff. Clerical workers received slightly lower monthly wages of between $90 and $185. Ward aides' salaries of $80 to $95 were matched by those paid to maids, cafeteria staff, seamstresses, and surgical supply staff. Alongside this female salary hierarchy existed a parallel scale for male staff. At the pinnacle of that hierarchy were professional men, like the pharmacists who earned between $200 and $300 per month. While nursing administrators managed to keep graduate nurse salaries above those of male attendants, to attract male-patient care personnel, and because subsidiary personnel were unionizing to demand improved wage scales, salaries for porters, orderlies, and morgue attendants had to compare favourably with those earned by men outside the hospital sector. For this reason, male patient-care personnel earned less than the 'professional' female staff of graduate nurses, physiotherapists, or dieticians, but consistently more than 'non-professional' female attendants. TGH male orderlies and porters earned between $105 and $125 per month, while the morgue attendant was paid $110 monthly, wages roughly equivalent to those of unskilled men employed by health-care institutions as cleaners and elevator operators, though substantially less than the many skilled tradesmen on hospital payrolls.[95]

By contrast, skilled female workers, such as telephone operators and clerical workers, and unskilled working women in the laundry and kitchen consistently earned less than their male counterparts. Table 6.1 provides a comparison of wages paid at Brandon General Hospital. Thus, two sex-specific labour markets operated within the hospital sector. They came together at the point of determining the wages of graduate nurses and the highest-ranking male 'non-professional' patient-care worker and from that point of intersection, wage levels ascended or descended. Throughout the 1942–68 years, it was

Table 6.1
Brandon General Hospital Staff Monthly Wages, 1947

Female Hospital Staff	Wage	Male Hospital Staff	Wage
Superintendent of nursing	$200	Medical superintendent	$375
Operating room nurse	$110.50	Chef	$125
General-duty graduate nurse	$100	Laundry worker	$121
		Fireman	$110
Licensed practical nurse	$ 75	Orderly	$ 65
Ward aide	$ 35		
Stenographer	$ 75		
Night telephone operator	$ 65		

SOURCE: Brandon General Archives, Box 51, 'Payroll Book', 1947.

relatively easy for graduate nurses to secure higher wages than female nursing assistants and aides, who averaged, according to census data, only $1,615 per year in 1961. It proved more difficult to stay ahead of 'non-professional' male attendants, who earned on average $2,681 in 1961, just $69 below the figure for female graduate nurses and $778 below that paid to male trained nurses.[96]

However small the wage differentials, the introduction of subsidiary patient-care attendants none the less substantially enhanced the professional standing of graduate nurses. Auxiliary workers constituted groups over whom general-duty ward nurses had positions of fixed authority. As they relegated certain tasks to those subsidiary personnel, RNs divested themselves of the labour-intensive personal care 'domestic' tasks that traditionally had blurred the boundaries between maternal or 'womanly' care and the specific skills offered only by trained nurses. Many practitioners and social commentators applauded these changes, using the language of liberation to celebrate nursing's new status. Charlotte Whitton articulated this position in 1950 when she characterized nursing aides as being able to 'free nursing of what is not nursing'.[97] National Department of Health and Welfare consultant Margaret McLean agreed that allocating certain functions to subsidiary personnel would 'free more nursing time for patient care'.[98] Implicit in such commentary was the celebration of nursing's victory in the long-running battle to distinguish the occupation from domestic labour. The RN 'class' of health-care providers in this era was defined, therefore, by the official content of their work as well as by the social privilege its members brought to the bedside and to the occupation. Just as changes in the content and allocation of nursing work seemed to be cementing nurses' status as professionals, competing forces appeared to be moving nurses closer to the experiences of other wage-earners. Like other workers, most nurses were employed by large third-party employers, for whom practitioners worked regular shifts. And because other occupations were offering attractive wages and working conditions, hospitals were forced to conform to post-war standards by reducing nurses' work week and improving nursing wages. By the 1960s, nurses and nursing students in all regions had finally achieved the eight-hour day, which they had been calling for since the 1930s, and the 40-hour work week.[99]

Working for a large, third-party employer also entailed new stresses, which in many ways contradicted the formal elevation of status represented by the introduction of subsidiary patient-care personnel. Hospitals continued to rely on nurses to 'fill in' where needed and thus many nurses had little control over their shift assignment. Retired nurses like Jessie Law believed: 'One of the worst things for nursing all through the years was the fact of not knowing when you were going to be working, you knew when you're going to be on days, afternoons or nights, but you don't know the actual day when its going to change . . . you could get phoned up in the middle of the day and told that you're coming to work that night when you thought you weren't.'[100]

The reduction of nurses' work week made staffing arrangements even more uncertain as hospitals scrambled to hire more nurses for the new scheduling system. Under this pressure, nursing and medical administrators once again turned to industry for suggestions regarding increased efficiency of existing staff. The benefits of time-and-motion studies and 'job analysis' were outlined in *CN* articles, while hospital administrators contracted consultants to survey existing conditions and recommend points of rationalization.[101] With such data in hand, administrators attempted to amalgamate wards and services, creating concentrations of patients with common afflictions.[102] Automated equipment such as motorized beds and pneumatic tube communication systems were heralded as 'time-saving innovation[s], of great usefulness to both patient and nurse'.[103] The labours of nursing staff were further reduced at hospitals like Winnipeg General when, in 1952, oxygen was piped directly to wards 'and the heavy cylinders no longer have to be trundled around from bed to bed'.[104] Certain procedures were also reduced in frequency. Unless otherwise ordered by a doctor, routine observations of temperature, pulse, and respiration continued to be recorded for the first 48 hours of patient stay, after which they were noted only once a day.[105]

Not surprisingly, nurses were encouraged to focus their energies on a specific number of highly skilled functions and to delegate all non-nursing tasks to other members of the health-care team. For example, nurses at WGH were instructed in 1965 to let physiotherapists teach patients how to walk with crutches. Centralization of supply services reduced the amount of time nurses spent preparing equipment, while also economizing on use of supplies. Sister Marie Irenaeus of Antigonish's St Martha's Hospital reported in 1942 that the centralized system of equipment and supplies reduced that institution's use of adhesive rolls, cellulose rolls, gauze rolls, and alcohol by up to one-half, while decreasing the amount of lysol used from 75 gallons per year to 26.[106]

Efforts to reduce nursing workload were accompanied by the creation of specialized nursing teams, such as the IV and drug administration teams.[107] For those nurses assigned to more general nursing functions, the team approach was also encouraged. A 'team' consisted of one or two graduate nurses and various subsidiary and student workers. Team nursing became particularly popular in the 1950s, promising not only efficiency of nursing time, but also a standardized method of supervising auxiliary staff. At WGH this system was labelled progressive patient care (PPC), wherein 'the professional nurses gave the intensive care required, and supervised and assisted the non-professional staff with the intermediate, and self care.'[108] In this way a formal distribution of duties was established, as was an official fragmentation of tasks.

While these efforts to focus nurses' energies on specific, skilled elements of patient care did ameliorate some of the pressures on their pace of work, other factors continued to press general-duty nurses to the limit. Granted, some older labour- and time-intensive treatments were marginalized in this era. For example, as late as 1961 fomentations were still on the list of nursing procedures at WGH, but that elaborate treatment, central to the experiences of third-generation practitioners, played little part in the daily practice of the fourth generation.[109] Jessie Law lived through the transition from manual treatment to pharmaceutical solutions. She observed: 'You could almost cure impetigo with one dose of penicillin ointment . . . and that's why you don't do hot fomentations any more either, because most of these infections are cured before they would erupt.'[110] Of course, as new medical interventions became integrated into daily practice, they, too, demanded their own kind of labour. Vancouver General's Grace Fairley informed the hospital community that 'modern medical methods in the prevention, treatment, and cure of disease inevitably has [*sic*] laid an increasingly heavy burden and a heavy responsibility on the members of the nursing staff' and reminded ratepayers that 'a successful method of preventing and combating certain types of disease' also required 'many added nursing hours day and night'.[111] Compounding this pressure on nurses' time and skills was the high rate of patient turnover administrators tried to achieve. Administrators laboured to reduce the number of days that each patient resided in the hospital, often by shifting 'long stay' chronic cases to other kinds of care facilities.[112] Winnipeg General reported an average stay for patients in 1943 of 14.1 days, but by 1964 this figure had been whittled down to 12.4 days. The hospital administration interpreted this decline as reflecting 'a better use of the hospital', but for nurses it meant they had to perform the elaborate procedures of discharge and admittance and the labour-intensive care involved in the first few days of patients' stays more often.[113]

Given the incessant pressures on daily work, efficiency measures were applauded as improving nurses' working conditions. In 1951, WGH authorities extolled the virtues of rationalization when they reorganized the operating room, proclaiming that the new system was not only 'more efficient service to patients and doctors' but 'more satisfying to nurses'. Statistics backed up these claims. The department experienced reduced staff turnover and increased the number of operations per annum by over 500. Nurses were the recipients of and participants in such reorganization. Their presence on hospital nursing committees or procedure committees helped those bodies generate strategies for standardization and rationalization.[114]

Sociologist Marie Campbell, who investigated similar (if more elaborate) efforts of the 1980s, has argued that strategies for reorganizing patient-care services had several phases. Administrators first compiled nursing knowledge, generated through experience at the bedside and on the ward, and then harnessed it to facilitate management restructuring and intensification of work. Such processes affected nurses negatively by increasing the pace of their work. Furthermore, because 'the system has provided officially sanctioned knowledge, built on what they themselves have reported . . . [nurses were] thus implicated in its production [and] that binds them to its . . . outcome.'[115] Important as Campbell's theoretical formulation is for conceptualizing the long-term effects of rationalization on nursing work, it is equally important to recognize that nurses at the time did not necessarily interpret rationalization as a negative process. For practitioners struggling to maintain standards of care in an industry suffering chronic staffing shortages, growing patient demand, and an explosion of new therapeutics, participating in the reorganization of work held a certain logic. Rationalization and efficiency were necessary for practitioners' daily survival on wards and in institutions. Under these conditions, some nurses doubtless were satisfied by any restructuring that allowed them to complete their patient load on time.

None the less, flashes of discontent were visible. In 1958, Winnipeg General officials, predicting greater 'automation' of hospital work, acknowledged that some considered standardization procedures were 'sometimes highly suspect' and therefore 'must be widely and sensibly introduced'.[116] A late 1960s study of Ontario nurses concluded that 'substantial ambivalence or disagreement' existed among nurses over how the RN position should be defined. Some were 'not at all reluctant to take over new cure functions from physicians'. Others, 'fearing that the nurse's job might be turned into that of an assistant doctor, composed of ever-increasing numbers of cure activities under the total control and supervision of the physician . . . resist the delegation by physicians of any more of their duties.' Both groups agreed that 'the nurse should be spending more time at the bedside' but could not agree as to 'which class of nurse should be there and what, exactly, each class should be doing'.[117]

This debate crystallized the differences that were emerging between nurses who provided direct patient care and those who performed administrative functions. At the same time that graduate nurses were assuming greater authority over new levels of subsidiary workers, among RNs a two-tier structure divided nurse-managers from nurse-workers, making general-duty nurses subordinate to administrative staff. Like second- and third-generation nurses, students in the post-1942 years moved through the strict hierarchy of the apprenticeship system, but unlike their predecessors who graduated into the 'rough equality' of private-duty work, most fourth-generation practitioners earned their living under the direct and permanent authority of other RNs. As a result, relations among nurses were reordered into a clearly stratified structure wherein some nurses cared for patients and others administrated.

Conflicts between nursing administration and general-duty nurses were frequently averted by the mobility the latter continued to enjoy and exercise. Tremendous turnover rates frustrated administrators' efforts at stable staffing, but indicated the degree to which rank-and-file nurses were determined to improve their lot. In 1957, nearly

2,000 of a work-force of 3,700 BC graduate nurses resigned during the year.[118] By far the highest turnover was among the general-duty group. In 1950, Winnipeg General coped with 135 resignations from the nursing staff, 88 per cent of which were from the general-duty staff. Most of the latter had worked there for less than a year. While some of that staff movement was attributed to the emergency health-care conditions created by Winnipeg's 1950 flood, similar figures were reported for other institutions across the nation and high turnover rates continued to plague institutional administrators throughout the 1950s.[119] For their part, nurses recognized that the labour market was in their favour. As Vancouver General graduate Jessie Law phrased it, getting work after graduation was like 'falling off a rock, it was not a problem . . . you went to bed one night as a senior student, you woke up the next morning as a graduate [on staff].'[120] Under these conditions, graduates could afford to be selective about the conditions of their labour.

While the chronic nursing shortage made changing jobs an easy way to resolve conflict, some practitioners pursued collective modes of pressing for better conditions and wages. Now working permanent shifts for large third-party employers in institutions that processed a high volume of patients, graduate nurses, like workers in other industries, learned that not only was collective action possible but in the new structures of employment it was necessary. Growing militancy and the changing relationships between general-duty and supervisory nurses prompted nurses in all regions of Canada to experiment with new forms of collective representation. As earlier chapters have demonstrated, trade unions and trade union tactics were not completely foreign to Canadian nurses. Previous generations had withdrawn or threatened to withdraw their labour, and nursing associations had traditionally served many 'trade union' functions, but the fourth generation was the first to establish permanent agencies designed to negotiate nurses' collective interests with employers. Nurses in Quebec City initiated this process when, in 1939, they formed Syndicat professionel des infirmières Catholiques (SPIC). In 1944, the Quebec Nurses' Act providing for collective bargaining for nurses was passed. At the federal level, in an effort to stabilize labour relations in the wartime economy, the Canadian government invoked a labour relations order, PC 1003, which encouraged the unionization of many Canadian workers, including nurses. Indeed, CNA inquiries into whether nurses as 'professionals' would be exempted from the federal legislation met with a negative reply: 'In the majority of provinces, nursing is not defined legally as a profession and that in order to have nursing so defined it would be necessary to have Nurse Practice Acts passed in each province.'[121]

Under these conditions the Quebec Federation of Labour took action to help Quebec nurses organize under the L'alliance des infirmières de Montréal.[122] In British Columbia, the successful unionization of subsidiary hospital employees prompted some nurses to explore the industrial union structure. As early as 1942, mass meetings were being held in the Vancouver General auditorium to organize hospital workers. Some members of the nursing staff attended these meetings, and shortly after the Hospital Employees' Federal Union (HEFU, now the HEU) was formed, the Vancouver General graduate nurses joined Local 180 and in 1947 negotiated their first contract.[123] The local did not last. The Registered Nurses' Association of British Columbia (RNABC), concerned over competition from rival organizations, established in 1946 a Labour Relations Committee (LRC) that set out 'recommended personnel practices' as endorsed by the British Columbia Hospital Association. The LRC was also responsible for collective bargaining on nurses' behalf and in 1946 negotiated an agreement with St Paul's Hospital. With these successes in place, the RNABC moved to convince the Vancouver General nurses that affiliation with the RNABC was preferable to membership in the HEFU.[124] As the BC case demonstrated, initial experiments with unionization did not necessarily result in the creation of discrete union structures, but they did alert occupational leaders that new forms of representation were needed.

Nurses elsewhere in the country shared the RNABC's concern that unionization would fracture the occupation. Alumnae associations, in which third-generation nurses were often active members, appeared particularly troubled by the threat of new representative vehicles. In Nova Scotia the Victoria General Nurses Alumnae met in January 1942 to discuss the recent formation by the hospital's general-duty nurses of 'an organization similar to a labour organization'.[125] In 1947, the president of the Toronto General alumnae, Dorothy Percy, expressed similar concerns when she wrote to members that 'Frankly, I don't think what we are doing is good enough, and I'm sure you don't think so either.' Percy enjoined her sister nurses to consider: 'What of the nursing situation in our own hospital? Is there something we could be doing to help improve it? We say, rather glibly, I am afraid, that we are "behind" the Superintendent of Nurses in her efforts for improved conditions of service. Is this anything more, at the moment, than a pious hope?' Calling for 'an informed membership' to consider conditions within their Alma Mater, Percy raised the question that would plague nursing's leadership and rank-and-file for the next 50 years: 'What is our opinion about the interest organized labour is taking in nurses as regards their possible membership in unions? Have we an opinion? Should we not have one?'[126]

Meanwhile, to deal with the 'problem of the affiliation of nurses with trades and labour unions' the CNA executive approved in 1943 'the principle of collective bargaining' and proclaimed the national and provincial associations as nurses' legitimate representatives at the bargaining table. That year the CNA's Labour Relations Committee was created to investigate the legal dimensions of collective bargaining. Recognizing that nurses employed by civil and civic associations or in industrial work might, by virtue of the larger workplace organization, be affiliated with trade unions, the CNA committee warned 'that no nurse should become a member of an association or a trade union under conditions that might call for the stoppage of necessary nursing service, in other words, to strike.'[127] The CNA's 1946 no-strike policy often convinced rank-and-file nurses that membership in trade unions, which well might vote to strike, was unprofessional.[128] Indeed, proclaimed the CNA leadership in 1946, unions lacked 'the advantage of long years of professional association with the public . . . [and therefore] would probably be forced to use stronger methods than collective bargaining to gain their objectives.'[129] For these reasons, argued CNA officials, the 'professional organizations' deserved rank-and-file support. As one *CN* editor declared:

> Should the nurses of Canada join unions? They already belong to a stronger body than any that could now be formed. It is up to the individual nurse to rally to the support of this emerging giantess— the Canadian Nurses' Association, the nine federated provincial associations, the local districts and chapters.[130]

The 'emerging giantess' did in fact dominate labour relations for graduate nurses until the late 1960s. In BC, for example, the RNABC began with one certified bargaining unit of RNs in 1946, and by 1966 represented 63 such bargaining units.[131] There, nurses' weekly hours of labour decreased from 48 in 1946 to 37.5 in 1968, while the basic monthly salary for hospital staff nurses grew fourfold over the same period, from $125 to $500.[132] The ARNPQ, although not the bargaining agent for Quebec nurses, became involved in the union process by running a two-day institute to inform nurses about the many acts and labour codes that shaped relations on the shop floor.[133] After the initial wave of union activity in British Columbia and Quebec during the 1940s, a second wave of union organizing occurred in the early 1960s. Between 1963 and 1968, nurses in Manitoba, Alberta,

Ontario, New Brunswick, Nova Scotia, Prince Edward Island, and Saskatchewan formed staff associations, which through their provincial associations' labour relations committees bargained with employers. Newfoundland nurses followed suit in 1971. In all provinces except Quebec, which had an autonomous nurses' union, and Prince Edward Island, where collective bargaining rights were established by the Nurses' Act, existing labour law mandated that nurses could not form certified bargaining agents.

Where provincial labour laws or local association politics prevented formal collective bargaining, the method of negotiation preferred by the registered nurses' associations was to establish personnel policies and then encourage hospitals to adhere to those guidelines. In this modified version of the BC system, recommended personnel policies advised employers on the importance of clearly delineated conditions of employment, orientation for new employees, a maximum work week of 44 hours, evening and night shifts of no more than two weeks in duration, and granting statutory holidays. Nurses expected to receive standardized provisions for vacation, sick leave and study leaves, pension plans, appropriate residence accommodation, and uniform pay rates. Included in this last item was the proviso that nurses with postgraduate training and experience should receive $10–$20 more per month than their counterparts without postgraduate preparation.[134]

These attempts to win improved working conditions through consultation and recommendation could not mitigate the growing tensions on the ward. 'Each year, the problems relating to working relationships between nurses and their employers—whether hospitals, public health agencies (governmental or private), private duty registries, or the public—continue to multiply', explained one speaker at a 1964 CNA Labor Relations Institute.[135] The CNA guidelines for wages and conditions of work could inspire nurses to act collectively to defend them, but, on their own, the traditional associations had little leverage with which to influence institutional personnel policy. Thus, while graduate nurses' wages did increase over the 1950s and 1960s, and while there were some indications that within regions some uniformity in wage scales applied,[136] nurses' salaries continued to lag behind those of other skilled workers. In 1961 the average annual earnings for professional and technical occupations were $5,448 for men and $2,996 for women. Male nurses earned on average only $3,459 per annum, while female graduate nurses averaged $2,752. These gendered wage rates reflected the greater presence of part-time workers in the female cohort. Most nurses, male or female, earned between $3,000 and $4,000. As a result, most male nurses earned substantially less than most professional men, the latter group earning between $5,000 and $6,000 per year. That most women professionals fell in the $2,000–$2,500 salary category reflected the variety of conditions female 'professions' offered. Women in male-dominated professions could expect substantially greater average salary rates than could their counterparts in female-dominated occupations. As in previous generations, fourth-generation nurses garnered incomes comparable to school teachers ($3,400) and clerical workers ($2,340) rather than such university-educated professionals as female engineers ($4,779 annual average), doctors ($4,316), and architects ($4,191). Wage disparities could be accounted for, in part, by the larger number (80 per cent) of all women professionals working more than 40 weeks per year, compared to only 70 per cent of nurses. In terms of hours worked per week, however, 65 per cent of all nurses worked more than 35 hours over seven days, as compared to other professional women who enjoyed higher average income with fewer members working full weeks. Only 60 per cent of all professional women clocked more than 35 hours per week, as did 71 per cent of clerical workers and 54 per cent of teachers.[137]

Even rudimentary statistics like these confirmed that whatever financial gains nurses made and whatever new authority they had gained in the workplace, the occupation remained firmly located within the 'women's' sector of professional life, with its lower wages and prestige. Nurses were working harder and their responsibilities had been amplified. Still, they could not win salaries commensurate with their skills or with women in male-dominated professions. Subsequent generations of nurses would develop more forceful means to improve their conditions, but in the 1942–68 era everywhere except Quebec, which had legal provisions for nursing's union structures, nurses entrusted their negotiations to the traditional, occupationally based organizations that represented all nurses, whether in management or general duty. This subtle shift in nursing's organizational structure masked the more dramatic changes occurring on the wards. Nurses' assumption of new, technical responsibilities, the extension of university and postgraduate educational programs, the introduction of subsidiary personnel, and the official reallocation of many personal-care functions all signalled the professional elevation of graduate nurses. At the same time third-party employers, intensification and rationalization of the work process, demands by nurses for improved working conditions, struggles to maintain wage levels commensurate with other workers, and the creation of a two-tiered

structure of nurse-workers and nurse-managers all appeared to constitute the proletarianization of the occupation. Given these contradictory impulses, it was perhaps inevitable that the compromise
solution whereby the existing nursing organizations assumed collective bargaining functions would prevail.

Continuities: Gender and Occupational Solidarity

The particular pattern of labour relations developed by fourth-generation nurses raises the question of why general-duty nurses did not
form autonomous union structures in the post-war era, as they would
in later decades. Such structures would have brought nurses into
closer communication with other female and male workers, who
themselves were forging a powerful white-collar union movement.
Part of the answer lay in loyalties to the existing registered nurses'
associations. The provincial associations had for several generations
intervened in the marketplace on behalf of nurses and had performed
many trade union-like functions. Another part of the answer lay in the
power of professional ideology, which continued to promise nurses
the autonomy and responsibility that membership in the working
class rarely entailed. Whether one agrees with authors such as Judi
Coburn, who considered professionalism an 'illusion' and thus an
inappropriate strategy for nurses, the fact that nurses would reject the
advances of union organizers speaks for their continued confidence in
the traditional, professional approach.[138]

Yet, loyalty and ideology cannot fully explain nurses' unwillingness to establish an alternative organizational forum or to participate
in the white-collar union movement more fully. Nurses' ambiguous
class consciousness, reflected in the compromise strategy of establishing labour relations committees within the traditional associations, was certainly a function of the contradictions of professional
advance and proletarianizing processes, but it was also a function of
specific continuities of labour experienced by nurses on the wards. To
comprehend fully the position and perceptions of rank-and-file
fourth-generation nurses, we need to turn our attention back to the
shop floor, to the bedside, where two traditional features of nursing
work mediated the effects of both the professional assumption of
greater technical and supervisory duties and the proletarianizing
effects of rationalization and intensification.

The first of these features was the persistence of overlapping
patient-care functions. In spite of the formal reallocation of duties to
subsidiary workers and of the efficiency measures designed to

concentrate graduate nursing time on complex and technical tasks, chronic shortages of institutional personnel often required 'high-level' nursing staff, whether graduate or licensed practical, to perform 'low-level' domestic and personal service functions. A BC study discovered that when in 1945–6 the 44-hour week was implemented in the provinces' small hospitals, 'no additional ward aides were employed and the nurses were "pinch-hitting" again.'[139] Winnipeg General's 1965 'Functional Activity Study' revealed that 22 per cent of nursing time was spent on non-nursing functions, in part because ward clerks did not work evenings or nights. When rationalization was implemented on hospital wards, it could only be accomplished where the physical layout and patient needs permitted. For this reason, on four WGH wards, changes to food provision were implemented, but elsewhere in the hospital ward design did not permit centralization so 'the nursing personnel continue to prepare in-between meal nourishments and wash these dishes plus all glasses and water carafes'.[140] Oral testimony confirmed the structural imperative to 'pitch in' and get the job done. Barbara Burr recalled that in the late 1950s nurses did assign work to the aides, but often the staff worked together, especially 'if you had heavy patients to do, you helped them.'[141]

Murray's 1968 study of Ontario nursing attempted to measure the frequency with which various levels of patient-care personnel engaged in activities 'below' their status. The study discovered that with respect to activities outside direct patient care, head nurses were especially prone to taking on RN, aide, and clerical duties, as were RNs to a lesser degree. The author admitted, however, that he could not adjudicate the appropriate distribution of functions in direct patient care, because 'professional and non-professional nursing levels' performed 'in the presence of the patient' could not be disentangled. In Murray's opinion, bedside nursing continued to demand that attendants perform whatever tasks were needed, regardless of the status of those tasks. The author explained:

> the reason for not distinguishing nursing *levels* in activities performed *at the patient's bedside* is that unless the nurse is observed continuously it is often difficult to determine the real skill requirements of an activity. With intermittent observations, a professional nurse might be observed straightening a patient's pillow, a simple activity that could be performed by a nursing assistant. However, a moment before this she might have been changing a patient's dressing, and then have straightened the pillow to make the patient comfortable after the dressing procedure. (italics in original)[142]

Murray concluded that for the sake of efficiency and quality patient care, registered staff should perform personal patient services in conjunction with a more technical and skilled treatment.

As the Ontario study illustrated, the difficulties administrators and nurses encountered trying to separate out technical and curative functions from domestic and caring ones were complicated further by the very nature of many new therapies and techniques nurses had assumed. For example, a 1942 *CN* article on 'Chemotherapy with Sulphonamide Drugs' reviewed nursing and medical procedure for administering these new pharmaceuticals. Since 'it may tax the resources of nurse and physician alike to persuade the patient to persist in a treatment which must sometimes seem worse than the disease', nurses were advised to use 'sedatives, encouragement, coaxing, and plain bullying' to convince patients that the nausea and vomiting caused by the drugs were 'normal'. Once administered, nurses had to measure fluid intake to ensure that blood drug levels did not become too high, and measure urinary output for reduction or cessation of 'urinary secretion'. Warning that other side-effects might occur, the article maintained that 'the early detection of these complications depends on observation of the patient, and their successful treatment depends, in turn, on their early detection.' For these reasons, throughout all new treatments 'careful nursing, supportive and symptomatic treatment have still to be carried out, and still constitute a major element in successful therapy of these diseases.'[143]

If the structure of patient-care services continued to require that graduate nurses perform a range of overlapping functions, so, too, did nursing education reinforce the need for practitioners to blend curing and caring. Although the apprenticeship system of staffing had been surpassed, the apprenticeship system of education remained. All but 2 per cent of fourth-generation practitioners learned their trade in three-year apprenticeship programs at the large, usually urban, hospitals that continued to function after many of the small schools had been closed. Those institutions that maintained their training programs were less constrained by institutional staffing needs than hospital schools in earlier decades. One key sign of this new autonomy was the introduction in the 1940s of the eight-hour day for students, a move that increased the amount of study and class time available.[144] None the less, during the hours they were on the wards, apprentices continued to supply substantial proportions of patient-care labour.

In 1947, the CNA recommended that graduate and student nurses each constitute 30 per cent of the nursing staff, yet the continued shortage of graduate nurses forced institutions such as Winnipeg

General to rely heavily on student labour. That year graduates constituted 12.2 per cent of the ward staffs and students made up 50 per cent.[145] By 1966, proportions had improved only slightly, with graduate nurses comprising 20 per cent of the female patient-care staff compared to the student contingent of 42 per cent.[146] Given these proportions, whenever a short-term staffing crisis erupted, it was met by shifting student nurses into the area of need. For instance, when, in 1954, the WGH operating room was threatened with closure due to lack of nursing staff, the crisis was managed 'by having five senior student nurses gain experience as scrub nurses'.[147] Oral testimony confirmed that for the many student nurses who continued to learn through labour on the wards, personal-care tasks were learned early. Barbara Burr recalled that as juniors at Windsor's Hôtel Dieu, she and her classmates 'answered bells, scrubbed bedpans, scrubbed urinals, cleaned any instruments that had to be autoclaved'. In other words, juniors 'got the "joe" jobs that the second and third years passed on to you.'[148] The result of this educational system was that graduate nurses learned, from their first days on the ward, that they were responsible for all facets of patient care, not as supervisors but by personally delivering those bedside services.

Because patient-care work was unpredictable, because the new therapies demanded that nurses possess a range of skills, and because as apprentices nurses learned all elements of patient services, the work of graduate nurses continued to be defined, at least informally, by a multiplicity of tasks and the simultaneous performance of curative and caring functions. True, the formal stratification of the patient-care work-force was erecting divides between nurse-managers, nurse-workers, practical nurses, aides, and clerks, but in practice the continued necessity for established patterns of patient care blurred such distinctions.

At the same time, gender continued to frame the distribution of power and resources within the health-care sector, thereby emphasizing the divide between female attendants and male physicians and administrators. Throughout the 1942–68 era, the medical profession remained male-dominated (in 1961, 93 per cent of doctors were men) and few, if any, women were promoted into non-nursing managerial roles. By contrast, more than 95 per cent of graduate nurses and 80 per cent of nursing assistants were female. It was not just the composition of the work-force and the persisting affiliation of nursing with femininity that created 'gender' in the health-care sector. The gender division of labour and authority also reinforced paternalist and heterosexual relations between nurses and male doctors or administrators.

Of these gendered relations, none were more influential than those between doctors and nurses. The old rule that female nurses 'stand at attention' when in the presence of medical men persisted through the post-war era (and in some circumstances well past 1968). Even though nurses were performing complex 'medical' tasks, doctors continued to wield final authority in decision-making over patient-care services. If anything, graduate nurses' new responsibilities to assume medical functions and provide sophisticated observations of patient progress served to reinforce the gendered patterns of interaction between doctors and nurses, not transform them. In 1967, a US psychiatrist termed these relations the 'doctor-nurse game'. The rules were hardly simple, but they were surely familiar. Nurses tried to provide doctors with critical information without appearing to assume too great a diagnostic role. Doctors relied on nursing knowledge but had to maintain the perception that they were in charge.[149] This 'game' was obviously built on the broader construction of heterosexual relations of the post-war era and was reinforced by the new claims to heterosexual complementariness being made in popular culture by and for nurses. The game played out in several contexts. With respect to nurses' assumption of technical procedures, nurses were made aware that doctors were 'letting them' provide particular patients services.[150] On the wards, doctors and nurses attempted to demonstrate appropriate levels of authority and subservience. For instance, at Vancouver General the doctors would arrive on the ward either to do a dressing themselves or to watch nurses perform it. In return, recalls RN Marjorie McLeod, nurses served as hostesses and facilitators for physicians on the ward: 'Usually you had to take the doctors around, they were very helpless when they needed supplies or anything.'[151] Like mothers and housewives, nurses wielded the power to empower. Like women in the domestic sphere, nurses adjusted their schedules and priorities to facilitate the actions of other members in the hospital 'household'. This division of labour and of etiquette reinforced nurses' traditional sphere of authority, outside medical control, even in an era when nurses were performing increasing numbers of 'medical' duties.

Relations between hospital administrators and nurses were also defined by paternalist cordiality, respect, authority, and deference. These relations were evident in institutional annual reports wherein once a year hospital superintendents publicly recognized nurses' 'sacrifices' and 'contributions'. When, in 1943, Winnipeg General authorized 'living-out allowances' for staff nurses, the superintendent reported: 'The privilege of living-out has been requested for a good many years, but financial difficulties have here-to-for prevented the granting of this step, which after all, is a most reasonable one.' In 1947, the superintendent acknowledged that the previous year 'provided the severest test yet experienced. It is with pride and gratitude that acknowledgement of our Nurses' devotion to duty, is made.' Such 'tributes' from senior administrators and boards of governors continued to be offered throughout the post-war years.[152] Similarly, the recommended personnel policies of nursing associations were premised on cordial and respectful relations between nursing and administrative bodies. When wage increases were granted, usually as a means to retain graduate nurse staff, administrators made a virtue out of a necessity by reporting the wage increase in institutional publications and celebrating the 'satisfaction' that being able to provide improved remuneration gave to administration and workers alike. Nursing administrators responded with equal measures of formality and deference. WGH Director of Nursing Margaret Cameron informed the hospital community in 1957 that 'the nursing staff appreciated the kindness of administration in providing gross salary for all nursing personnel. . . . The $20.00 overall increase for all nurses . . . was also much appreciated.'[153]

Within this gendered system of power, nursing administrators occupied a contradictory position. Often members of the third generation who had graduated in the 1920–42 era, supervisory nurses held on to an earlier understanding of their position, which included serving as benefactresses for their 'girls'. The maternalist position was sometimes underscored by the generational difference between many supervisors and recently graduated general-duty personnel.[154] Although supervisory nurses were officially part of management, their own training in the apprenticeship system and their occupational affiliation and professional ambitions for nursing inspired them to use their position to win improved conditions for their nursing staffs. In 1943 Brandon General Superintendent of Nursing Christina Macleod informed her board of directors that a staff nurse, with one year of experience, had been offered the night supervisor job at a Winnipeg hospital at the same wage that BGH was paying to its night supervisor of 20 years' experience. Macleod took advantage of the opportunity to press the board into rectifying low salary levels. 'Such things are upsetting when apparently no thought is being given for faithful service. The employment situation is grave and no one can afford to let employees go for the sake of a few dollars.'[155] The benevolence of nursing supervisors could have material significance for working nurses. When Violet McMillan became her family's sole support in 1959, she immediately started looking for nursing jobs.

I went around town a little bit. I went to offices, doctors' offices, and places . . . they would be very kind, but . . . I was 52 years old at that time . . . and they would be very kind and say, 'I think we're looking for someone a little younger'. . . . So I went to my training school [WGH] and told them my story, and they took me on at the [Maternity] Pavilion.

Later, when McMillan experienced back problems, nursing administrators transferred her to a ward that required less heavy lifting. Such administrative benevolence allowed McMillan to work for 15 years until her retirement.[156]

At the same time that their institutional positions permitted superintendents to dispense patronage of this kind, the changing nature of hospital work challenged the benevolent and maternalist role of nursing administrators. When nurses began to press for collective bargaining, tensions between general-duty nurses and nurse supervisors emerged. One Vancouver General graduate recalled the time in the mid-1940s when the staff met to discuss joining the hospital union: 'I remember having this mass meeting and Miss Fairley being so upset that her nurses would feel they had to form a union to get things they wanted. She thought she had slipped, that her nurses had formed a union.'[157]

Changing relations between administrative and rank-and-file nurses did not completely undermine the sense of common bond between the two tiers. Nurse-workers and nurse-managers shared gender, training, and occupational affiliation, as well as an organizational structure that appeared flexible enough to encompass the new responsibility of collective bargaining. On the wards, nurses slowly were acquiring experience with fixed relations of female dominance and subordination, but few social models existed upon which nurses might have based those relations.[158] For these reasons, the social distance between general-duty nurses and nurse administrators was not as great as it might have been, or would become. By contrast, hierarchical relations between nurses and doctors or administrators, all too familiar to rank-and-file nurses, were constructed according to biological and social difference that was reinforced on the ward but also underscored by the broader structures of patriarchal society.

The strength of occupational relationships was tested in this era, revealing the resiliency of paternalist gender relations and of maternalist relations among nurses, but also the fissures that were beginning to emerge. A conflict that erupted on 23 October 1950 at Toronto General Hospital illustrated the continuities and contradictions informing relations at the bedside. That day, 73 graduate nurses from the hospital's seven floors, labour room, relief staff, and blood bank submitted a petition to the superintendent and board of trustees of the TGH. The complaint was twofold: the nurses believed the 'salaries and working conditions of the general duty nurses in the Private Pavilion' required adjusting and they were convinced that the committee appointed to investigate working conditions there had failed to suggest any corrective measures. The petition promised that the 73 signatories would resign as of 23 November unless the hospital met the nurses' demands. The 11-point program for change included specifications regarding the hours nurses could work, the number of patients they would be required to attend, the number of staff on duty, length of holidays and daily rest periods, and basic salary rates. Their demands built on the RNAO's 'Recommendations on Personnel Practices, 1950', which among other things established the base salary for a general-duty nurse at $165 per month. The TGH salary range for these workers started at $150 and peaked at $170 for an experienced employee.

The TGH superintendent and board of trustees responded by relaying the problem to Nursing Superintendent Mary Macfarland and Assistant Superintendent Jennie Ives. Ives generated data regarding current working conditions and formulated her suggestions for readjusting the pay scale.[159] With this information in place, Macfarland drafted a letter to be sent to the petitioners. The letter acknowledged the 23 October 'communication'. It then asserted: 'I think you should know that prior to the receipt of this communication, nurses' salaries and other adjustments were under consideration by the Chairman of the Board and the Superintendent preparatory to making recommendations to the Board on your behalf.' Given that Ives's report was dated 29 October, it was unlikely that the administration was in fact ready to take action before the conflict erupted. None the less, having insisted that collective action was not needed, Macfarland went on to inform her dissatisfied staff members that in order for the board to continue on with its deliberations regarding working conditions, the pugnacious nurses had to withdraw their threat of resignation by 10 November 'so that we may continue to deal with the recommendations which were under consideration prior to the receipt of your communication'.[160]

Responses from the nurses were mixed. On 6 November, the committee representing the Private Patients Pavilion requested a meeting with the superintendent and the board before they would consider any action. They must have had some success because on 14 November the nurses reported to the administration that 'it has been decided by the General Duty Nurses to withdraw their resignations on your assurance that adjustments are to be made in the near future and on your assurance that a committee appointed by the General Duty Nurses will be granted a hearing by the Board of Trustees to state their grievances.' In the meantime, 13 individuals had already rescinded their resignation. Several of these nurses recanted entirely. One petitioner told Macfarland that she regretted signing the 'communication' and assured her superior that she had been 'most happy in my work, always giving any patient under my care the very best of my ability'. She concluded her note by writing that 'I also realize the hard task of you all at this time. . . . Believe me yours faithfully'. Another found that she 'did not agree with the petition with the exception of a raise in pay.' A colleague withdrew her name because 'I am a Christian, and as such realize that I have taken the wrong action.' One petitioner claimed that her signature had been forged by a colleague who thought she would 'want it so'. Another staff nurse pleaded ignorance: 'I know nothing of [the petition's] meaning and wish to have no part in it.' One staff nurse decided that she disagreed with the tactics of the 'radical dictatorial group' of the staff nurses' leadership committee and so withdrew her withdrawal.

Not all nurses were prepared to recant. One staff member withdrew her resignation on 3 November, only to reconsider her decision on 4 November, saying, 'I have signed the petition and I feel as if I should stick by it.' Most touching was the letter submitted by an older nurse who claimed to be ashamed at having signed the petition because she had not read it carefully first. Having not worn her eyeglasses that day, the nurse signed before realizing the meaning of the petition. She tried to remove her signature and, when unsuccessful, voiced her concerns to her peers that 'we will all be lucky if we do not get fired right away'. In spite of her hesitation over tactics, the nurse did agree that the wage demands were reasonable. Stating that 'we really do work hard', the nurse maintained that living expenses were high, and even though she rarely socialized, she still found saving for the future difficult. She pointed out that she had had no increase in salary since 1947, saying: 'I know some of the others have. Can you explain this?' The older practitioner defended her younger colleagues, stating: 'One cannot blame them if they want to live and still have something for the future.' The nurse concluded: 'Now Miss Macfarland, I do not want you to get the impression that I am blaming anyone else for my having signed the paper. I did a foolish thing in putting my name on a paper without reading it through myself', and stated that she would like to rescind her resignation if possible, but only if the other nurses had the same chance. If not, 'having foolishly gotten into this thing, I would have to see it through with the rest, if they did not have the same chance. I could not be a piker, even if it was only a foolish one.'[161]

TGH records do not reveal the precise outcome of this conflict, though some resolution must have occurred because salaries were soon raised to $165 per month for a 44-hour work week, and several of the signatories were still on staff two years later.[162] Regardless of the outcome, this conflict illuminates several of the key tensions that conditioned workplace relations for general-duty nurses. The nurses' collective action revealed a solidarity and sense of shared position around 'bread and butter' issues of pay and conditions. That nurses would insist on adhering to associational wage scales indicated the possibilities for collective action against a third-party employer that had not been realistic within private-duty work. The conflict also suggested that the presence of older nurses was providing some leadership around workplace issues. A note attached to one of the nurses' letters, perhaps penned by the author or by Assistant Superintendent Ives, concluded: 'The young nurses do not know what it is all about. This is the work of older graduates.'

But it was the position of Mary Macfarland that was most contradictory, and most telling. The general-duty nurses did not address their collective proposals to Macfarland, their superintendent of nursing, but instead communicated directly to the superintendent of the hospital and the board of trustees. This could be interpreted as a statement of lack of faith in Macfarland and a rejection of her position as benefactress and maternal authority figure. Or, it could be read as an effort on the part of the general-duty nurses to keep Macfarland safely out of the line of fire. At the same time, in spite of the nurses' pointed avoidance of communicating with Macfarland, the hospital superintendent insisted that the senior nursing administrator resolve the matter. This could have been a strategy on the part of the board to pit nurse against nurse and capitalize on older relations of female benevolence. Or, Macfarland could have insisted on resolving the conflict to protect her sovereignty over nursing issues.

Whatever the scenario, Macfarland demonstrated her ability to act with administrative force and to place a wedge in the solidarity of her staff. Her efforts to reassert her position as benefactress and nursing representative to the TGH senior administration worked in so far as she was able to get a number of the nurses to request clemency on an individual basis. But the response of the older nurse who 'could not be a piker' also revealed that maternalism could cut both ways. In appealing to Macfarland's sense of humour and sympathy for human error, their shared understanding of the difficulty of saving for their futures, and their common bond as 'older' nurses, and in delivering a gentle reproof that Macfarland had used her maternalism unevenly, giving some nurses raises and not others, the older nurse subtly reminded Macfarland where her loyalties should lay. The nurse's decision that she 'could not be a piker' stood as warning to Macfarland of how powerful the alliances forged at the bedside could be.

Conclusion

The fourth generation of Canadian nurses encountered a paradoxical set of structures defining their work and workplace relations. Tremendous changes seemed to be transforming nursing work, but whether those changes were causing an increase or decrease in nurses' class status was not entirely clear. At the same time, nursing remained closely identified with women's work. Most practitioners, whether 'professional' or 'non-professional', were female, and powerful ideological forces insisted that nursing's sex-typing was part of the 'natural' gender division of labour. Like housewives and mothers, nurses were expected to adjust their daily activities to meet the unpredictability of patient care; like housewives and mothers, nurses were expected to supervise subordinates and facilitate the needs of male authorities. Gender was important not just because it defined who would become a nurse, but because relations of authority and subordination were constructed and negotiated around it. This gendered paradigm was by no means new, but for fourth-generation nurses it was highlighted in new ways, both by the rearticulation of heterosexual complementariness in popular culture and by the redefinition of nursing as a suitable job for married women. Thus within the changing health-care system, gender helped to solidify relations among nurses at the same time that those relations were being tested.

Theoretical and historical analyses of nursing work in this era must, therefore, account for the complex intersections of contradictions and continuities that shaped nurses' experiences within the emerging health-care bureaucracy of the post-war years. Scholarly studies that emphasize ambiguous class status and consciousness provide an important starting point for such a reconceptualization, but those scholars underestimate the powerful gendered traditions within nursing and within women's work that continued to resonate throughout the fourth generation of Canadian nursing. Further research into the experiences of immigrant and minority nurses is also needed to understand fully the significance of race and ethnicity in shaping the division of labour within the health-care system and the meaning of 'whiteness' in defining the status of RNs at the bedside and on the wards. Exploring the interplay of class, gender, and ethnicity promises to provide nursing historians with avenues through which they can investigate power relations within the occupation and within the health-care hierarchy.

7

'The Price of Generations':
Canadian Nursing Under Medicare,
1968–1990

In the spring of 1989, the fifth generation of Canadian nurses was writing a new chapter in its occupation's history.[1] Frustrated with inadequate staffing, an intensified pace of work, insufficient salaries, and dramatic outmigration of their co-workers from the province and the occupation, nurses in British Columbia went on strike. On 14 June, when negotiations between the British Columbia Nurses Union (BCNU) and the Health and Labour Relations Association (HLRA) broke down, nurses took action, shutting down all but essential services of the health-care delivery system.[2] Allied workers in the Hospital Employees Union (HEU) soon joined the walkout.[3] Within two weeks the HLRA had proposed a contract, offering a 29.5 per cent wage increase over three years, which the BCNU bargaining committee tentatively accepted.[4]

Such strike action was not unprecedented, for in recent years growing militancy among Canadian nurses had been manifest in bitter strikes and work-to-rule campaigns across the nation.[5] Events in British Columbia took a radical turn, however, when dissident union members challenged their own bargaining committee and mounted a determined campaign to convince nurses to reject the proposed contract. Between 26 June and 12 July leaders of the dissident group, Vancouver General Hospital's Bernadette Stringer and Debra McPherson, drove 1,600 kilometres to meet with nurses throughout the province and to convince them that the contract would not solve nurses' problems. Their efforts paid off. On 12 July, 65 per cent of BCNU members—including 85 per cent of the Vancouver General staff—supported McPherson and Stringer's 'vote no' campaign and rejected the HLRA offer.[6]

The rationale for dissent was clear. BCNU members believed that greater financial incentives—greater than even the 29.5 per cent— were necessary to attract and keep enough new nurses to reduce the overwork, stress, and 'burn out' debilitating the existing work-force. Over 2,000 additional nurses were required if BC health-care workers were to provide adequate patient care, but the province's health-care system could not attract or retain sufficient practitioners. Many registered nurses agreed with student nurse Marcia Weir's sentiments: 'I want to stay and work in BC when I graduate, but I will not stay where I am taken for granted.'[7] Only drastic measures would protect and defend the interests of patients and practitioners in BC's health-care system. As primary caregivers responsible for patients' health, nurses believed that the long-term goals of quality service demanded a withdrawal of that service in the short term. In the words of BCNU president Pat Savage: 'ethically [nurses] see themselves as patient advocates and are obliged to speak out.'[8] Savage herself, although sensitized to the militancy of her membership, did not anticipate that nurses' commitment to quality care would lead them to 'speak out' both against employers and, if necessary, against their own union leadership.

For some nurses, their experiences in other provinces convinced them of the necessity to persevere until a satisfactory settlement was won. Vancouver General nurse Cheryl Davis, a veteran of the 19-day strike in Alberta in 1988, declared: 'I think we should have stayed out longer [in Alberta]' and encouraged her peers in BC to stand firm, maintaining that 'we have to suffer now but I think in the long run it will be to our benefit.'[9] As elsewhere, striking did not come easily to most BC nurses. Operating room nurse Brenda Kormin articulated the ambivalent feelings that withdrawal of service evoked in many nurses. 'I support the strike all the way. But I was born in this hospital. So were my two kids. We have to take this action but it's the complete opposite of everything we do, everything we trained for.'[10] That nurses like Kormin would take so militant a stand signified the extent of their frustration, as well as a more fundamental transformation occurring in nurses' collective consciousness. Two factors informed that transformation. The first was the feminist critique of society's devaluation of women's work.[11] The second was the increasing presence of female service workers within the union movement.[12] Together these social forces prompted nurses to question the concepts of femininity and professionalism that had been central to their occupational identity and organizational form.[13]

For many, answers lay in the history and traditions created by their predecessors. Debbie Oliver, nurse and daughter of a nurse, explained: 'I think about leaving the profession but it is part of my soul, my very being. As my mother before, I will always be a nurse. My spirit was broken long ago but every once in a while, I feel the old enthusiasm coming back. Lately, those feelings are harder to hold onto.'[14] Looking back over her mother's career, Oliver concluded that 'this nursing crisis has been with us for many years' and that only when public recognition was won for the 'bedside nurse . . . the most important care-giver in the system' would solutions be found. For this 16-year veteran of the Canadian health-care system, the British Columbia strike alone would not resolve nursing's problems: 'I don't know what the answer will be, but for a brief moment in Canadian history, we felt we were important.'[15]

As such commentary reveals, the contemporary crisis has revitalized nurses' interest and awareness of their place in Canadian history and has raised new questions about the persistent difficulty nurses have experienced in winning social value and economic reward for their work. Clearly, the portrait of progress depicted in conventional nursing history does not speak to the emerging frustration and disillusionment being manifest through strikes and walkouts. In seeking new interpretations of their occupational history, nurses are not alone. In the past decade, academic researchers from a range of disciplines have joined rank-and-file nurses in re-examining nursing's place in the health-care system and in the female labour force. Sociologists, historians, and economists, writing from feminist, Marxian, and anti-racist perspectives, have demonstrated the continued importance of the categories of gender, ethnicity, and class in shaping the experiences of nurses at work, in educational institutions, in organizations, and in the community. While these researchers do not always agree on the trajectory of change in nursing or on the appropriate strategies for future struggles, they do concur that in the years after the implementation of Medicare, Canadian nurses became more willing to defend their collective needs and aspirations. Identifying persistent forces of oppression within the occupation, scholars have challenged profoundly the older belief that nursing is best understood as being, or becoming, professional. In the past, such assertions would have been rejected immediately by many nurses, but recent developments within the occupation have made élite and rank-and-file practitioners more willing to critique professional gains and question nurses' continued difficulty in winning social authority. Nurse-scholars, often teachers in university nursing schools, have facilitated this process by embracing new perspectives and presenting diverse analyses in their publications.

The heightened militancy and political awareness of the fifth generation of Canadian nurses, as displayed in the BC strike and in recent nursing scholarship, was the result of the particular combination of unionization, feminism, and professional development that occurred in the post-1968 era. Critical to this process was the emergence of new forms of collective representation. For most of the previous generation, except in Quebec and Prince Edward Island, nurses by law could not form certified bargaining agents. In the late 1960s, however, when labour laws were liberalized to permit 'professionals' to join other workers' bargaining units, the door was opened for the provincial associations to become certified bargaining units. The progression from associational labour relations committees to bargaining units was disrupted in the early 1970s when hospital nurses in Nipawin, Saskatchewan, began to organize. At that point, the Saskatchewan Registered Nurses' Association (SRNA) labour relations committee had successfully negotiated collective agreements with roughly 50 per cent of the province's hospitals. But under revised labour codes, when the SRNA tried to organize the Nipawin nurses, the Service Employees International Union (SEIU) challenged the SRNA position, petitioning to the provincial labour relations board that as a 'professional association' the SRNA 'should not be allowed to act as a trade union since its Board of Directors had nurse managers as members'. The labour relations board agreed with the SEIU, as did the Supreme Court of Canada. The 1972 Supreme Court ruling reverberated throughout the provincial associations. Fearing lengthy and expensive court challenges of their own, between 1972 and 1977 the other eight provinces joined Quebec and Saskatchewan in establishing autonomous union structures.[16]

While the Supreme Court ruling of 1972 was the catalyst that inspired the nationwide move to distinct union structures, the formation of new organizations cannot be understood merely as an extension of the older associations, or only as a response to legal imperatives. Other forces were also providing an impetus to create stronger, more aggressive modes of representation. In particular, the political economy of health care was inspiring greater degrees of worker dissatisfaction. Under Medicare, hospitals and the medical profession were guaranteed a secure funding base, but federal financing of health services also generated new pressures to make health-care dollars stretch to ensure 'universality'. Hospital nursing was one important target of the new efficiency measures implemented by health administrators.[17]

Marie Campbell's research into the changing structure of nursing work has revealed the stress and dissatisfaction efficiency measures provoked. Rationalization techniques such as patient classification systems served to standardize the amount of time nurses spend on particular tasks and particular types of patients, but also created 'objective' staffing decisions based on those patient 'needs'. According to Campbell, rather than relying on the experience of nurses and administrators to adjust staffing to patient demand, the new documentary system produced knowledge away from the ward. Because how and when nursing care was performed remained the prerogative of the nurse, nursing was not 'deskilled' in the classic sense. Instead, standardized times for specific tasks were established, but the extra time nurses needed to complete the 'indeterminate work' or 'untimed background work'—such as communicating with physicians, patients, and families or organizing the work of subsidiary personnel—was not adequately factored into the staffing formula. The professional commitment to patient care and the gender-specific tendency of women to absorb the extra tasks combined to ensure that nurses intensified their pace of work. They had to work harder to meet the standardized time allocation for specific tasks but also to make time to complete the necessary 'extra' duties. As Campbell explained: 'Policing how nurses spend their time is not really necessary, as long as they maintain their high level of professional commitment to their patients.'[18]

Efforts to systematize nursing care and to insist that nurses adhere to a standardized and predictable, if often unrealistic, pace of work were accompanied by intensified workloads, either through an increase in patient population or a decrease in nursing staff. Overtime and extra shifts became routine. By 1989 the Fédération québécoise des infirmières et infirmiers was reporting that 78 per cent of nurses surveyed claimed they had worked overtime, either staying late after a shift or working through breaks and mealtimes, extra work for which they received no extra remuneration.[19]

Shortages of nurses that developed periodically in the post-1968 years were both cause and effect of the intensification of the pace of work. In both the 1970s and 1980s, the inadequate supply of nurses being reported at the beginning of each decade lifted by the middle years and then developed again by the end of the decade.[20] Inquiries into the erratic pattern of supply and demand for nursing revealed that nurses often withdrew from the nursing work-force because of poor working conditions. A 1979–80 study of Alberta nurses reported that 30 per cent of respondents lacked job satisfaction. Of that 30 per cent, the most frequently cited reason for dissatisfaction was working conditions, and the second was inappropriate administrative policies.

In the years between 1973 and 1983 the number of graduate nurses employed increased from 73 per cent to 81 per cent, but over the same years the percentage of part-time nurses also increased, from 28 per cent to 38 per cent. Difficulties in hiring and retaining practitioners for full-time duty were exacerbated by the constant drain of Canadian nursing resources to the United States.[21]

Given these conditions, the rise of autonomous nursing unions must be seen not only as a response to changing labour law, but also as a rank-and-file response to intensification of nursing work. After all, the impetus to form provincial bargaining units preceded the 1972 Supreme Court decision. As well, some of the pressure to form more powerful bargaining bodies stemmed from the fact that nurses represented by non-nurse unions, such as government employee unions, had achieved substantial salary increases over their institutional counterparts. Whatever the reasons that nurses reformulated their organizational vehicles, members soon demonstrated that they were ready to use radical measures to improve their position. Strike action by nurses in Amherst, Nova Scotia, in 1971, by members of l'Alliance des Infirmières et Infirmiers du Québec in 1972, and by the United Nurses of Alberta in 1977, 1980, and 1982 reflected the growing militancy of rank-and-file nurses.[22] At the same time, other patient-care personnel, organized within national unions such as the Canadian Union of Public Employees (CUPE), were also withdrawing their labour and demanding improved working conditions.[23]

In joining the union movement, nurses participated in the larger trend towards white-collar unions and increasing militancy in late twentieth-century Canada. Although women's participation in unions was not new, the growth of the service sector and of white-collar unions brought large numbers of female workers into the labour movement and, with them, a new critique of women's place within organized labour. The feminist critique of gender relations within unions facilitated larger numbers of women assuming leadership positions and placed 'women's issues' such as day care on the bargaining table. These new connections between the union movement and the women's movement also began to influence nurses' collective consciousness. In many ways, rank-and-file militancy within nursing was fuelled as much by a growing awareness and acceptance of feminism as by traditional working-class consciousness.[24]

That nurses and feminists would become allies was not immediately apparent. Despite nurses' close relationships with feminism in the early twentieth century, by the 1960s nursing's public image as heterosexually complementary and as subservient to doctors stood as a barrier to sororal relations. Early feminist critiques of women in the professions focused on encouraging women to break into male-dominated professions like medicine, not remain in subservient 'women's' occupations like nursing. When, in the 1970s, feminists turned their attention to the private sphere, the socialist-feminist analysis of women's household production developed. The 'domestic labour debate', as it became known in Canadian academic circles, maintained that personal and domestic care provided by women had not only psychological value to individual family members, but also that in producing and reproducing healthy workers, women's household labour was a vital element of the capitalist economy.[25] However empowering for women working in the home, this reclamation of maternal and domestic work held little appeal for nurses, who were trying to distance themselves from the very personal services the domestic labour debate celebrated. The growing women's health movement found it equally difficult to incorporate nurses in their strategies for change. In her 1986 essay 'On the Importance of Being a Nurse', feminist sociologist of health Ann Oakley confessed: 'In a lengthy career as a medical sociologist studying medical services, I have to admit to a certain blindness with respect to the contribution that nurses make to health care. Indeed, over a period of some months spent observing healthcare work in a large London hospital, I hardly noticed nurses at all.'[26] For these reasons, feminist activity in the 1970s served to alienate nurses more than to build alliances with them.[27]

By the 1980s some of those tensions dissolved. At the workplace, their growing dissatisfaction with the intensification of work and persisting low pay prompted nurses to rethink personal-care services. Increasingly, nurses were insisting that interaction with patients was an important part of nursing care and of the healing process, and therefore should be factored in as a crucial element in nurses' daily work. Jerry White's analysis of the 1981 strike in Ontario hospitals revealed that for female employees the erosion of direct patient services and hospitals' unwillingness to value those services had alienated and angered all levels of patient-care personnel. One registered nursing assistant proclaimed: 'The world was becoming backward. Budgets and timetables meant more than patients.' Hospital housekeeping staffs also defended the significance of direct patient care. One such worker reported: 'Some of the younger girls say "why spend your time chatting up all the patients?" I tell them that if the most exciting thing that happens in the day is rolling over then you need some talk. You almost be a mother I guess—and it does wonders.'[28] These grassroot defences of the value of bedside care now appeared consistent with feminist analyses that celebrated women's domestic labours.

The renewed emphasis on the value of personal patient care was also linked to feminist calls for equal pay for work of equal value. In 1973, the CUPE local at the Winnipeg Health Sciences Centre (formerly the Winnipeg General Hospital) initiated a program to evaluate the equity of existing wage scales. The job evaluation concluded that 936 women workers, over 98 per cent of the female staff, were being undervalued for their labours. When the Anti-Inflation Board (AIB) decreed that the salary readjustment process at the Health Sciences Centre could not be implemented, CUPE, women's groups, and NDP leader Stanley Knowles all condemned the AIB decision as perpetuating sex discrimination.[29] Pay equity would continue to function as a radicalizing force within the health-care sector. In the 1980s, feminist sociologist Pat Armstrong conducted a study for the Ontario pay equity commission. Her research documented the overwork and lack of recognition still experienced by working nurses.[30] The persistence of such problems, along with the critique of the medical profession mounted by activists and academics in the women's health movement, widened the chasm between nurses and the medical profession, the latter of whom had enjoyed dramatic salary increases under Medicare.[31]

The degree to which basic feminist claims to pay equity and the valuation of women's work had infiltrated rank-and-file nurses' attitudes was reflected in the results of a survey conducted by sociologists William Carroll and Rennie Warburton. Examining 'Feminism, Class Consciousness and Household-Work Linkages Among Registered Nurses in Victoria', the authors reported that 'at least 93 per cent agreed that the most blatant male prerogatives in the workplace and household should be eliminated. These include pay inequities, priority for jobs in periods of high unemployment, final authority over children and unequal division of domestic labour.'[32]

The 'male prerogatives in the workplace' became clearly visible to nurses in 1981 when nurse Susan Nelles was arrested for the murder of four children at Toronto's Hospital for Sick Children (THSC). Between June 1980 and March 1981, 32 children had died on the THSC cardiology wards where Nelles worked. Staff nurses had repeatedly expressed concern over the deaths, but hospital authorities and medical staff could find no explanation for them. In March 1981, when outside authorities were called to investigate, the police decided that at least four of the babies had been killed by an overdose of a heart medication called digoxin and that the perpetrator was staff nurse Nelles. Police believed their suspicions were correct when, upon her arrest, Nelles neither protested her innocence nor broke down in tears, but rather called a lawyer. Court proceedings against Nelles commenced in January 1982, but, in spite of police opinion, by May the charges had been dropped for lack of evidence or motive.

The ensuing public pressure to investigate the infant deaths prompted the Ontario government to establish a Royal Commission of Inquiry, led by Mr Justice Samuel Grange, to probe not only the deaths of the babies but also the police treatment of Nelles. That mandate, combined with the fact that the medical witnesses consulted could not provide concrete answers as to the pharmacology of digoxin, meant that the focus of the inquiry and of its media coverage was on the nurses. TSCH staff nurses and representatives of provincial nursing associations were examined and cross-examined in front of Judge Grange and, through daily television coverage, before all of Canada. The treatment nurses received at the hands of the Grange Commission has led Elaine Buckley Day to call it a 'twentieth century witch-hunt'. Still convinced that foul play had occurred, inquiry attorneys aggressively interrogated the testifying nurses. Any expertise nurses might have offered to unravel the mysterious deaths was not sought out, while medical testimony was actively recruited and respectfully received. For more than nine months, Day argues, Canadian cable TV viewers watched nursing authority and expertise devalued or brought under suspicion.[33]

The Grange Commission thus crystallized nurses' sense of vulnerability that, as the first suspected and least protected of the health-care 'team', nurses were granted substantial responsibility for patient health and for the work of subsidiary workers, but none of the authority or financial reward that other professionals enjoyed. Years later, Kathy Coulson, night supervisor at TSCH, recalled to journalist Sarah Jane Growe how the deaths at Sick Children's Hospital and the Grange Commission had politicized her. Growe explained that Coulson 'never saw herself as a feminist; now she finds feminism is not as negative a term as she had thought. Looking back, she realizes nurses lacked credibility at the Grange inquiry because they are women.'[34]

As feminism and unionism were gaining greater rank-and-file support among fifth-generation practitioners, a distinctive feminist critique of nurses' position within the health-care system was also being promoted by the occupation's élite. Still committed to the goals of professionalization, nursing leaders in registered nurses' associations and in the university and college systems increasingly integrated analyses of gender asymmetry into their professional struggles. This was evident in strategies such as primary nursing, a system of assigning nursing duties to ensure that one nurse was responsible for a patient's care throughout her/his hospital stay. 'One nurse on each shift provides total care for the same group of patients day after day. Round-the-clock care is coordinated for each patient by the nurse designated as the primary nurse for that patient.' In this way, hospital-based RNs co-ordinated the totality of a patient's care and could assume the position of patient advocate.[35] This approach maintained RNs' place of authority, while retaining some direct patient care for them and combating the fragmentation of their work. The nurse-practitioner movement promised similar results. Introduced unsuccessfully in the early 1970s and then again in the early 1990s, the position of nurse-practitioner was designed to allow nurses, especially those in poorly served health-care markets like the North, to expand their scope of practice without losing the bedside skills that were their occupation's trademark.[36] Both primary nursing and the primary care dispensed by nurse-practitioners promised to reintegrate the caring and curing functions of nursing and secure for nursing a distinct body of knowledge and authority that professional status demanded.

Claims to professional rights were also buttressed by the decline of hospital apprenticeship training schools and the establishment of nursing education institutes of higher learning. By the late 1960s, many hospital schools of nursing were closing, a pattern that continued for the next two decades to the point that in the early 1990s even large schools such as those at Vancouver General, the former Winnipeg General, and Halifax's Victoria General Hospital either closed or faced substantial integration with university programs. Over the same period, community college nursing education programs were established offering two- and then three-year diploma programs. However much the creation of these signalled the demise of hospital reliance on student labour, many nursing leaders were still not satisfied and pinned their hopes for professional status on baccalaureate education. During the 1960s and 1970s, existing university nursing schools expanded their size and scope, while other universities created four-year baccalaureate programs for the first time. The Canadian Nurses' Association and its provincial affiliates have now decreed that by the year 2000 the category RN (and the community college diploma programs that produced RNs) will be eliminated and all 'professional' nurses will have bachelor degrees. University schools have also encouraged the pursuit of nursing research and, with it, the formation of master's and doctoral programs in nursing. Although much of the scholarship generated thus far has focused on clinical research, a significant number of nursing scholars now pursue social research, many using feminist frameworks of analysis.[37]

At the same time that nurses were struggling over the meaning of unionization and proletarianization, of feminism and patriarchy, and of professionalism, the fifth generation of Canadian nurses also experienced greater ethnic diversification and identification. Liberalization of Canadian immigration policy after 1967 facilitated wide-scale immigration of Caribbean nurses to Canada.[38] Nursing schools accepted greater numbers of visible and ethnic minority students and curricula now include units on 'transcultural nursing'. Due in part to the broader social emphasis on multiculturalism and to the continued immigration of nurses from non-European nations, some Canadian nurses began to identify ethnically specific needs of themselves and of their patients. These needs were articulated within specific political contexts of race and nation. As Quebec's sovereignty debate sharpened, in 1985 that province's nurses withdrew from the CNA. First Nations nurses developed a collective voice in 1974 when the Registered Nurses of Canadian Indian Ancestry was formed. In 1983 the name was changed to Indian and Inuit Nurses of Canada (IINC). Initially opposed to the organization, in 1987 the CNA agreed to grant IINC special interest group status. The national group now lists 276 members of Canadian Indian and Inuit ancestry and works not only to support First Nations students in their RN careers but also to represent Native health issues to appropriate governmental bodies.[39]

Similar associations emerged in the 1980s when Black nurses organized in Toronto and Montreal.[40] In 1992 the long-standing issue of racism was confronted directly by a group of African-Canadian nurses who appealed to the Ontario Human Rights Commission over the discriminatory promotion and disciplinary practices of their employer, the North York Hospital. Fourteen Black nurses had been 'dismissed or suspended indefinitely' by the hospital, and nine 'filed complaints of racial discrimination, harassment, and reprisals against the hospital'. The nurses were successful in their bid for justice.[41]

This incident revealed that nursing must join the rest of Canadian society in addressing racism and ethnocentrism. But the question of ethnic and racial privilege as well as class and gender divisions will continue to have particular meaning for nursing as the political economy of health undergoes further changes in Canada. As hospitals seek to cut costs by reducing patient stay and as patients are released from institutional care shortly after procedures or treatments are completed, the relative importance of institutional versus home nursing care may undergo another shift. The sixth generation of Canadian nurses, now receiving their education in universities across the nation, faces a health-care market in which hospitals employ a core of practitioners but many others work in domestic health-care services. In home nursing, RNs and BNs, who are relatively expensive members of the nursing team, find themselves sharing patient care with subsidiary workers, some of whom are trained and registered, such as RNAS, others of whom may be home helpers with minimal specific training. In these conditions, the economic incentive to assign RNs, BNS, and RNAS supervisory positions, directing patient care and performing only the most specialized of tasks, is great. As was the case for the fourth and fifth generations of Canadian nurses, patient care will be subdivided, but now in isolated domestic workplaces, patients' homes. In many cases, bedside care will be provided by home helpers who are often drawn from the least powerful social groups, including immigrant and ethnic minorities, and who therefore occupy weak bargaining positions.

As long as unionized hospital nurses remain the majority, the private nursing sector will continue to benefit from wage and working condition standards won by unionized institutional nurses. If and when hospital-sector jobs become harder to find, private-care nurses will face the same challenges as did their predecessors in private duty to define the parameters of nursing work and defend their definition of quality care. Unlike second- and third-generation nurses, who negotiated directly with a patient or doctor or used nurse-run registries, private-care practitioners in the late twentieth century will be hired by large multinational and national corporations, whose primary mandate is to generate profit. Will private nurses be able to defend wages, conditions, and even union structures on their own? Will trained and registered staff be able to defend their position *vis-à-vis* less trained, unregistered staff, especially when confronting powerful corporate employers? Can bonds be developed between levels of patient-care personnel in the face of class and ethnic differences?

Within the new health-care structure, there may be sufficient supervisory and educational positions available to absorb those practitioners who are able to acquire university training. In fact, BNs may find their status elevated within the health-care hierarchy to a position akin to medicine's general practitioner, but such elevation begs the question, who will provide bedside patient care and who will defend the value of that work? Simply moving into management and leaving technical or personal-care tasks to technicians or home helpers may secure a position for university-trained nurses within the health-care hierarchy, but this does not resolve what Susan Reverby has termed

nursing's 'dilemma' of valuing personal-care duties. With these contradictions to confront, the sixth generation of Canadian nurses may
well want to cast their vision backwards to consider how previous generations coped with the contradictions of gender, class, and ethnicity
at the bedside, on the ward, on the streets, and in the labour market.

This study provides one such perspective on that past, by exploring the experiences and relationships of working nurses in twentieth-
century Canada. As the preceding chapters have demonstrated, each
generation of trained nurses in this century has encountered a distinctive political economy of work. The second generation, trained during the 1900–20 era of dramatic hospital expansion, plied their trade
in the buoyant private-duty market. By the 1920s, overproduction of
nurses and more generalized economic stagnation created high levels
of unemployment and underemployment for the third generation of
hospital graduates. These conditions were alleviated in the post-
World War II years when hospital employment of graduate nurses for
'general duty' superseded private duty as the dominant occupational
sector. The introduction of Medicare in 1968 has provided a stable
funding base for the medical system, but pressure to increase services
in an era of inflationary health-care costs has prompted hospital
administrators to rationalize and intensify the work performed by
fifth-generation nurses. Further restructuring of health care indicates
that the sixth generation is now facing the resurgence of private-duty
nursing, similar to that experienced by their predecessors of the early
twentieth century but with greater corporate involvement.

Throughout these many changes nurses have coped, and continue
to cope, with two sets of relationships, each structured by class, gender, and ethnic difference. The first set of relationships was created as
nurses drew occupational boundaries between themselves and the
other actors on the health-care stage—doctors, untrained nursing personnel, and patients. Nursing's relationship to medicine was determined by class in that doctors were empowered to conceptualize and
organize health services while nurses were expected to execute medical orders. That fundamental hierarchical division of labour was naturalized by, and in fact rested upon, gender asymmetry. By contrast,
class and ethnicity, rather than gender, determined nurses' hierarchical relationship with less-trained patient-care personnel. The certification nurses boasted and the ethnic and racial composition of the
nursing work-force made graduates of hospital training programs relatively more privileged and powerful than the women who worked as
untrained community nurses or as hospitals' subsidiary nursing staff.
Positioned between doctors and less-skilled bedside attendants,

nurses' relationship to their patients depended on the latter's social status. Private patients might enjoy superior class status compared to their nurses, whereas public health or charity patients might occupy class or ethnic positions below nurses on the social hierarchy. In both scenarios, gender commonality might forge a cross-class or cross-ethnic bond among women that narrowed the gap dividing practitioner and patient.

At the same time that nurses were negotiating the appropriate boundaries between themselves and other citizens at the bedside, a second set of tensions internal to nursing were at play. Relations between working nurses performing direct patient care and the nurses who assumed supervisory roles created a significant 'class' divide between what Barbara Melosh has termed 'nurse-workers' and 'nurse-managers'. Differences between the two lay not only in the fact that one group supervised the other, but also in their understanding for what mattered in nursing. While administrative nurses valued managerial skills, educational credentials, and developing a scientific knowledge base through which to achieve professional standing, nurse-workers tended to value bedside skills, decent wages and hours of work, credentials based in on-the-job performance, and their occupationally specific 'technique'.

Conflict between the two groups was mitigated by several factors. For most of the century, the apprenticeship system of training, with its mobility through the ranks, served to diffuse permanent antagonisms among nurses. The shared experience of apprenticeship training bridged the gap between supervisors and staff, and across generations. This commonality of interest was underscored in decades when nurses united to define the boundaries between themselves and the other players in the health-care system. Even during the 1920s and 1930s, when economic dislocation intensified divisions among nurses on subjects like the scientific underpinning of nursing work or the appropriate feminine image for nurses, substantial points of accommodation could be forged between administrative and bedside nurses.

Divisions among nurses were reflected in but also resolved within the organizational structures they supported. The associations created by second-generation nurses struggled to achieve 'professional' legal authority and social status throughout the century, but in each generation these organizations were also compelled to defend members' workplace interests. As such, associations fulfilled numerous 'trade union' functions ranging from supporting employment registries in the inter-war years to engaging in collective bargaining in the 1950s and 1960s. Nursing associations combined trade union and professional organizational duties and strategies as a means to maintain occupational solidarity, a solidarity built in part on the gender of its members. Nursing's leadership, often drawn from the administrative group, vigorously defended what they knew was one of the few skilled occupations available to women. Even in the fifth generation, when autonomous nursing unions were formed, feminist analyses of women's place in the work-force and in the labour movement fuelled rank-and-file discontent.

Indeed, understanding the trajectory of change in nursing work necessitates that gender be a critical variable. For this reason, nurses do not fit neatly into either framework of professionalization or proletarianization. Analyses that emphasize the former fail to consider the difficulties women have had in gaining the social legitimation necessary for professional status, while advocates of the proletarianization thesis underestimate the privilege that nurses have enjoyed relative to other female health-care providers and over the subsidiary personnel that they supervise. As well, nurses have been able to defend the value of their labour, in some instances even against managerial efforts at rationalization, by drawing on traditions of female caring.

Neither truly professional nor completely proletarianized, the occupation of nursing has, none the less, provided generations of skilled health services to Canadians. That contribution demands recognition and appreciation, not only to credit the women who made it but also to ensure that future generations of Canadian continue to receive quality health services. However besieged the current generation feels, nurses possess a powerful voice for insisting that patient-care services remain a priority. Recognizing the important occupational traditions of nursing as skilled women's work constitutes an important starting place for defending the Canadian health-care system and the nurses who helped to build it.

Notes

Abbreviations

ARNPQ	Association of Registered Nurses of the Province of Quebec
BGH	Brandon General Hospital
BGHA	Brandon General Hospital Archives
BGNA	Brandon Graduate Nurses' Association
CBMH	*Canadian Bulletin of Medical History*
CN	*Canadian Nurse*
CNA	Canadian Nurses' Association
DBS	Dominion Bureau of Statistics
JHA	*Journal of the House of Assembly* (Nova Scotia)
MARN	Manitoba Association of Registered Nurses
MGH	Misericordia General Hospital (Winnipeg)
MGHNAAA	Misericordia General Hospital Nurses Alumnae Association Archives
MHHC	Massachusetts-Halifax Health Commission
MSNM	Margaret Scott Nursing Mission (Winnipeg)
MUA	McGill University Archives
NSH	Nova Scotia Hospital
OIIQ	Ordre des infirmiers et infirmières du Québec
PABC	Provincial Archives of British Columbia
PAM	Provincial Archives of Manitoba
PANS	Provincial Archives of Nova Scotia
PAO	Provincial Archives of Ontario
RNABC	Registered Nurses' Association of British Columbia
RNANS	Registered Nurses' Association of Nova Scotia
RNAO	Registered Nurses' Association of Ontario
TGHA	Toronto General Hospital Archives
TGHNAA	Toronto General Hospital Nurses Alumnae Association
UBCA	University of British Columbia Archives
VanGH	Vancouver General Hospital
VanGHNAA	Vancouver General Hospital Nurses Alumnae Association

VanGHNAAA   Vancouver General Hospital Nurses Alumnae Association
            Archives
VCA   Vancouver City Archives
VicGH   Victoria General Hospital (Halifax)
VicGHNAA   Victoria General Hospital Nurses Alumnae Association
VicGHNAAA   Victoria General Hospital Nurses Alumnae Association
            Archives
VON   Victorian Order of Nurses
WGH   Winnipeg General Hospital
WGHNAA   Winnipeg General Hospital Nurses Alumnae Association
WGHNAA   Winnipeg General Hospital Nurses Alumnae Association
            Archives

Chapter 1

1. Monica E. Baly's *Florence Nightingale and the Nursing Legacy* (London, 1986) is the most recent in a long line of Nightingale biographies. See also F.B. Smith, *Florence Nightingale: Reputation and Power* (London, 1982); Marion Royce, *Eunice Dyke: Health Care Pioneer* (Toronto, 1983).

2. See Barbara Melosh, 'Doctors, Patients, and "Big Nurse": Work and Gender in the Postwar Hospital', in Ellen Condliffe Lagemann, ed., *Nursing History: New Perspectives, New Possibilities* (Philadelphia, 1983); Margaret Ann Jensen, *Love's Sweet Return: The Harlequin Story* (Toronto, 1984), p. 87.

3. For a discussion of the nurses' war memorial in the Canadian Parliament buildings, see Natalie Riegler, 'The Work and Networks of Jean I. Gunn, Superintendent of Nurses, Toronto General Hospital 1913–1941: A Presentation of Some Issues in Nursing During Her Lifetime, 1882–1941', Ph.D. diss. (Univ. of Toronto, 1992), ch. 9. See also Anne Hudson Jones, ed., *Images of Nurses: Perspectives from History, Art, and Literature* (Philadelphia, 1988), for further articles on American nursing imagery.

4. This fact has been driven home to me by the frequency with which discussions of my thesis work have provoked stories of family members who were/are nurses. See also David Macfarlane, 'Her Brothers' Keeper', *Saturday Night* (Apr. 1991), pp. 21–8, an excerpt from his *The Danger Tree*, for an example of the position of a graduate nurse, Great-Aunt Kate, in the Goodyear family's collective memory.

5. Carol Gino, *The Nurse's Story* (New York, 1982), presents a personal account of the horrors and agonies of nursing work. See also Zane Robinson Wolf, *Nurses' Work: The Sacred and the Profane* (Philadelphia,

1988), p. 139, for an analysis of contemporary nurses' reaction to the 'dirty work' of nursing.

6. For instance, American historian Charles Rosenberg acknowledged that 'in 1800, as today, nurses were the most important single factor determining ward and room environment' but then proceeded to discount nurses as minor forces in shaping the modern hospital. Charles Rosenberg, *The Care of Strangers: The Rise of America's Hospital System* (New York, 1987), p. 9. Canadian scholars such as David Gagan have likewise paid only cursory attention to the influence of nursing. David Gagan, *'A Necessity Among Us': The Owen Sound General and Marine Hospital, 1891–1985* (Toronto, 1990).

7. See George M. Torrance, 'Hospitals as Health Factories', in David Coburn, Carl D'Arcy, Peter New, and George Torrance, eds, *Health and Canadian Society: Sociological Perspectives* (Don Mills, Ont., 1981); Veronica Strong-Boag and Kathryn McPherson, 'The Confinement of Women: Childbirth and Hospitalization in Vancouver, 1919–1939', in *Vancouver's Past: Essays in Social History* (Vancouver, 1986), examines the impact of hospitalization on one area of health care. Colin Howell, 'Reform and the Monopolistic Impulse: The Professionalization of Medicine in the Maritimes', *Acadiensis* 11, 1 (Autumn 1981), pp. 3–22, provides an insightful analysis of the role of hospitals in the professionalization process. Scholarly studies of modern hospitals are few in number. For instance, Charles G. Roland, ed., *Health, Disease, and Medicine: Essays in Canadian History* (Toronto, 1984), does not contain a single article on institutional services. Those monographs that do exist often chronicle administrative and financial growth without placing those developments in a wider social context. See, for example, W.G. Crosbie, *The Toronto General Hospital 1819–1965: A Chronicle* (Toronto, 1975).

8. For discussions of the growth of Canadian asylums, see Daniel Francis, 'The Development of the Lunatic Asylum in the Maritime Provinces', *Acadiensis* 6, 2 (Spring 1977), pp. 23–38; Thomas E. Brown, 'The Origins of the Asylum in Upper Canada, 1830–1939', *CBMH* 1, 1 (Summer 1984), pp. 27–58; Barry Edginton, 'Moral Treatment to Monolith: The Institutional Treatment of the Insane in Manitoba, 1871–1919', *CBMH* 5, 2 (Winter 1988), pp. 167–88; S.E.D. Shortt, *Victorian Lunacy: Richard M. Bucke and the Practice of Late Nineteenth Century Psychiatry* (Cambridge, 1986).

9. See DBS, *Census of Canada*, 1921, 1931, 1941 (Ottawa, 1929, 1936, 1946). For a discussion of one nurse's experiences as an industrial nurse in Pinawa, Manitoba, see Ingibjorg Cross, tape-recorded interview by author, Vancouver, BC, 20 July 1988, PAM, 'Nurses and Their

Work', Oral History Collection. (Hereafter, unless indicated otherwise, copies of all tape-recorded interviews are deposited in the PAM Oral History Collection.)

10. See, for example, Charlotte Searle, *Professional Practice: A South African Nursing Perspective* (Durban, 1986); Josephine Castle, 'The Development of Professional Nursing in New South Wales, Australia', in Christopher Maggs, ed., *Nursing History: The State of the Art* (London, 1985); Glenda Strachan, 'The Third Sex: Women and the Colonisation of White Collar Jobs: The Case of Nursing in Australia', paper presented to Australian Historical Association Conference, June 1991; Strachan, 'Sacred Office, Trade or Profession? The Dilemma of Nurses' Involvement in Industrial Activities in Queensland, 1900–1950', in Raelene Frances and Bruce Scates, eds, *Women, Work and the Labour Movement in Australia and Aotearoa/New Zealand* (Sydney, 1991); Brian Abel-Smith, *A History of the Nursing Profession* (London, 1960).

11. John Murray Gibbon in collaboration with Mary S. Mathewson, *Three Centuries of Canadian Nursing* (Toronto, 1947), p. v.

12. Linda B. McIntyre, 'Towards a Redefinition of Status: Professionalism in Canadian Nursing, 1939–45', MA thesis (Univ. of Western Ontario, 1984), concluded that wartime shortages provided nurses with an opportunity to develop professional aspirations and at the same time prove their worth as 'co-partners, not subordinates' to a collegial medical community.

13. Barbara Melosh's review of the literature on professionalism is especially useful on this question. See Melosh, *'The Physician's Hand': Work Culture and Conflict in American Nursing* (Philadelphia, 1982), ch. 2.

14. See, for example, Rondalyn Kirkwood, 'Blending Vigorous Leadership and Womanly Virtues: Edith Kathleen Russell at the University of Toronto, 1920–52', CBMH 11, 1 (1994), pp. 175–206; Lee Stewart, *'It's Up to You': Women at UBC in the Early Years* (Vancouver, 1990). On the importance of university credentials for professionals, see Robert Gidney and Wyn Millar, *Professional Gentlemen: The Professions in Nineteenth Century Ontario* (Toronto, 1995).

15. Amitai Etzioni, ed., *The Semi-Professions and Their Organization* (New York, 1969). Writing from a very different perspective, Jo Anne Ashley termed nurses 'second-class professionals' because of their subordination as women. Ashley, *Hospitals, Paternalism and the Role of the Nurse* (New York, 1976), p. 126. Bernard R. Blishen labelled nursing a 'dependent profession' that relies on doctors 'for the initiation of their activities, but [nurses] are waging a continuing struggle for professional autonomy.' See Blishen, *Doctors in Canada: The*

Changing World of Medical Practice (Toronto, 1991) p. 107; also see ch. 6, esp. pp. 107–10, for Blishen's discussion of nursing's dependent status.

16. Mary Kinnear, *In Subordination: Professional Women, 1870–1970* (Montreal, 1995). Kinnear rejects sociological definitions of professionalism and relies instead on the more traditional definition that emphasizes service provision, post-secondary education, certification, and 'a degree of self-regulation' (p. 7). Kinnear asserts that nurses, like the female doctors, lawyers, university professors, and teachers that she studied, boasted sufficient workplace autonomy to qualify as professionals. Unfortunately, her analysis does not consider how that autonomy was shaped by nurses' daily interactions with members of the medical profession, or the divisive impact professionalizing strategies had on nurses themselves.

17. Celia Davies, 'Professionalizing Strategies as Time- and Culture-Bound: American and British Nursing, Circa 1893', in Lagemann, ed., *Nursing History: New Perspectives, New Possibilities*, p. 49. Jo Ann Whittaker uses Davies's model to assess British Columbia nurses' professional strategies. See Whittaker, 'A Chronicle of Failure: Gender, Professionalization and the Graduate Nurses' Association of British Columbia, 1912–1935', MA thesis (Univ. of Victoria, 1990).

18. Nursing textbooks also address the question of professional successes. See, for example, Alice J. Baumgart and Jenniece Larsen, eds, *Canadian Nursing Faces the Future: Development and Change* (St. Louis, 1988); Janet Ross Kerr and Jannetta MacPhail, *Canadian Nursing: Issues and Perspectives*, 2nd edn (St Louis, 1991).

19. Similar models have been employed to conceptualize the class status of other white-collar or service workers, such as teachers. See Glen Filson, 'Ontario Teachers' Deprofessionalization and Proletarianization', *Comparative Education Review* 32, 3 (1988), pp. 298–317. Authors such as Filson, in his study of Ontario teachers since the 1930s, have stressed the declining wages and standard of living, changes in the labour process, and the working-class consciousness of white-collar workers, all of which define them as part of the proletariat.

20. David Wagner, 'The Proletarianization of Nursing in the United States, 1932–1946', *International Journal of Health Services* 10, 2 (1980), p. 283. For an overview of this process as it occurred within American nursing, see Susan Reverby, *Ordered to Care: The Dilemma of American Nursing 1850–1945* (New York, 1987), esp. chs 9, 10. See also Paul Bellaby and Patrick Oribabor, 'Determinants of the Occupational Strategies Adopted by British Hospital Nurses', *International Journal of Health Services* 10, 2 (1980), pp. 291–309.

21. Wagner, 'The Proletarianization of Nursing in the United States', p. 283.

22. Barbara Ehrenreich and Deirdre English, *Witches, Midwives, and Nurses: A History of Women Healers* (Old Westbury, NY, 1973), p. 4.

23. Ashley's *Hospitals, Paternalism and the Role of the Nurse*, p. v, begins with the statement: 'The book you are about to read could as well be titled "sexism is dangerous to your health."' See also Sheila Bunting and Jacquelyn C. Campbell, 'Feminism and Nursing: Historical Perspectives', *Advances in Nursing Science* 12, 4 (1990), pp. 11–24.

24. Baumgart and Larsen, eds, *Canadian Nursing Faces the Future*, p. 9.

25. Melosh, *'The Physician's Hand'*.

26. Reverby, *Ordered to Care*. In her introduction (p. 6) Reverby stated: 'I share much of Melosh's perspective but have cast my study back into the nineteenth century and within a broader historical framework of the political economy of the hospital's development.'

27. Darlene Clark Hine, *Black Women in White: Racial Conflict and Cooperation in the Nursing Profession 1890–1950* (Bloomington, Ind., 1989), pp. 188–9.

28. See also Nona Glazer, 'Between a Rock and a Hard Place: Women's Professional Organizations in Nursing and Class, Racial, and Ethnic Inequalities', *Gender and Society* 5, 3 (Sept. 1991), pp. 351–72.

29. Shula Marks, *Divided Sisterhood: Race, Class and Gender in the South African Nursing Profession* (New York, 1994).

30. Sociologists have been more willing to consider the interplay of social forces. See Pat Armstrong, 'Women's Health-Care Work: Nursing in Context', in Armstrong, Jacqueline Choiniere, and Elaine Day, *Vital Signs: Nursing in Transition* (Toronto, 1993). David Coburn's research assesses the relative importance of professionalization and proletarianization, and while he makes reference to social forces such as occupational segregation by sex and feminism, he does not integrate gender as an analytic category in any substantive way. Coburn, 'The Development of Canadian Nursing: Professionalization and Proletarianization', *International Journal of Health Services* 18, 3 (1988), pp. 437–56. See also William K. Carroll and Rennie Warburton, 'Feminism, Class Consciousness and Household-Work Linkages Among Registered Nurses in Victoria', *Labour/Le Travail* 24 (Fall 1989), pp. 131–45. Meryn Stuart's research on Ontario's public health nursing program in the post-World War I years explores the intersection of class, gender, and region. It examines public health work in northern communities as nurses negotiated their way through the conflicting needs of southern politicians, local governments, and physicians, and women needing and wanting improved medical care. See Stuart, '"Half a Loaf is Better

than No Bread": Public Health Nurses and Physicians in Ontario, 1920–1925', *Nursing Research* 41, 1 (Jan./Feb. 1992), pp. 21–7; Stuart, 'Shifting Professional Boundaries: Gender Conflict in Public Health, 1920–1925', in Dianne Dodd and Deborah Gorham, eds, *Caring and Curing: Historical Perspectives on Women and Healing in Canada* (Ottawa, 1994).

31. Judi Coburn, '"I See and Am Silent": A Short History of Nursing in Ontario', in Janice Acton *et al.*, eds, *Women at Work: Ontario, 1850–1950* (Toronto, 1974).

32. Suzann Buckley, 'Ladies or Midwives? Efforts to Reduce Infant and Maternal Mortality', in Linda Kealey, ed., *A Not Unreasonable Claim: Women and Reform in Canada 1880s to 1920s* (Toronto, 1979).

33. Coburn, 'The Development of Canadian Nursing', p. 453.

34. Martha Vicinus, *Independent Women: Work and Community for Single Women, 1850–1920* (Chicago, 1985). See also Brian Abel-Smith, *The Hospitals 1800–1948: A Study in Social Administration in England and Wales* (Cambridge, Mass., 1964).

35. Pauline Jardine, 'An Urban Middle-Class Calling: Women and the Emergence of Modern Nursing Education at the Toronto General Hospital 1881–1914', *Urban History Review* 17 (Feb. 1989), pp. 179–90. As evidence of nursing's elevated class status, Jardine cites superintendents' appeals for a 'better class' of recruit and the rising educational backgrounds of students over the 1881–1914 period. While it is true that the old-style working-class nurse was eradicated in those years, it was possible for single, working-class women to achieve the necessary educational requirements.

36. Harry Braverman, *Labor and Monopoly Capital: The Degradation of Work in the Twentieth Century* (New York, 1974). On the medical profession's authority over the division of labour in health care, see Eliot Freidson, *Profession of Medicine: A Study of the Sociology of Applied Knowledge* (New York, 1970).

37. For midwives, chiropractors, homeopaths, and other 'irregulars', medicine's legal authority has resulted in long-standing conflicts, which, current developments notwithstanding, medicine has usually won. David Coburn and C. Leslie Biggs, 'Limits to Medical Dominance: The Case of Chiropractic', *Social Science and Medicine* 22, 10 (1986), pp. 1035–46. For physiotherapists, occupational therapists, dietitians, and pharmacists, medicine's legal authority has resulted in subcontracting, in which the former are responsible for certain services but only under the benevolent supervision of the medical profession.

38. The four western provinces define a special category of registered psychiatric nurses, whereas psychiatric nursing is a subspecialty of

general nursing in the rest of Canada. See Baumgart and Larsen, eds, *Canadian Nursing Faces the Future.*

39. Mick Carpenter's criticism of nursing history for conflating a complex set of practices into one category of 'nurse' is well placed. He writes: 'Other branches [of nursing] receive scanty, if any, attention. . . . When we say "nurse",. . . everyone knows a general hospital nurse is signified.' See Carpenter, 'Asylum Nursing Before 1914: A Chapter in the History of Labour', in Celia Davies, ed., *Rewriting Nursing History* (London, 1980).

40. Marg Gorrie, 'Nursing', in E. Shorter, ed., *TPH: History and Memories of the Toronto Psychiatric Hospital* (Toronto, forthcoming).

41. I make this argument in Kathryn McPherson, 'Nurses and Nursing in Early Twentieth Century Halifax, 1900–1925', MA thesis (Dalhousie Univ., 1982). See also Susan Riddell, 'Curing Society's Ills: Public Health Nurses and Public Health Nursing in Rural British Columbia, 1919–1946', MA thesis (Simon Fraser Univ., 1991).

42. Clio Collective, *Quebec Women: A History* (Toronto, 1987), pp. 218–19.

43. Marta Danylewycz, *Taking the Veil: An Alternative to Marriage, Motherhood, and Spinsterhood in Quebec, 1840–1920* (Toronto, 1987).

44. The Montreal General Hospital established its training school in 1875, while the first program for French laywomen was initiated in 1897 at the Hôpital Notre-Dame. Clio Collective, *Quebec Women*, pp. 220–1. Johanne Daigle, 'Devenir infirmière: les modalités d'expression d'une culture soignante au XXe siècle', *Recherches féministes* 4, 1 (1991), pp. 67–86, examines the work culture developed within the apprenticeship system at one francophone and Catholic hospital school, l'école Jeanne Mance de l'Hôtel-Dieu in Montreal. Daigle analyses the nursing system at the Hôtel-Dieu in the context of the transformation of hospitals in Western industrial nations.

45. Edouard Desjardins, Eileen Flanagan, and Suzanne Giroux, *Heritage: History of the Nursing Profession in Quebec from the Augustinians and Jeanne Mance to Medicare* (Quebec, 1971). Relations among nursing organizations are discussed in ch. 6.

46. For example, Quebec nurses were the first to engage successfully in collective bargaining, in 1939, followed by British Columbia nurses in 1946. Phyllis Jensen, 'The Changing Role of Nurses' Unions', in Baumgart and Larsen, eds, *Canadian Nursing Faces the Future*, pp. 461–2.

47. Yolande Cohen and Michèle Dagenais, 'Le métier d'infirmière: savoirs féminins et reconnaissance professionnelle', *Revue d'histoire de l'Amérique française* 41, 2 (automne 1987), pp. 155–77; Johanne

Daigle, 'L'émergence et l'évolution de L'alliance des infirmières de Montréal: 1946–1966', MA thesis (Université du Québec, 1983).

48. For example, Elizabeth Medeiros's initial research into nursing at two Toronto Catholic hospitals run by the Sisters of St Joseph, St Michael's Hospital and St Joseph's, suggests that nuns who undertook nursing training were offered the most prestigious administrative postings, while graduate nurses who became nuns were placed as ward heads. Lay graduates of the two programs rarely earned hospital appointments. As well, nun-administrators of these Catholic hospitals used their religious communities and connections to develop an extensive network and mutual support system. Elizabeth Medeiros, 'Catholic Nursing in Toronto—1920s–1940s', unpublished paper, York University, 1990. See also Pauline Paul, 'The Contribution of the Grey Nuns to the Development of Nursing in Canada: Historiographical Issues', CBMH 11, 1 (1994), pp. 207–17.

49. Christian prayers and hymns were part of the daily morning ritual and annual graduation exercises of large lay hospitals such as the WGH, VanGH, and Halifax's VicGH. All nurses were expected to attend, regardless of their personal religious beliefs. Anne Ross, tape-recorded interview by author, Winnipeg, 4 Aug. 1988.

50. Agnes Calliste, 'Women of "Exceptional Merit": Immigration of Caribbean Nurses to Canada', Canadian Journal of Women and the Law 6, 1 (1993), pp. 85–103.

Chapter 2

1. NSH, *44th Annual Report*, 1900–1, *JHA*, vol. 1 (Halifax, 1901).

2. The 1901 census lists only 280 women, and no men, in the category of 'nurses and midwives', although the number of practising midwives especially probably was undercounted. In 1911, the newly defined census category 'nurses and nurses-in-training' listed 5,600 members, nearly 20 times the number of nurses and midwives counted in the 1901 census report. Of those 5,600, 124 or 2.2% were males. Between 1911 and 1921, the Canadian contingent of student and graduate nurses continued to increase, reaching 22,385 by 1921. This figure included 223 male nurses, who constituted 1% of the total nursing population but only .008% of the total male work-force. The 21,162 female nurses represented 4.3% of the female work-force, which itself had increased by one-third during the previous decade. See DBS, *Census of Canada*, 1901, 1911, 1921 (Ottawa).

3. The story of the old-style nurses has been retold so often that it has assumed mythic proportions. More concrete research is needed to learn

about the women who tended the sick in such mid-nineteenth-century hospitals as the Toronto General Hospital and Halifax's Victoria General Hospital, as well as in the Catholic institutions that had long relied on 'respectable' religious women to staff the wards. For an analysis of this transition in the English context, see Carol Helmstadter, 'Old Nurses and New: Nursing in the London Teaching Hospitals Before and After the Mid-Nineteenth-Century Reforms', *Nursing History Review* 1 (1993), pp. 43–70. See also Vicinus, *Independent Women: Work and Community for Single Women, 1850–1920* (Chicago, 1985), pp. 85–7. For the original character, see Charles Dickens, *The Life and Adventures of Martin Chuzzlewit* (Boston, n.d.).

4. Cited in H.E. MacDermot, *History of the School of Nursing of the Montreal General Hospital* (Montreal, 1940), pp. 7–8.

5. H.L. Scammell, 'History of the Victoria General Hospital', PANS, RG 25, C, vol. 45.

6. On nuns outside Quebec, see Pauline Paul, 'The Contribution of the Grey Nuns to the Development of Nursing in Canada: Historiographical Issues, *CBMH* 11, 1 (1994), 207–17. For discussions of religious nurses in Quebec, see André Petitat, *Les infirmières. De la vocation à la profession* (Montreal, 1989); Nicole Laurin, Danielle Juteau, and Lorraine Duchesne, *À la recherche d'un monde oublié, les communautés religieuses de femmes au Québec de 1900 à 1970* (Montreal, 1991). The contributions made by Catholic sisters to the development of American anaesthetics are discussed in Marianne Banckert, *Watchful Care: A History of America's Nurse Anesthetists* (New York, 1989).

7. Florence Nightingale letters to Maria Machin, 1873–9, MUA, MG 3046.

8. At WGH the number of graduates each year for the 1889–1900 years ranged from 3 to 13. WGHNAA, *Nurses' Alumnae Journal*, 1974.

9. Vancouver Trades and Labor Council, *Minutes*, 23 June 1893, 329, UBCA. I would like to thank Randy Wick for sharing this research with me.

10. This includes women like the widows who listed nursing as a part-time occupation on their applications for Manitoba homesteads in the 1890s–1910s. For example, see Government of Canada, correspondence with Susanna Hastings, 1905, PAM, GR 2060.

11. vicGH, *37th Annual Report*, 1902–3, JHA, vol. 1 (Halifax, 1903), stated that the extension of the hospital's nursing home, when completed, 'will satisfy an urgent need, and enable the management to meet the growing necessities of the Hospital in the nursing department.'

12. For a recent example of a Canadian hospital history, see David Gagan, *'A Necessity Among Us': The Owen Sound General and Marine Hospital, 1891–1985* (Toronto, 1990). Insightful American studies include Morris Vogel, *The Invention of the Modern Hospital: Boston,*

1871–1930 (Chicago, 1980); Charles Rosenberg, *The Care of Strangers: The Rise of America's Hospital System* (New York, 1987).

13. Available sources suggest that 57 of the 70 Canadian schools were three-year programs. John Murray Gibbon and Mary S. Mathewson, *Three Centuries of Canadian Nursing* (Toronto, 1947), p. 155.

14. Of this group, 72 had graduated before 1910, whereas the remaining 306 trained in the following decade when construction of new wards increased staffing needs. Anne S. Cavers, *Our School of Nursing, 1899–1949* (Vancouver, 1949).

15. The implication from these figures, that the ratio of nurses to beds was declining, is somewhat misleading. Unless factors like the number of special-duty nurses hired by patients or the rate of patient turnover could be measured precisely, any firm conclusions about staff/patient ratios cannot be drawn. vanGH, *Annual Reports*, 1905, 1920, vca, Add mss 320, series A.

16. vicGH, 'By-Laws and Regulations', *40th Annual Report*, 1905–6, p. 83. In 1918 the wGH reported 394 days of 'special nursing' by pupil nurses. wGH, *Reports and Accounts*, 1918, p. 38.

17. 'Social Service Information Hospitals', *Henderson's Directory* (Winnipeg, 1920).

18. See, for example, bGH, *Rules and Regulations for Nurses*, 1906, bGHA, box 55.

19. vicGH, *35th Annual Report*, 1900–1.

20. bGH, *Rules and Regulations for Nurses*, 1906; 'House Rules for Nurses', wGH House Committee, *Minutes*, 25 Aug. 1920, pam, mg 10, B, 2.

21. *cn* 10, 10 (Oct. 1914), pp. 573, 576.

22. Evelina Adams, 'Diary of a Nurse', *Manitoba History* 14 (Autumn 1987), pp. 23–8.

23. Mary Poovey, *Uneven Developments: The Ideological Work of Gender in Mid-Victorian England* (Chicago, 1988).

24. Ibid., p. 14.

25. Vicinus presents a more complex pattern of historical change in *Independent Women*, ch. 3, 'Reformed Hospital Nursing: Discipline and Cleanliness'.

26. vicGH, 'Report of Commissioners Appointed to Enquire into Management', *jha*, App. no. 15, 1896.

27. wGH, *Student Register*, 1903–6, wGHNAA, uncatalogued. See also vicGH, *Chronological Record of Ward Service*, Mar. 1912–Mar. 1920, pans, mg 20, vol. 1000, no. 1.

28. Historian of fashion Elizabeth Wilson argues that 'By the 1890s it had become customary for maid-servants to wear black, and, like nurses at

the same period, to have women's caps from an earlier period.' *Adorned in Dreams: Fashion and Modernity* (London, 1985), p. 36. Irene Poplin demonstrates that within German nursing the 'brilliant strategy to make the attire worn by Kaiserswerth nurses central to the strategy for reforming nursing and women's public role the nurse uniform acquired singular importance. It became an instrument for change.' 'Nursing Uniforms: Romantic Idea, Functional Attire, or Instruments of Social Change?' *Nursing History Review* 2 (1994), p. 164.

29. Nora Kelly, *Quest for a Profession: The History of the Vancouver General Hospital School of Nursing* (Vancouver, 1973), p. 36. At the Royal Jubilee in Victoria one student lost the right to wear her cap for a week when she failed to report a patient's death right away. Anne Pearson, *The Royal Jubilee Hospital* (Victoria, n.d.), p. 24.

30. vanGH Board of Directors, *Minutes*, 23 Apr. 1914, VCA, add MSS 320, Series A, vol. 2, listed salary scales for all hospital staff. The superintendent was paid $250 per month and the staff anaesthetist $225. The 'lady superintendent' received $150 and her staff between $50 and $75.

31. Annmarie Adams, 'Rooms of Their Own: The Nurses' Residences at Montreal's Royal Victoria Hospital', *Material History Review* 40 (Fall 1994), pp. 29–41.

32. For data on VicGH male nurses' wages, see VicGH, *Payroll Accounts*, PANS, RG 25, B, VI and VicGH, *Annual Report*, 1915–16. The Winnipeg General also tried a short-lived experiment with male nurses. In 1909–10 the WGH hired two male nurses, 'one on duty in the isolated ward for syphilitic cases and one in the men's ward for chronic tuberculosis.' No explanation was given for the termination of those nurses' employment, and male nurses were never again mentioned. See WGH, *Reports and Accounts*, 1900–40, and WGHNAA, *Nurses' Alumnae Journal*, 1974. The Vancouver General Hospital discussed the possibility of establishing a training school for male nurses, but that plan was never acted on. vanGH House Committee, Minutes, 5 Dec. 1907, VCA, MSS 320, series A, vol. 15.

33. While there is no evidence of any students being forced or encouraged to mask their ethnic origin, in 1920 *CN* published a report of the 1919 Canadian National Conference on Character Education, at which Jean Browne represented the CNA. *CN* reprinted a resolution submitted at that conference: 'That immigrants having non-British names be required to change their spelling or adopt new names, in order that none might know their original origin.' *CN* 16, 1 (Jan. 1920), p. 13.

34. See, for example, Coburn, '"I See and am Silent"', pp. 127–63; Alice J. Baumgart and Jenniece Larsen, 'Overview: Issues in Nursing Education', in Baumgart and Larsen, eds, *Canadian Nursing Faces the*

Future, pp. 316–17; Nora Kelly, *Quest for a Profession*. Susan Reverby makes a convincing argument for the oppressive educational methods employed in early twentieth-century American hospitals. She claims that 'emergencies and understaffing were the rule rather than the exception. Students frequently had to provide care in situations for which they were ill prepared.' The result was a teaching method of learning by rote. Susan Reverby, *Ordered to Care: The Dilemma of American Nursing* (New York, 1987), pp. 64–5.

35. Barbara Melosh, *'The Physician's Hand': Work Culture and Conflict in American Nursing* (Philadelphia, 1982); Tom Olson, 'Apprenticeship and Exploitation: An Analysis of the Work Pattern of Nurses in Training, 1897–1937', *Social Science History* 17, 4 (Winter 1993), pp. 559–76; Charles Rosenberg, *The Care of Strangers: The Rise of America's Hospital System* (New York, 1987), p. 221.

36. A.T. Frampton to secretary of the Labour Commission, letter, 3 Nov. 1913, PABC, RG 684, file 5, box 4. I would like to thank Linda Kealey for sharing this research with me.

37. In centres like Halifax, the proportion of women in manufacturing decreased over the 1911–21 years from 23% to 13% of the female work-force. DBS, *Census of Canada*, 1911, 1921. On the rise of clerical work for Canadian women, see Graham Lowe, *Women and the Administrative Revolution: The Feminization of Clerical Work* (Toronto, 1987). For studies of specific groups of women in factory and domestic work, see Acton *et al.*, *Women at Work*; Ruth Frager, *Sweatshop Strife: Class, Ethnicity, and Gender in the Jewish Labour Movement of Toronto, 1900–1939* (Toronto, 1992); Joy Parr, *The Gender of Breadwinners: Women, Men and Change in Two Industrial Towns, 1880–1950* (Toronto: 1990).

38. VicGH, *Nurses Register*, 1900–26, p. 1, PANS, RG 25, B, vol. X.

39. Between 1907 and 1912, WGH accepted one student for every 10 letters of inquiry, and VanGH reported similar figures. In 1915, perhaps inspired by the prospects in military nursing, 624 women requested applications for the WGH school. Only 172 completed the form and 81 were accepted. Of those, 17 never appeared at the school and, of the 64 who did begin their training, only 38 survived the probationary period. Some of those who failed to complete the first three months were asked to leave, but others quit of their own accord. WGH, *Reports and Accounts*, 1905–12, 1915.

40. Susan Reverby's data from the Boston City, Somerville, and Long Island hospitals revealed that during the 1900–19 years nearly 28% of the students entering training were born in the Maritimes. A further 5% had been born elsewhere in Canada. Some American institutions

actively recruited Nova Scotia women. The Somerville Hospital in particular relied on Maritimers, who represented 51% of that hospital's students from 1878 to 1939. Reverby, *Ordered to Care*, pp. 80–1.

41. Adams, 'Diary of a Nurse', p. 28.

42. WGH, *Student Register*, 1903–6. Olson calculated that at St Luke's Hospital in Minnesota non-graduates averaged only six months on duty before leaving the school, while graduates averaged 3.01–3.04 years in the 1897–1923 era. He concludes that 'The St Luke's data cast doubt on one of the most abusive practices with which hospital training has been charged, that nurses were used to meet labor demands and then dismissed when no longer needed.' 'Apprenticeship and Exploitation', pp. 564–5.

43. vicGH, *Records*, 1903–6, p. 27, PANS, RG 25, B, vol. 5.

44. Ibid., p. 79. Sometimes parents got involved. In October 1915, the vanGH board of directors discussed a letter from a Mr Thirdle 'complaining of his daughter being dismissed from the Training School for Nurses and asking for an appointment to meet the Board'. Dr MacEachern reported that Superintendent of Nurses Helen Randal had informed the irate father 'that his daughter was not dismissed, but her extended probation had not been satisfactory and as her whole service as a probationer had not been up to the standard she was not accepted'. vanGH Board of Directors, *Minutes*, 28 Oct. 1915.

45. Cited in F. Madeline Perry, *BGH—100: A History of the Brandon General Hospital 1883–1983* (Brandon, n.d.), p. 39.

46. *Vancouver Daily World*, 18 Aug. 1902, from 'Copied from Files Supplied by Mr Fish 1886–1945' (1945), VCA, MSS 320.

47. This story is apocryphal as Johns and Stewart both went on to establish international reputations in nursing, Stewart as professor of Columbia University's nursing program and Johns as editor of *Canadian Nurse* and as commissioned researcher for the Rockefeller Foundation's studies of nursing in Europe and the United States.

48. Ethel Johns, manuscript of unfinished autobiography, cited in Margaret M. Street, *Watch-fires on the Mountains: The Life and Writings of Ethel Johns* (Toronto, 1973), p. 26.

49. Ibid., p. 33.

50. See, for example, the recollections of Margaret Gemmell's first job in charge of the Victorian Order Hospital in Shoal Lake, Manitoba. Margaret Gemmell, *Memoirs*, n.d., BGHA, uncatalogued. Note that even small-town hospitals like that in Neepawa, Manitoba, hosted a nursing training school. See Adams, 'Diary of a Nurse'.

51. vanGH, *Annual Reports*, 1906, 1920. Ratios elsewhere were sometimes higher. At WGH in 1919 the staff of 23 graduate nurses supervised the work of 167 apprentices. WGH, *Reports and Accounts*, 1919, pp. 33–5.

52. A.T. Frampton, in his letter to the secretary of British Columbia's Board of Labour, appended the postscript: 'at night it is often the case that one Nurse has sole charge of 17 to 20 patients and in the day time the conditions are not vastly different.' Frampton, letter, 3 Nov. 1916.

53. vicGH, *Rules for Patients*, May 1904, PANS, RB 25, B, vol. 5, no. 8. The rules specified that patients were forbidden from gambling, loitering in hallways or washrooms, missing meals, spitting, making 'undue' noise, using profane language, or visiting with patients of the opposite sex. Nurses were expected to enforce these rules.

54. 'Guide for New Head Nurses' and 'Nurses in charge of Pavillion Floors', VicGH, Register of Nurses (c. 1920), PANS, RG 25, B, section X.37.

55. vanGH, *Annual Report*, 1908.

56. vanGH Board of Directors, *Minutes*, Special Meeting re: Salary Schedule, 23 Apr. 1914.

57. Domestic workers at the Victoria General Hospital earned $8–$10 per month in 1908. vicGH, 'Payroll Accounts', PANS, RG 25, B, VI, 13–15.

58. Ibid. In March of 1905, the superintendent of Victoria General Hospital earned $100, exactly twice that of the $50 per month the superintendent of nursing received. In 1915 this salary ratio was still in effect, as the superintendent of nursing earned $75 compared to the $158.33 earned by her male superior. The gap began to close somewhat in the post-World War I years, so that by 1920 the superintendent of nursing's salary had risen to $100 as compared to the $183.33 the head administrator received.

59. Edouard Desjardins, Eileen Flanagan, and Suzanne Giroux, *Heritage: History of the Nursing Profession in Quebec from the Augustinians and Jeanne Mane to Medicare* (Quebec, 1971), p. 86, argue that nuns 'received a remuneration that was kept at an extremely modest level to make good their vows to work for eternal salvation rather than worldly recompense.'

60. vanGH, Board of Directors, *Minutes*, Special Meeting, 10 Apr. 1916.

61. Linda White, 'Who's In Charge Here? The General Hospital School of Nursing, St. John's, Newfoundland, 1903–30', *CBMH* 11 (1994), pp. 91–118.

62. vanGH, House Committee, *Minutes*, 9 Jan. 1919.

63. Ibid., 23 Jan. 1919.

64. vicGH, *44th Annual Report*, 1909–10, p. 9. In 1912, the superintendent again asserted graduate nurses' 'desire to go into private practice or take special courses'. vicGH, *46th Annual Report*, 1911–12, p. 41.

65. In 1908 and 1912 the wGH *Reports and Accounts* listed the employment status of the women who had graduated since 1900: 42% of the 125

names in the 1908 report were categorized as 'private nurse', as were 36% of the 230 graduates cited in 1912.

66. MARN, *Registry Cards*, WGHNAAA, uncatalogued. Initially, provincial organizations used the term 'graduate nurse' in their titles, such as the Manitoba Association of Graduate Nurses. When registration legislation was passed, the term 'registered nurse' was incorporated into the title. For the sake of clarity the subsequent organizational title of 'Registered Nurses Association' is used throughout here, but please note that the original sources are often formally listed as from a province's 'Graduate Nurses Association' (GNA).

67. BGNA, Minutes, 6 Aug. 1918, BGHA. During World War I, the RNANS reduced its standard rates to $18 per week for general nursing and $21 for contagious cases. By 1919 a $3.75 per day fee had been reasserted. *CN* 13, 12 (Dec. 1917), p. 767; Ethel Redmond interview by author, Halifax, July 1981.

68. At $25 per week, nurses working 40 weeks earned $1,000 per year. Census figures for 1921 show that nurses in Quebec City earned, on average, $420 per annum while practitioners in Edmonton averaged nearly $750 per year. DBS, *Census of Canada*, 1921.

69. Peter Lambly, 'Toward a Living Wage: The Minimum Wage Campaign for Women in Nova Scotia, 1920–1935', honours thesis (Dalhousie Univ., 1977), p. 31; Michèle Dagenais, 'Itinéraires professionnels masculins et féminins en milieu bancaire: Le cas de la Banque d'Hochelaga, 1900–1929', *Labour/Le Travail* 24 (Fall 1989), pp. 62–3; see also Linda Kealey, 'Women and Labour during World War I: Women Workers and the Minimum Wage in Manitoba', in Mary Kinnear, ed., *First Days, Fighting Days: Women in Manitoba History* (Regina, 1987); Wayne Roberts, *Honest Womanhood: Feminism, Femininity and Class Consciousness Among Toronto Working Women, 1893–1914* (Toronto, 1976). Ruth Frager reports that in 1921, female garment workers averaged $620 per year. Frager, *Sweatshop Strife*, p. 20.

70. Ethel Redmond interview, July 1981. Redmond recalled that nurses 'had to do it all'. See also *CN* 11, 2 (Feb. 1915), pp. 73–5, which asserted that 'no medicine or disinfectant can take the place of nutritious food as a factor of recovery.'

71. WGH, 'Guide for Special Nurses on Duty in the Winnipeg General Hospital', Dec. 1912, PAM, MG 10 B 2.

72. *Might's Directory*, 1910 (Toronto). *CN*, 1909–20, contains many reports of nurses visiting sick family members.

73. WGH, *Reports and Accounts*, 1908. See also VicGH, *Annual Reports*, 1912–25, which reveal that of 159 students who worked as nurses after graduation, 26% worked in New England at some point. An even

greater proportion of Nova Scotia Hospital graduates took advantage of employment opportunities in American psychiatric institutions. Nearly 50% of the 1907–15 working graduates found work in New England institutions. NSA, *Annual Reports*, 1907–16.

74. Ethel Johns and Beatrice Fines, *The Winnipeg General Hospital and Health Sciences Centre School of Nursing 1887–1987* (Winnipeg, 1988), p. 47.

75. See Ruth Brouwer, *New Women for God: Canadian Presbyterian Women and India Missions, 1876–1914* (Toronto, 1990); Rosemary Gagan, *A Sensitive Independence: Canadian Methodist Women Missionaries in Canada and the Orient, 1881–1925* (Montreal, 1992).

76. RNANS, 'Report of the Registry from Sept. 1st to Aug. 31st 1918', PANS, MG 20, box 1.

77. MARN, *Registry Cards*, 1911–21.

78. 'Don'ts for Nurses', CN 16, 3 (Mar. 1920), p. 167.

79. For example, in 1917–18, the Halifax registry investigated rumoured complaints about registry nurses being slow to respond to calls. A registry official 'called up some of the doctors in the town and asked them if they had any fault to find with the way it was conducted. They all assured me they were quite satisfied . . . .' Helen F. Uniake, letter to Mrs Doyle, PANS, MG 20, box 1.

80. RNANS, *Report of the Registry Committee*, 16 Oct. 1918–16 Oct. 1919, PANS, MG 20, box 1. In 1926 the former registrar of the Winnipeg Nurses' Registry provided the WGH medical superintendent with information about Miss Sullivan. She had been listed with the Registry prior to 1921, 'her character was good and no complaints were ever received against her from either the doctors with whom she had cases or their patients . . . .' S.D. MacIntyre, letter to G.F. Stephens, 8 Jan. 1926, MARN, *Registry Cards*.

81. Sister Eva, *Private Nurse's Own Note Book* (London, c. 1905), pp. 17, 19, 21, 23, 25, 27.

82. WGH, *Rules for Special Duty Nurses*.

83. MARN, *Registry Cards*, 1910–21.

84. Mrs George Cran, *A Woman in Canada* (Toronto, 1916), p. 250.

85. Adriana R. Layton, letter to Miss Burgoyne, 15 Jan. 1920, PANS, MG 20, box 1.

86. Cran, *A Woman in Canada*, pp. 252–3.

87. RNANS, *Report of the Registrar*, 1918–19. In 1917 the RNANS had only 30 nurses on its registry. CN, 13, 10 (Oct. 1917), pp. 653–5.

88. 'Nurses Make Big Increase in Fees: Registry Announces Immediate Advance in Accord with Dominion-Wide Movement', *Winnipeg Free Press*, 11 May 1920. See also BGNA, *Minutes*, 15 Sept. 1918, which established the same hours of duty.

89. Dr Harry Watson, letter, 11 Feb. 1919, MARN, *Registry Cards*. The respected Dr Neil John Maclean, of Winnipeg's Maclean Mission, testified to the work of Mrs Newman, who 'has nursed for me and has given entire satisfaction. I wish to recommend her as a splendid nurse though not certified.' Ibid., 17 July 1911.

90. John Murray Gibbon, *Victorian Order of Nurses for Canada 1897–1947* (Montreal, 1947).

91. Denyse Baillargeon, 'Care of Mothers and Infants in Montreal between the Wars: The Visiting Nurses of Metropolitan Life, Les Gouttes de lait, and Assistance maternelle', in Dianne Dodd and Deborah Gorham, eds, *Caring and Curing: Historical Perspectives on Women and Healing in Canada* (Ottawa, 1994), pp. 163–81.

92. Katheryn McPherson, 'Nurses and Nursing in Early Twentieth Century Halifax, 1900–1925,' MA thesis (Dalhousie University, 1982), ch. 4.

93. The most innovative of the rural public health programs was that instituted by the United Farmers of Ontario government in 1920. See Meryn Stuart, 'Ideology and Experience: Public Health Nursing and the Ontario Rural Child Welfare Project, 1920–1925', *CBMH* 6, 2 (Winter 1989), pp. 111–31. On British Columbia's rural health project, see Susan Riddell, 'Curing Society's Ill's: Public Health Nurses and Public Health Nursing in Rural British Columbia, 1919–1946', MA thesis (Simon Fraser University, 1991). 'Curing Society's Ills'. See Alan Artibise, *Winnipeg: A Social History of Urban Growth, 1874–1914* (Montreal, 1975), for a review of Winnipeg's public health programs in the pre-World War I era.

94. Ethel Johns, 'Ideals of Public Health Nursing', *CN* (Mar. 1918), p. 909, cited in Riddell, 'Curing Society's Ills', p. 49.

95. For instance, in the years after 1907 the fee per visit for Halifax VONS was 50 cents, but nearly half the clientele did not pay. Agnes Dennis, 'Report of the Victorian Order, Halifax', *CN* 5, 8 (Aug. 1909), p. 426.

96. The original nursing staff of one was expanded to four in 1905, in which year alone over 7,000 home visits were made. A year later, a mutually beneficial affiliation with the Winnipeg General Hospital supplied the Mission with senior student nurses and permitted Mission work to grow substantially, to which the 1913 service record of 28,830 home visits attested. See Artibise, *Winnipeg*, pp. 191–2.

97. Meryn Stuart, 'Shifting Professional Boundaries: Gender Conflict in Public Health, 1920–1925', in Dodd and Gorham, eds, *Caring and Curing*. Such conflict continued throughout the inter-war years, as the fate of Eunice Dyke revealed. See Marion Royce, *Eunice Dyke: Health Care Pioneer* (Toronto, 1983).

98. MHHC, *Minutes*, 12 Nov. 1920, PANS, MG 20, vol. 199.

99. Buckley, 'Ladies or Midwives?' For a discussion of disillusionment among British Columbia's public health nurses, see Riddell 'Curing Society's Ills', esp. ch. 3.
100. Riddell, 'Curing Society's Ills', p. 8.
101. Dennis, 'Report of the Victorian Order, Halifax', Aug. 1909, p. 426; Jean S. Forbes, *History of the VON Halifax Branch, 1898–1947* (Halifax, 1947).
102. The company boasted that between 1911 and 1918 the mortality rate of policyholders had dropped by 18%. See Baillargeon, 'Care of Mothers and Infants', p. 165.
103. See Ina J. Bramadat and Marion I. Saydak, 'Nursing on the Canadian Prairies, 1900–1930: Effects of Immigration', *Nursing History Review* 1 (1993), pp. 105–7.
104. Mariana Valverde, *The Age of Light, Soap and Water: Moral Reform in English Canada, 1880–1925* (Toronto, 1991).
105. Dennis, 'Report of the Victorian Order, Halifax', Aug. 1909.
106. Kari Delhi, 'Health Scouts for the State: School and Public Health Nurses in Early Twentieth Century Toronto', *Historical Studies in Education* 1, 2 (1990), p. 260.
107. Stuart, 'Shifting Professional Boundaries', p. 54.
108. Riddell, 'Curing Society's Ills', pp. 31–3.
109. VON Halifax Branch, *List of Nurses*, 1917, PANS, MG 20, vol. 759, no. 1.
110. For an analysis of the complex, and often gendered, relationships between clients and social workers in the United States, see Linda Gordon, *Heroes of Their Own Lives: The Politics and History of Family Violence* (New York, 1988). Gordon (p. 297) argues that 'the whole welfare state, including particularly its regulatory organizations, derived to a significant degree from the feminist agenda of the late nineteenth and early twentieth centuries.' Relations between female nurses and patients under the Sheppard-Towner Act are explored in Molly Ladd-Taylor, *Mother Work: Women, Child Welfare, and the State, 1890–1930* (Urbana, Ill., 1994), pp. 177–82.
111. See Gordon, *Heroes of Their Own Lives*; Seth Koven and Sonya Michel, eds, *Mothers of a New World: Maternalist Politics and the Origins of Welfare States* (New York, 1993).
112. Julia Stewart, 'The Inception and Development of the Graduate Nurses' Association, Ontario, 1904–1926', *CN* 24, 2 (Feb. 1928), p. 66.
113. Dorothy G. Riddell, 'Nursing and the Law: The History of Legislation in Ontario', in Mary Quayle Innes, ed., *Nursing Education in a Changing Society* (Toronto, 1970), p. 19. Canadian women called this group the 'Society for Superintendents of Training Schools in United States and Canada'.

114. CNA, *The Leaf and the Lamp: The Canadian Nurses' Association and the Influences which Shaped its Origins and Outlook during its First Sixty Years* (Ottawa, 1968), p. 36.

115. Listed in CNA, *A Brief History of the Canadian Nurses' Association, founded 1908* (Winnipeg, n.d.), p. 6.

116. *Canadian Nurse* became the property of the CATN in 1916, when Miss Helen Randal was named national editor. Stewart, 'The Inception and Development of the Graduate Nurses Association', p. 67.

117. Quoted in Street, *Watch-fires on the Mountains*, p. 2.

118. When the St Boniface Hospital graduates established their alumnae association in 1905 the superintendent of the school was named honorary president. 'History of St Boniface School of Nursing', n.d., St Boniface School of Nursing Archives, uncatalogued.

119. For a more detailed discussion of alumnae association activities, see Kathryn McPherson, 'Skilled Service and Women's Work: Canadian Nursing, 1920–1939', Ph.D. diss. (Simon Fraser Univ., 1990). See also Ethel Johns, *The Winnipeg General Hospital School of Nursing, 1887–1953* (Winnipeg, 1953).

120. For instance, beginning in 1920, the WGHNAA honoured each graduating class with a dinner and took an active part in commencement exercises. WGHNAA, *Journal* (1962), pp. 33–4.

121. VanGH, *Nurses' Annual*, 1920.

122. CNA, *A Brief History*.

123. McDermott, *History of the School for Nurses of the Montreal General Hospital*.

124. Florence Paulson, tape-recorded interview by author, Winnipeg, 1 July 1987.

125. 'Summary of History of the Graduate Nurses Association of Ontario, 1904–1925' (1926), pp. 1–2, RNAO Library, History File #1.

126. Ibid., p. 5.

127. Desjardins, Flanagan, and Giroux, *Heritage: History of the Nursing Profession in Quebec*.

128. For example, in Brandon, Manitoba, Mrs B.A. Bigelow, wife of a prominent local doctor, remained on the BGNA 'Membership Register and Roll Call' through the 1918–20 years, occasionally hosting the monthly meetings. BGNA, *Minutes*, 4 Feb. 1919, and 'Membership Register and Roll Call', 1918–20, BGHA. Agnes Pafford, the moving force behind the Graduate Nurses Association of Ontario, was also a married woman who was not actively working but was actively organizing on behalf of her sisters. See Stewart, 'The Inception and Development of the Graduate Nurses' Association', p. 65.

129. Frances M. Moss, *A Brief History of the Years from the Beginning of the Associations in 1909 through 1934* (Halifax, 1979) p. 2.

130. Jo Ann Whittaker, 'A Chronicle of Failure: Gender Professionalization and the Graduate Nurses' Association of British Columbia, 1912–1935', MA thesis (University of Victoria, 1990), pp. 86, 164.

131. The RNANS registry was originally housed at Restholme and then moved to the Children's Hospital. CN 13, 1 (Jan. 1917), p. 742. When the BGNA founded its registry, BGH Superintendent of Nurses Christina McLeod served as registrar. BGNA, Minutes 6 Aug. 1918.

132. VicGHNAA, *Minutes*, 16 Nov. 1921.

133. In 1927 MARN gained control over graduates of 18-month training programs in mental, contagious, and obstetrical hospitals. MARN, 'Registration Act, Constitution and By-Laws', 1927, MARN Library, uncatalogued.

134. The 1913 Act respecting 'The Manitoba Association of Graduate Nurses', first assented to on 15 Feb. 1913, determined that 'Every person registered under this Act shall be known as a registered nurse, and any person not being registered under this Act assuming such title, or using the abbreviation "Reg.N." or in any manner representing that he or she is a registered nurse, or by false or fraudulent declaration attempting to procure registration under this Act, shall be liable . . . to a fine of twenty-five dollars, and in default of payment to imprisonment for a period not exceeding six months' (pp. 9–10).

135. For an analysis of the 1922 registration act in Ontario, see Lauretta Hazzard, 'Towards Professionalization: Ontario Nursing 1874–1925', MA thesis (Univ. of Western Ontario, 1991), pp. 93–114; Coburn, '"I See and Am Silent"'. On the BC campaign, see Whittaker, 'A Chronicle of Failure'.

136. 'Evolution of the Nurse', *Maritime Medical News* 18, 5 (May 1906), pp. 167–8.

137. CN 15, 6 (June 1919), pp. 16–17.

138. Whittaker, 'A Chronicle of Failure', pp. 58–63; Hazzard, 'Towards Professionalization', pp. 40–1.

139. Stewart, 'The Inception and Development of the Graduate Nurses' Association', p. 66.

140. Margaret MacKenzie, 'State Registration for Canadian Nurses', CN 7, 10 (Oct. 1911), p. 252.

141. Stewart, 'The Inception and Development of the Graduate Nurses' Association', p. 66.

142. The MARN registry in Winnipeg listed a variety of levels of nurses who boasted a range of qualifications and experience. The BGNA discussed the status of Voluntary Aid Detachment nurses who had returned to civilian nursing after garnering significant practical experience in military work. Members concluded that VADs 'who have done bedside nursing should be allowed one month for each year of Overseas service if they take hospital training.' BGNA, Minutes, 6 May 1919.

143. *CN* 7, 11 (Nov. 1911), p. 162.
144. *CN* 10, 4 (Apr. 1924), p. 232.
145. Street, *Watch-fires on the Mountains*, p. 42.
146. Beverly Boutilier, 'Helpers or Heroines? The National Council of Women, Nursing, and "Woman's Work" in Late Victorian Canada', in Dodd and Gorham, eds, *Caring and Curing*, examines the National Council of Women's decision, in 1900, to support professional nursing organizations. For an analysis of the relationship between American nurses and feminists, see Sandra Beth Lewenson, *Taking Charge: Nursing, Suffrage and Feminism in American, 1873–1920* (New York, 1993).
147. Histories of nursing emphasized the important interconnections between nurses and feminists. See, for example, Riddell, 'Nursing and the Law', p. 20.
148. *CN* 13, 4 (Apr. 1917), pp. 210–11. When suffrage was achieved, the RNANS proudly reported to their sisters across the country that 7,000 women had entered their eligibility for voting at City Hall. *CN* 13, 4 (Apr. 1919), pp. 1704–5.
149. Stewart, 'The Inception and Development of the Graduate Nurses Association', reviews this difficult process in Ontario, the last province to win nurses' legislation. Describing the bill presented to the Ontario legislature, Stewart wrote: 'No serious opposition was met till the bill came up for its third reading when it was violently opposed by representatives from ten boards of some of the small hospitals, as well as some of the larger ones. . . . The public press assailed the measure as "Trade Unionism" of the worst type, and members of the House heretofore friendly to it, became either indifferent or actively hostile. When the Committee of the House, which had the matter in hand, made its final report, the bill had been altered to such an extent as to nullify what the organization had in view.' For further discussion of medical and political opposition to nursing legislation, see Jo Ann Whittaker, 'The Search for Legitimacy: Nurses' Registration in British Columbia, 1913–1935', in Barbara K. Latham and Roberta J. Pazdros, eds, *Not Just Pin Money: Selected Essays on the History of Women's Work in British Columbia* (Victoria, 1984); McPherson, 'Nurses and Nursing in Early Twentieth Century Halifax'.
150. Melosh, *'The Physician's Hand'*, pp. 5–6.

Chapter 3

1. In part, the dearth of scholarly literature addressing nurses' daily practice reflects the particular emphasis educators have placed on program development and curricular reform. See, for example, Helen M.

Carpenter, *A Divine Discontent: Edith Kathleen Russell: Reforming Educator* (Toronto, 1982).

2. Nora Kelly, *Quest for a Profession: The History of the Vancouver General Hospital School of Nursing* (Vancouver, 1973), p. 11, states that 'The slowly-growing conviction that knowledge and understanding are required even to follow orders competently, and more that it was making but poor use of the nurse's potential abilities to keep her in ignorance, is perhaps the most important theme in the history of nursing education. The expanding knowledge and functions of the nurse and her evolving relationship with the physician and other health workers are the live issues in nursing today.'

3. Rondalyn Kirkwood, 'Blending Vigorous Leadership and Womanly Virtues: Edith Kathleen Russell at the University of Toronto, 1920–52', *CBMH* 11, 1 (1994), pp. 175–206.

4. Edith Kathleen Russell, 'A half century of progress in nursing', *New England Journal of Medicine*, 22 March 1951, pp. 1, 4.

5. Tony Cashman, *Heritage of Service: The History of Nursing in Alberta* (Edmonton, 1966), p. 215.

6. Donna Lynn Smith, 'Nursing Practice in Acute Care Hospitals', in Alice Baumgart and Jenniece Larsen, eds, *Canadian Nursing Faces the Future: Development and Change* (St Louis, 1988), p. 99.

7. S.E.D. Shortt, '"Before the Age of Miracles": The Rise, Fall and Rebirth of General Practice in Canada, 1890–1940', in Charles Roland, ed., *Health, Disease, and Medicine: Essays in Canadian History* (Toronto, 1984), pp. 123–52.

8. Barbara Keddy et al., 'Nurses' Work World: Scientific or "Womanly Ministering"?' *Resources for Feminist Research* 16, 4 (1987), p. 38. In another article Keddy asserts that 'the role of every nurse in that era was primarily that of housekeeper', an unusual conclusion given her evidence. See Keddy, 'Private Duty Nursing Days of the 1920s and 1930s in Canada', *Canadian Woman Studies* 7, 3 (1984), p. 102.

9. For an example of the discussion generated within academic nursing, see Helen K. Mussallem, '2020: Nursing Fifty Years Hence', in Mary Quayle Innes, ed., *Nursing Education in a Changing Society* (Toronto, 1970), pp. 209–24. Mussallem (p. 217) argues that 'the body of scientific knowledge of nursing is derived from and based on the principles of the behavioural, biological, and physical sciences.'

10. Margaret Connor Versluysen, 'Old Wives' Tales? Women Healers in English History', in Celia Davies, ed., *Rewriting Nursing History* (London, 1980), pp. 188–9.

11. Judi Coburn, '"I See and Am Silent": A Short History of Nursing in Ontario,' in J. Acton et al., eds, *Women at Work: Ontario, 1850–1930* (Toronto, 1974), p. 128.

12. Marianne Gosztonyi Ainley, ed., *Despite the Odds: Essays on Canadian Women and Science* (Montreal, 1990). While it is true that a contribution dealing with nursing may not have been available for this collection, nursing is not mentioned in the introductory essay as an area needing study or even theoretical consideration. Such exclusion is not unusual in the Canadian literature. For example, see *Canadian Woman Studies/les cahiers de la femme* 5, 4 (Summer 1984). This issue on 'Science and Technology' focuses on women in male-dominated occupations and the struggles for equal education, funding, and recognition in those fields. It also includes essays on the effects of technology on women, such as in clerical work. A recent contribution to the feminist journal *Women's Studies* reclaims nursing as a 'women's science' but focuses only on the scientific content of nursing work since World War II. See Celine Marsden and Anna Omery, 'Women, Science, and a Women's Science', *Women's Studies* 21 (1992), pp. 479–89.

13. Bryan Palmer, *Working-Class Experience: Rethinking the History of Canadian Labour, 1800–1991*, 2nd edn (Toronto, 1992), is one of the few surveys of Canadian labour history to mention nurses in discussion of work before 1950. Palmer's revised second edition states that 'while a minority of skilled female workers, such as stenographers and nurses, might command as much as $20 weekly, there were instances in the sweated or outwork situations of women earning fifty-three cents a week (in 1895) or the equivalent of two cents an hour (in 1901).' Most other labour histories, like Palmer's first edition, include nurses only when discussing late twentieth-century developments such as the new forms of managerial control nurses in the 1980s and 1990s have faced and nurses' use of strikes to gain improved working conditions. For an example of how a popular labour history depicts public health nurses ministering to working-class children, see, Craig Heron *et al.*, *All That Our Hands Have Done: A Pictorial History of Hamilton Labour* (Oakville, Ont., 1981).

14. Susan Reverby, 'A Legitimate Relationship: Nursing, Hospitals and Science in the Twentieth Century', in D. Long and J. Golden, eds, *The American General Hospital* (Ithaca, NY, 1989); Reverby, *Ordered to Care*; Melosh, *'The Physician's Hand'*.

15. The following categorization of nursing duties is based on interviews with retired nurses as well as on student notebooks, into which apprentices transcribed the various procedures they learned. See 'Senior Lecture Notes', 1 Oct. 1910–16 Jan. 1911; Furby Thorolfson, 'Notebook', 1924–7; Ruby Bowman, 'Notebook', 1925–8; Dorothy Nicholson, 'Notebook', 1926–9; Myrtle Bowman, 'Notebook', 1928–31; and Violet Erickson, 'Notebook', 1929–33, and 'Lecture Notes', 1929–33,

WGHNAAA, uncatalogued. See also Dorothy L. Brewster, 'Hygiene and Sanitation', 'Nursing Notes', *c.* 1925, MUA, MG 3084; Annie W. Buchanan, 'Diary', 1928, BGHA, uncatalogued.

16. 'Winnipeg General Hospital School of Nursing', WGH Alumnae *Annual*, 1928, pp. 70–2, WGHNAAA, lists the 'practical experience and theoretical instruction' given as tabulated from the year 1924–5. Nurses' oral testimonies and popular culture make frequent references to the various stages of apprenticeship, probationer or 'probie', junior, intermediate, and senior.

17. VICGH, 'By-Laws and Regulations for the Management of the Victoria General Hospital, Halifax, Nova Scotia', 1909, PANS, RG 25 B, vol. 5, no. 6, legislated that 'regular lectures shall be delivered and practical instruction given in the wards and at the bedside by the Attending and Resident Staff', but shortage of medical and nursing personnel meant that lectures were often cancelled during World War I. The 1917 Halifax explosion further disrupted the educational system at VICGH so that 'the lectures and classes of the Training School were greatly disorganized'. VICGH, *Annual Report*, 1917–18, JHA, vol. 1. Lecture schedules could also be disrupted when individual members of the medical house staff refused to participate. For example, BGH Superintendent of Nurses Birtles had to rearrange the lecture schedule for the fall of 1911 because one doctor 'preferred not to lecture this season'. BGH Board of Directors, *Minutes*, 12 Oct. 1911, BGHA, box 1, book 3.

18. Nurses were required to account for patients' belongings, and when a patient died they had to close out that record by ensuring that belongings were returned to the patient's family. VICGH, *Death Register: Patients Records, 1902–1906*, PANS, RB 25, B, 2–20.

19. Samples of lecture notes reveal instructors' initials and occasional comments, as do some of the student notebooks consulted. Erickson, 'Lecture Notes'; M. Bowman, 'Notebook'.

20. Erickson, 'Lecture Notes'.

21. Beryl Seeman, tape-recorded interview by author, Winnipeg, 8 July 1987.

22. Harriet Pentland, tape-recorded interview by author, Winnipeg, 13 June 1986, possession of author.

23. Some procedures, such as samples and smears, were sent to the hospital laboratory for analysis; other tests, such as the Wasserman, Dye, Ewald Breakfast, Reigal Meal, and Functional Renal Mosenthal tests, were performed on the ward. M. Bowman, 'Notebook'; Erickson, 'Notebook'; R. Bowman, 'Notebook'; Thorolfson 'Notebook'.

24. Seeman interview. See also the following tape-recorded interviews by author in PAM, Oral History Collection: Mary Duncan, Winnipeg,

22 June 1987; Violet McMillan, Winnipeg, 23 June 1987; Vera Chapman, Winnipeg, 2 July 1987. See Keddy, 'Private Duty Nursing Days of the 1920s and 1930s in Canada', pp. 99–102.

25. Pentland interview. See also McMillan interview; Thorolfson, 'Notebook'; Erickson, 'Notebook'. If being boiled for sterilization, gloves had to be covered with water and weighted down, dried inside and out, and examined for punctures. Unless requiring repair, they were then powdered and wrapped for transfer to the autoclave. Silk Guyon Catheters were damaged by Lysol or boiling and thus required disinfecting in 'Bichloride of Mercury 1–1000 or in Formalin 1/2%' followed by rinsing with sterile cold water before using. Other rubber articles—mackintoshes, medicine droppers, duodenal, stomach, and rectal tubes and catheters—and glassware all demanded specific regimens for cleaning and storing.

26. Pentland interview.

27. Erickson, 'Notebook', states that post-operative genital care was required as follows: 'After urination and defecation following repair of perinium, scraping and washing out of uterus childbirth and abortion'.

28. Ibid.

29. McMillan interview; Seeman interview.

30. In 1926 the WGH House Committee allocated $55 per floor to equip the private wards with flat silver. WGH House Committee, *Minutes*, 4 Jan. 1926, PAM, MG 10, B 2. Helen Smith recalled a reduced patient/nurse ratio on private wards, and the china cups in which private patients were served their tea, Helen Smith, tape-recorded interview by author, Winnipeg, 3 Aug. 1988. Myrtle Crawford stated that private patients had a choice of menus, and their food trays were set attractively, with cloth tray covers and cloth napkins. Myrtle Crawford, tape-recorded interview, Winnipeg, 2 Aug. 1988.

31. WGH House Committee, *Minutes*, 22 Oct. 1928.

32. WGH, *Blue and White*, 1923, p. 27, WGHNAAA.

33. For instance, VanGH introduced the eight-hour day for students in 1919, but persisting staff shortages prevented administrators from putting the 'new' schedule into effect until 1942. VanGH, *Annual Reports*, 1919 and 1942, VCA, add MSS 320, series A.

34. Jessie Law, tape-recorded interview by author, Vancouver, 7 Oct. 1986, possession of author.

35. Ethel Johns, WGHNAA, *Journal*, March 1925, pp. 5, 7.

36. R. Bowman, 'Notebook'.

37. B.W. Payton, 'Medicinal Leeching: The Golden Age', *CBMH*, 1, 1 (Summer 1984), p. 86, maintained that 'even respectable 20th century medical texts continued to mention [leeches'] use' and cited a 1949

British nursing text that instructed students 'of the correct way for preparing a trolley for leeching'. Leeches have been resurrected in modern medical practice.

38. VICGH, 'By-laws and Regulations', 1898.

39. As the English historian of nursing Anne-Marie Rafferty explained: 'control of disease implied control of the "environment", and this was interpreted broadly to include the physical and spiritual, human, hospital and external environments. Nursing was concerned with regulating those environments and placing the body in the best circumstances for nature to act upon it.' Anne-Marie Rafferty, 'Decorous Didactics: Early Explorations in the Art and Science of Caring, Circa 1860–90', in A. Kitson, ed., *Nursing: Art and Science* (London, 1993). Rafferty was summarizing the argument about post-Nightingale nursing made in Charles Rosenberg, 'Florence Nightingale on Contagion: The Hospital as Moral Universe', in Rosenberg, ed., *Healing and History* (New York, 1979).

40. 'Senior Lecture Notes', 1 Oct. 1910–16 Jan. 1911. At BGH the Ladies Hospital Aid Society proposed to purchase a new sterilizing plant in 1910. BGH Board of Directors, *Minutes*, 14 Apr. 1910.

41. Wilhelmina Mowat (Mowie) Waugh, ARRC, 'White Veils, Brass Buttons and Me: Memoirs of a Nursing Sister in World War I in the Canadian Army Medical Corps. 1915–1920', manuscript, n.d., BGHA, box 87.

42. In 'Listerim Unmasked: Antisepsis and Asepsis in Victorian Anglo-Canada', *Journal of the History of Medicine and Allied Sciences* 49, 2 (Apr. 1994), pp. 207–39, J.T.H. Connor argues that many medical practitioners were pragmatic about integrating elements of Lister's antiseptic surgical techniques without necessarily embracing the theoretical underpinning of Lister's procedures. Pointing to the parallel notions of a pure society and a pure operation, he writes (p. 238): 'the new operating amphitheatre of the 1890s may be viewed as the symbolic paragon of purity of the age . . . here was an environment—an inner sanctum in the temple of science—that typified the purity being sought in the outside world.'

43. Brewster, 'Hygiene and Sanitation'.

44. Given the complex debate regarding the changing historical definition and practice of 'science', a note of clarification is required here. John Harley Warner reminds us that '"science" always has been a freighted term'. Historians of science have viewed the biological sciences as vague and imprecise compared to the 'mathematically-grounded physical sciences', and believed that medical practice often failed to meet the criteria of scientific inquiry at all. On the other hand, the medical profession did win, in the late nineteenth century, the right to serve as

arbiter of scientific knowledge with respect to health care. Whether that right was based on the ideological authority of science or the efficacy of treatment, physicians wielded their social and political power with might. For the purposes of this paper, medical science refers to the body of knowledge developed and employed by the medical profession in the late nineteenth and early twentieth centuries. This definition is used here to measure nurses' engagement with 'science' as it was defined at the time. See Warner, 'History of Science and History of Medicine', *Proceedings: Conference on Critical Problems and Research Frontiers in History of Science and History of Technology* (Madison, Wis., 1991), pp. 395–422.

45. Erickson, 'Lecture Notes'.
46. See Ella M. Forrest, Supervisor, Infectious Disease Department, vanGH, 'Medical Aseptic Technique', *CN* 25, 12 (Dec. 1929), pp. 715–18. Mary Anderson left her home in North Sydney, Cape Breton, to train as a nurse in New York during the early 1920s. She recalls her bacteriology course and learning how to 'catch' bacteria in agar. Mary Anderson, interview with Anne Warren, Vancouver, Feb. 1989, BC Women's History Collection, Simon Fraser University Archives, Burnaby, BC.
47. R. Bowman, 'Notebook'.
48. Thorolfson, 'Notebook'.
49. R. Bowman, 'Notebook'.
50. See Braverman, *Labor and Monopoly Capital*, pp. 113–14, for a discussion of the distinction between conception and execution.
51. See Thorolfson, 'Notebook'.
52. Cali Dunsmuir, tape-recorded interview by author, Vancouver, Sept. 1986, possession of author.
53. While rules guiding the behaviour of nurses on and off duty did not entirely cloister the young women enrolled in the various schools, feminine respectability was demanded and parallels to female religious orders were not accidental. At the same time, the regular practice within hospital nursing schools of uniform inspection and standing at attention drew on the military model to instil obedience and discipline. As well, anthropological studies have emphasized the cross-cultural importance of ritual in the healing process. I would like to thank Kathleen McMillan and the members of the Ontario Society for the History of Nursing for bringing this latter point of comparison to my attention.
54. One nurse tells of a patient requiring a doctor's order to sleep with the blankets untucked. McMillan interview.
55. wGH, *Reports and Accounts*, 1920–39, PAM, MG 10, B 2.
56. Ibid., 1921, p. 16.
57. Reverby, *Ordered to Care*; Melosh, *'The Physician's Hand'*.

58. Percy S. Brown, 'A Few Facts about Scientific Management in Industry', *CN* 23, 11 (Nov. 1927), pp. 568–77.

59. Forrest, 'Medical Aseptic Technique'.

60. VicGH, *Chronological Record of Ward Service*, 2 Aug. 1912–Mar. 1920, PANS, MG 1000, no. 1; *Ward Nursing Register*, 1920–4, PANS, RG 25, B, X.10. For similar evaluations of students at WGH, see WGH, *Student Register*, 1903–6, WGHNAAA, uncatalogued. Like their hospital counterparts, VON supervisors boasted that VON training produced 'nurses with superior qualifications and marked executive ability'. VON, 'Report', *CN* 5, 12 (Dec. 1909), p. 769.

61. Ibid. Similar combinations of adjectives were used to describe Margaret Spence, recipient of VicGH's 1923 Gold Medal for General Excellence.

62. Thomas Olson, 'Laying Claim to Caring: Nursing and the Language of Training, 1915–1937', *Nursing Outlook* 41, 2 (Mar./Apr. 1993), pp. 68–72.

63. WGH, *Student Register*, 1903–6.

64. VON Halifax Branch, *List of Nurses*, 1917, PANS, MG 20, vol. 759, no. 1.

65. Hospital administrators constantly bemoaned the fact that they could not retain RNs in staff positions. Graduates might accept a staff position for a short time, but then quit to seek work in the private health-care market. In 1920 Superintendent of Nurses Charlotte Powell reported that she had received 37 requests from other institutions seeking staff nurses, 'but owing to the fact that so many of our graduates are interested in private duty nursing we were unable to supply very many.' WGH, *Reports and Accounts*, 1920, p. 39.

66. McMillan interview; Erickson, 'Notebook'; Thorolfson, 'Notebook'.

67. McMillan interview. In 1930 the average residence for patients at WGH was 16 days. For the next decade that figure hovered between a low of 13.4 days and a high of 15.2. 'Comparative Statistical Statement for the Past Ten Years', WGH, *Reports and Accounts*, 1940, p. 24.

68. R. Bowman, 'Notebook'.

69. Every graduate nurse interviewed insisted that a massage and a cup of hot milk before bed accomplished what sedatives now do for hospital patients. See, for example, McMillan interview.

70. Waugh, 'White Veils, Brass Buttons and Me'.

71. *CN*, 1932, p. 246.

72. For a discussion of the difficulties facing rural nurses, see Kathryn McPherson, '"The Country is a Stern Nurse": Rural Women, Urban Hospitals and the Creation of a Western Canadian Workforce, 1920–1940', *Prairie Forum* 20, 2 (Fall 1995), pp. 175–206.

73. MSNM, *Nursing Procedure in District Work* (c. 1935), PANS, MG 10, B 9, file 1673. Even Montreal General Hospital students, who received extensive training in obstetrical care at the progressive Montreal

Maternity Hospital, were denied direct instruction in delivery techniques. See Brewster, 'Nursing Notes'.

74. Isabel Cameron, tape-recorded interview by author, Winnipeg, 1 July 1987.

75. Letter, 13 Apr. 1924, PANS, MG 20, box 1.

76. Isabel Cameron knew enough to slap a newborn she had just delivered, but that was all she knew. Cameron, interview. Other nurses shared similar experiences. For example, Grace Parker was called to attend a birth during her training at the Margaret Scott Mission, only to arrive and discover the woman did not have a doctor. By the time the interns from WGH arrived, the baby was born. Grace Parker, tape-recorded interview by author, Winnipeg, 25 June 1987. Olive Irwin regretted not receiving better obstetrical instruction when, as a VON nurse, she alone had to deliver a baby with its umbilical cord wrapped around its neck. Olive Irwin, tape-recorded interview by author, Winnipeg, 3 Aug. 1988. See also Florence Paulson, tape-recorded interview by author, 1 July 1987.

77. Paulson interview. Margaret Scott Nursing Mission staff learned that upon entering a patient's house: 'Cuffs are then removed, and the sleeves rolled above the elbows and apron put on. After opening the bag and removing one serviette, soap and towel (serviette being placed on a table protected by newspapers), the nurse washes her hands and then removes other necessary articles from the bag, arranging them on paper serviette . . . .' MSNM, *Nursing Procedure in District Work*. See also *History of the VON Halifax Branch*, PANS, BM 20, vol. 893, for a description of the absorbent cotton, baby clothes, pillow cases, flannelette nightgowns, cheesecloth handkerchiefs for tuberculosis patients, and other supplies for maternity, medical, and surgical nursing that VON nurses carried with them in 1907.

78. James Crampton, 'It's been a healthy 75 years: Pioneer public health nurses remember the old days', *Winnipeg Free Press Weekly*, 17 Dec. 1991, p. 4. This story, based on an interview with retired public health nurses Mary Wilson and Jessie Williamson, includes a photograph of the two women holding a public health nurse's black bag, with its contents laid out on a sterile apron.

79. Marjorie Leonard, 'Memoirs' and 'Patent Certificates', PABC, Add MSS 2308, box 1.

80. Erickson, 'Notebook'; R. Bowman, 'Notebook'.

81. See, for example, Ann M. Forrest, Lady Superintendent, The Queen Alexandra Sanatorium, Long, Ont., 'Increase of Tuberculosis Among Nurses', CN 27, 11 (Nov. 1931), pp. 578–81; H.B. Cushing, MD, Montreal, 'Erythema Nodosum Among Nurses', CN 23, 6 (June 1928), pp. 286–7.

82. Erickson, 'Lecture Notes'.

83. vicGH, *Ward Nursing Registers*, 1920–42, PANS, RG 25, B, vol. IX, lists the many health problems afflicting student nurses.

84. Crawford interview.

85. Paulson interview; Irwin interview; Anne Ross, tape-recorded interview by author, Winnipeg, 4 Aug. 1988.

86. Susan Porter Benson, *Counter Cultures: Saleswomen, Managers and Customers in American Department Stores, 1890–1940* (Urbana, Ill., 1986), p. 6.

87. Martha Riggs, interview by author, Halifax, May 1982.

88. Ruth Freygood, letter to Nursing Service Bureau, 2 Mar. 1938, OIIQ Archives, box 5, folder 3.

89. Wilfred V. White, letter to Secretary of the Registered Nurses Association, Halifax, 23 Jan. 1933. The Brandon General Hospital received a similar request in 1940 when a Moose Jaw man complained to BGH officials about a private-duty nurse who had attended his wife at the BGH the previous year. He demanded that the nurse in question be 'struck off the register', but also took the opportunity to 'condemn the Brandon General Hospital' for treatment he received some years previously. BGH Board of Directors, *Minutes*, 9 Feb. 1940.

90. Cross interview.

91. Crawford interview.

92. Dunsmuir interview. Given the danger of anaesthetics, nursing technique for 'Putting an Anaesthetized Patient to Bed' was time-consuming: 'Take and record pulse every fifteen minutes for the first hour, then hourly to the fourth hour. . . . Then every four hours until normal.' Violet Erickson, 'Notebook'.

93. Shepherd interview.

94. Crawford interview.

95. Another WGH graduate, Beryl Seeman, recalled that every 11 November, McGillvray, a World War I veteran, 'used to get into her army regalia and sell poppies. She was quite a character and we were very fond of her.' Seeman interview. In smaller training schools, the superintendent of nursing could also win the favour of students by pitching in to complete the ward work. See Buchanan, 'Diary', for description of BGH Superintendent Birtles's ward work.

96. E. Johns, letters to M. MacEachern, 22, 25 June 1921, VCA, Add MSS 320, vol. 10, file 94.

97. Pentland interview.

98. vanGH House Committee, *Minutes*, 20 Aug. 1918, VCA, Add MSS 320, series A, vol. 19. Other records reveal that burns and mistakes with medications were constant concerns for hospital administrators. See

Ibid., 12 June 1919. See also WGH, *Student Register*, 1903–6. For example, WGH student Bess Cooper 'Gave Mr E. a hypo of [morphine] by mistake.' Maryann Dunn burned a baby with a hot-water bag and also gave a patient hydrogen peroxide instead of magnesium sulphate and then 'carelessly left bottle of 1/25 Bicholoride on delirious patient's table.' Sally O'Connor 'let' an elderly patient fall out of bed, did not report the fall, and the next morning the patient was diagnosed with a broken leg.

 99. Crawford interview; Duncan interview.
100. President, RNANS, correspondence with C.H.L. Sharman, Chief, Narcotic Division, Dept. of Health, 15 Nov. 1927, 16 Oct. 1935, and 25 Feb. 1936, PANS, MG 20, box 2.
101. Dr Bigelow, letter to W. Mitchell, June, 1937, private collection, W. Nichol.
102. Nurses' own records of patient care could also provide a measure of protection. A BGH grad of 1925, Jean Campbell Poynter, donated a blank set of notes to the BGH Archives, the type 'we used to buy from the drug stores when we were on private duty in homes in town or in the country.' Crawford's Drug Store, *Bedside Notes* (n.d.), BGHA, uncatalogued.
103. Letters to Miss Fraser, RNANS, 5 July 1928, 15 Feb. 1929, PANS, MG 20, box 1.
104. Braverman, *Labor and Monopoly Capitalism*. For a review of the deskilling of male clerical workers, see D. Lockwood, *The Black Coated Worker* (London, 1966); Marjery Davies, *Woman's Place is at the Typewriter: Office Work and Office Workers 1870–1930* (Philadelphia, 1982).
105. For a discussion of the feminization of deskilling of clerical work in Canada, see Graham Lowe, *The Administrative Revolution: The Feminization of Clerical Work* (Toronto, 1987).
106. As Barbara Melosh argues in her critique of nursing professionalism, 'as professional leaders strove to distinguish their work from women's unpaid domestic nursing, they had to disassociate themselves from the sentimental conception of womanly service.' Melosh, *'The Physician's Hand'*, p. 25.
107. This was especially true given the early twentieth-century efforts to make housework scientific. For a description of the domestic science programs in Canada, see Barbara Riley, 'Six Saucepans to One: Domestic Science vs the Home in British Columbia, 1900–1930', in Barbara K. Latham and Roberta J. Pazdro, eds, *Not Just Pin Money: Selected Essays on the History of Women's Work in British Columbia* (Victoria, 1984).
108. Seeman interview.

109. Crawford interview.
110. Riggs interview.
111. WGH, *Blue and White*, 1936, p. 36.
112. Ibid., 1927, p. 62.
113. VanGH, *Nurses Annual*, 1928, VGHNAAA, uncatalogued.
114. M.R. Gay, 'Scrubs', ibid., 1926, p. 34.
115. WGH, *Blue and White*, 1923, p. 20.
116. Ibid., 1928.
117. Ibid., 1926, p. 53.
118. MGH, *Blue and Gold*, 1931, p. 25, MGHNAAA, uncatalogued.
119. See Ainley, *Despite the Odds*. See also Veronica Strong-Boag 'Canada's Women Doctors: Feminism Constrained', in L. Kealey, ed., *A Not Unreasonable Claim: Women and Reform in Canada, 1880s to 1920s* (Toronto, 1979).
120. This of course was a primary reason for many nursing educators and leaders to battle for university schools of nursing wherein a discrete body of knowledge, and therefore professional status, could be developed.
121. Manitoba, Provincial Board of Health, *Regulations Respecting Public Health Nurses* adopted at a meeting of the board held on 12 June 1919, pp. 10, 13, WGHNAAA.
122. George Weir, *Survey of Nursing Education in Canada* (Toronto, 1932).
123. Londa L. Schiebinger, *The Mind Has No Sex? Women in the Origins of Modern Science* (Cambridge, Mass., 1989).
124. The best-known example of this orientation is Elizabeth Fox Keller, *A Feeling for the Organism: The Life and Work of Barbara McClintock* (New York, 1983). The term 'different voice' was coined by Carol Gilligan: *In a Different Voice: Psychological Theory and Women's Development* (Cambridge, Mass., 1982). For a review of the various approaches to women and science, see Sue V. Rosser, 'Feminist Scholarship in the Sciences: Where Are We Now and When Can We Expect a Theoretical Breakthrough?' in Nancy Tuana, ed., *Feminism and Science* (Bloomington, Ind., 1989).
125. See, for example, Riley, 'Six Saucepans to One'.
126. Thomas Kuhn, *The Structure of Scientific Revolutions* (Chicago, 1970) presented a powerful argument for thinking about science as a paradigm rather than an absolute truth. Kuhn asserted that scientific paradigms are accepted, or rejected and replaced, as the best available explanation for the natural world according to the beliefs and values of the day. As beliefs change, so, too, are new explanatory paradigms of 'science' introduced. This has led many historians to emphasize the legitimizing function that science has played, particularly in areas such as medicine. Authors such as Sam Shortt and Colin Howell have

claimed that medical professionalization was based on claims of scientific knowledge more than on any proven record of treatment. See S.E.D. Shortt, 'Physicians, Science, and Status: Issues in the Professionalization of Anglo-American Medicine in the Nineteenth Century', *Medical History* 27, 1 (1983), pp. 51–68. See also Colin Howell, 'Reform and the Monopolistic Impulse: The Professionalization of Medicine in the Maritimes', *Acadiensis* 11, 1 (Autumn 1981), pp. 3–22; Howell, 'Elite Doctors and the Development of Scientific Medicine: The Halifax Medical Establishment and 19th Century Medical Professionalism', in Roland, ed., *Health, Disease and Medicine*.

Chapter 4

1. DBS, *Census of Canada*, 1921, 1931, 1941 (Ottawa). The few men who did define themselves as graduate nurses to the census takers were never reported by other sources, neither in hospital records nor in nursing association reports.

2. G. Weir, *Survey of Nursing Education in Canada* (Toronto, 1932); DBS, *Census of Canada*, 1941. In 1941, 90% of non-military nurses were unmarried, while 5% were married, 4% widowed, and 1% divorced or separated. In 1941, only 80% of working women (not including active service) were single, 10% married, 7% widowed, and 3% divorced or separated.

3. Veronica Strong-Boag, *The New Day Recalled: Lives of Girls and Women in English Canada, 1919–1939* (Toronto, 1988), pp. 94–5. In her study of American working women during the 1930s, Lois Scharf discovered that in 1940 'nurses constituted the smallest proportion of working wives in any group of professional women', a trend caused both by discrimination and by the structure of nursing work. 'Nurses associated with hospitals were sometimes expected to live on the premises, and private duty nurses often worked longer than average hours. . . . Both conditions made work combined with marriage difficult.' Lois Scharf, *To Work and to Wed: Female Employment, Feminism, and the Great Depression* (Westport, Conn., 1980), p. 103. For a discussion of the contributions made by women married to doctors, see Audrey Peterkin and Margaret Shaw, eds, *Mrs Doctor: Reminiscences of Manitoba Doctors' Wives* (Winnipeg, 1976), pp. 143–9.

4. Few married women, less than 0.4%, were admitted into hospital schools of nursing. Weir, *Survey of Nursing Education*.

5. This point was made clear to me by a number of female interview participants, and one husband, during an interview with his wife, volunteered the information that he had expected her to stop working after

their wedding. She did stop working regularly for pay, but clearly enjoyed her occasional terms substituting for absent nurses at the local Red Cross Hospital, Genesta McMullan, interview by author, Hantsport, Nova Scotia, Apr. 1982. Reminiscences collected by the WGH class of 1928 include several stories of women returning to nursing when marital finances necessitated. Mary Shepherd, ed., 'The 1928 Class: 28 Years Later', WGHNAAA. The same claim was made for British Columbia by F. Eaton in *Report of the Advisory Committee*, p. 7. 'In most sections of the province it is possible to secure temporary and part time help in the immediate district for the reason that graduate nurses, married and resident are often available for temporary work.' For a discussion of doctors' wives who used their nursing training to assist in their husbands' medical practices, see Peterkin and Shaw, eds, *Mrs Doctor*.

6. Weir, *Survey of Nursing Education*, pp. 69, 97; DBS, *Census of Canada*, 1941.

7. See, for example, data on ages of working women presented in DBS, *Census of Canada*, 1931.

8. Weir, *Survey of Nursing Education*. Entrance standards for most Canadian hospitals included minimum age of 19 years and maximum age of 30–5 years; minimum education of grade 10 or 11; certification from a physician that the applicant was in good health; and a letter from a clergyman or medical practitioner testifying to the applicant's 'character' or 'personality'. See McPherson, 'Skilled Service and Women's Work', pp. 142–4.

9. For a discussion of women teachers in Canada, see Alison Prentice, 'The Feminization of Teaching', in Susan Mann Trofimenkoff and Alison Prentice, eds, *The Neglected Majority: Essays in Canadian Women's History* (Toronto, 1977); Susan E. Houston and Alison Prentice, *Schooling and Scholars in Nineteenth-Century Ontario* (Toronto, 1988), pp. 67–9, 179–83; Marta Danylewicz, Beth Light, and Alison Prentice, 'The Evolution of the Sexual Division of Labour in Teaching: A Nineteenth-Century Ontario and Quebec Case Study', *Histoire sociale/Social History* 16, no. 31 (May 1983), pp. 81–109.

10. RNAO, no title, Toronto, 4 Apr. 1923, RNAO Archives, uncatalogued.

11. See Strong-Boag, *The New Day Recalled*, ch. 1, for a discussion of girls' increased educational opportunities at the public school level during the inter-war years.

12. DBS, *Census of Canada*, 1941. An even greater proportion of student nurses, 63%, fell into the 9–12 years of school category, while another 35% had over 13 years of education.

13. Mary Shepherd, tape-recorded interview by author, Winnipeg, 18 June 1987; Mabel Lytle, tape-recorded interview by author, Winnipeg,

30 June 1987; Olive Irwin, tape-recorded interview by author, Winnipeg, 3 Aug. 1988; Ingibjorg Cross, tape-recorded interview by author, Vancouver, 20 July 1988; Isabel Cameron, tape-recorded interview by author, Winnipeg, 1 July 1987; Grace Parker, tape-recorded interview by author, Winnipeg, 25 June 1987; Anne Ross, tape-recorded interview by author, Winnipeg, 4 Aug. 1988; Beryl Seeman, tape-recorded interview by author, Winnipeg, 8 July 1987.

14. DBS, *Census of Canada*, 1921, 1931, 1941.

15. Ibid., 1931.

16. From at least 1917, VanGH had acknowledged that women of Chinese and Japanese descent were entitled to enrol, although the first students were not admitted until 1932. For the details of the long-running debate regarding the admission of Chinese and Japanese women to the VanGH nursing program, see VanGHNAA, *Minutes*, 1908, May 1910, May 1917, 1932, VanGHNAAA. For a discussion of the experiences of Chinese women in British Columbia, see Tamara Adilman, 'A Preliminary Sketch of Chinese Women and Work in British Columbia 1858–1950', in Barbara K. Latham and Roberta J. Pazdro, eds, *Not Just Pin Money: Selected Essays on the History of Women's Work in British Columbia* (Victoria, 1984).

17. Letter to G. Roberts, President, Toronto Coloured Liberal Association, 14 July 1940, PAO, RG 10-107-0-166, container 23, file #1, 'Nurses (Training) etc.' 1939–40.

18. Miss A.M. Munn, RN, Director, Nurses' Registration, Letter to Dr B.T. McGhie, deputy minister of health, 2 Oct. 1940, ibid.

19. I would like to thank Margaret Gorrie for sharing this research with me. G. Roberts, president, Toronto Coloured Liberal Association, letter to Hon. Harold Kirby, minister of health, 19 July 1940, and B.T. McGhie, MD, deputy minister, letter to G. Roberts, president, Toronto Coloured Liberal Association, 26 July 1940, ibid.

20. The breadth of some of Weir's categories weaken the usefulness of his data, particularly with respect to the 'business and clerical worker' grouping, which included a range of employees (from foremen to office staff) with diverse socio-economic statuses. As well, his category 'farmers' included ranchers and fruit growers as well as family farmers and homesteaders, occupations requiring very different kinds of labour and capital. There is also evidence to suggest that Weir's survey inadequately represented French-speaking nurses everywhere but especially in Quebec. The fact that Weir was unable to administer his intelligence tests in French and that, while his results were translated from English, the Quebec association informed the CNA that 'there is very little demand for the French copy of the Survey Report' brought into question

the representation of French-speaking nurses in his sample. Of the 2,280 sent out to Quebec nurses, only 764 questionnaires were returned completed (33% as compared to 34% in Ontario, 46% in the Maritime provinces, 59% from the prairie provinces, and 64% from BC).

21. *Henderson's Directory* (Winnipeg, 1929–33).
22. Jean Ewen, *Canadian Nurse in China* (Toronto, 1981), p. 10.
23. See Ross Hamilton, ed., *Prominent Men of Canada, 1931–32* (Montreal, 1932), p. 595, for a brief biography of Farmer.
24. *Henderson's Directory*, 1931. This directory listed 204 unmarried nurses who lived with their families. Of the 118 whose fathers were currently employed, 34% were clearly working class, 12% were employed in unspecified capacities in various companies, 28% were in white-collar managerial or administrative postings, and 25% were either professional or businessmen.
25. Ibid. I would like to thank Margaret McPherson for tabulating these results for me.
26. Ibid.
27. Calculated from WGH, *Blue and White*, 1924–39, WGHNAAA. Most years, the yearbook included under their photographs the home towns of graduates.
28. Calculated from MGH, *Blue and Gold*, 1921–33, MGHNAAA, uncatalogued. For a day-by-day account of the experiences of one farm girl in the Brandon General Hospital school, see Annie W. Buchanan, 'Diary', 1928, BGHA, uncatalogued.
29. Calculated from VanGHNAAA, *Annuals*, 1925–50.
30. Calculated from VicGH, *Annual Reports*, 1934–41, PANS, RG 25 B.
31. Joy Parr, *Labouring Children: British Immigrant Apprentices to Canada, 1869–1924* (London, 1980), pp. 128–9.
32. For a discussion of the difficulties faced by women in the prairie West who remained in rural economies, see Veronica Strong-Boag, 'Pulling in Double Harness or Hauling a Double Load: Women, Work and Feminism on the Canadian Prairie', *Journal of Canadian Studies* 21, 3 (Fall 1986), pp. 32–52; Eliane Leslau Silverman, *The Last Best West: Women on the Alberta Frontier, 1880–1930* (Montreal, 1984); Paul Voisey, *Vulcan: The Making of a Prairie Community* (Toronto, 1988), pp. 31–2, 158–9.
33. Paul Voisey discovered that the sex ratio 'never balanced completely, not in new rural communities like Vulcan, not even in the century-old ones of Ontario . . . neither rural frontiers nor settled rural areas anywhere offered single women many opportunities to earn a living', and despite small-town demand for teachers, secretaries, store clerks, hotel waitresses, and telephone operators, between 1931 and 1936 females

'constituted more than half of those leaving the Vulcan area . . . while males accounted for over half of those entering it. . . . More often than men, single women fled to cities, where a variety of options abounded.' Voisey, *Vulcan*, p. 20.

34. Florence Polson's father was an employee of the general store in the Icelandic community of Gimli. Florence Polson, tape-recorded interview by author, Winnipeg, 1 July 1987; Shepherd interview; Mary Duncan, tape-recorded interview by author, Winnipeg, 22 June 1987; Harriet Pentland, tape-recorded interview by author, Winnipeg, 13 June 1986, possession of author.

35. Weir, *Survey of Nursing Education.*

36. See, for example, McMillan interview.

37. DBS, *Census of Canada,* 1921, 1931, 1941.

38. Martha Riggs was pleased to get accepted by the VicGH School of Nursing because, as she explained it, she was not good at secretarial work and only had the options of nursing, domestic service, or marriage remaining. Martha Riggs, interview by author, Halifax, May 1982. It is also worth noting that nurses from middle-class and agricultural families may have found that family enterprises in business or office work may not have produced obvious economic options for girls in the same way that connections in industry aided working-class women in securing paid employment.

39. Strong-Boag, 'Canada's Women Doctors'; Carlotta Hacker, *The Indomitable Lady Doctors* (Halifax, 1984). For numbers of women in selected professional occupations, see DBS, *Census of Canada,* 1931.

40. Between 10 and 50 nursing students per year were enrolled at the UBC School of Nursing during the 1920s and 1930s, compared to the average of 62 students per year who graduated from the VanGH school each year. Lee Stewart, *'It's Up to You': Women at UBC in the Early Years* (Vancouver, 1990), ch. 3. For an analysis of gender and administrative power at the University of Toronto, see R. Kirkwood, 'Blending Virtues of the Good Woman with Powers of Leadership', *CBMH* 11, 1 (1994), pp. 175–206.

41. In an earlier era, one of Winnipeg's most famous graduate nurses, Ethel Johns, chose nursing because of the influence of an older woman. Johns's father, the schoolteacher on the Ojibway reserve at Wabigoon, died when Johns was a teenager. Ethel pursued nursing education when E. Cora Hind persuaded the younger woman to enrol at WGH. See Margaret Street, *Watch-fires on the Mountains: The Life and Writings of Ethel Johns* (Toronto, 1973), pp. 16–19.

42. Seeman interview.

43. Cross interview. Cross recalled that she and her teammates were paid

$5 per player when they won a district baseball game. At other sports days she won cash prizes in the various sprints.

44. Parr, *Labouring Children*, p. 129.

45. Jo Mann, tape-recorded interview by author, Abbotsford, BC, 22 July 1988.

46. Ibid.

47. Chapman interview.

48. McMillan interview.

49. Mann interview. See also Shepherd, ed., 'The 1928 Class: 28 Years Later, 1956', to which graduates of the class of 1928 submitted short life histories. Stories such as that of one graduate who, after a military posting with the Canadian forces, married. She and her husband 'set out to make our fortunes on a mink ranch', but when in 1950 'we found ourselves with all our dollar signs on the wrong side of the ledger' she returned to nursing. See also 'Biography of Edna Wilson', n.d., author's personal collection, for the work history of a Dauphin General Hospital graduate of the 1916 class whose husband died suddenly, leaving Edna to support her two daughters. This she did, first serving as a superintendent of a small rural hospital, then returning to Regina where she 'had no difficulty in securing steady work at the Regina General Hospital and Grey Nuns Hospital'.

50. Calculated from VicGH, *Annual Reports*, 1925–30. At VanGH two-thirds of all graduates from the 1920–9 years were single in 1930. While the most recent graduating classes had very low rates of matrimony, even those classes that had graduated in the early 1920s listed nearly half their members as single in 1930. Calculated from VanGH, *Nurses Annual*, 1930. A report in 1922 to the Hospital Association from Dr Charles H. Mayo, Rochester, Minn., cited a study of St Mary's Hospital in Rochester showing that 31% of the nurses graduated from that school over the previous 10 years had married. 'Hospital Association, 1922: Round Table', *CN* 18, 12 (Dec. 1922), p. 764.

51. Weir, *Survey of Nursing Education*, pp. 75–7.

52. DBS, *Census of Canada*, 1931; Weir, *Survey of Nursing Education*. Data from Halifax in the early 1920s exemplify the division of the nursing work-force. The 1923–4 Halifax Nurses' Directory listed 204 registered nurses. Of those, 63 were employed on institutional staff, 8 worked for public health agencies, and 132 had private addresses. RNANS, *Registrar's Report*, 1924. In Ontario in 1923, 675 nurses 'have availed themselves of the privilege of registration in Ontario.' Of that number, 356 were in private duty, 237 in institutional work, 54 in public health, and 28 were housewives (presumably married women not actively seeking work but desiring to maintain their registration).

Of those, 53 had been registered elsewhere. RNAO, 'Untitled', 4 Apr. 1923.

53. DBS, *Census of Canada*, 1931. The census report also revealed that nearly one-half of graduate nurses lived and worked in Montreal and Toronto.

54. RNAO, *Registrar's Report*, 1924.

55. Lucy Hatch, RN, 'Private Nursing in Alberta', *CN* 16, 5 (May 1920), p. 200.

56. Maureen Carley, 'My Most Interesting Case', *CN* 25, 5 (May 1929), p. 249.

57. 'The Nurses' Registry', *CN* 23, 4 (Apr. 1927), pp. 196–8.

58. Buckley, 'Ladies or Midwives?'; Veronica Strong-Boag and Kathryn McPherson, 'The Confinement of Women: Childbirth and Hospitalization in Vancouver, 1919–1939', in Robert A.J. McDonald and Jean Barman, eds, *Vancouver Past: Essays in Social History* (Vancouver, 1986).

59. Annie C. Lawrence, 'Nursing in Rural Ontario', *CN* 18, 7 (July 1922), pp. 409–11.

60. Catherine De Nully Fraser, 'A Few Thoughts on Private Nursing', *CN* 21, 1 (Jan. 1925), pp. 21–2.

61. Weir, *Survey of Nursing Education*, p. 80. Weir reported that public health nurses also considered the hospital work schedule 'too regular'.

62. Mary A. Catton, 'Special Nursing in the Hospital', *CN* 18, 5 (May 1922), pp. 293, 291.

63. John Herd Thompson and Allen Seager emphasize the instability of the Canadian economy during the 1920s, as it varied over time and region, and contrast that reality with the image of the 'Roaring 20s' often borrowed from American literature. John Herd Thompson with Allen Seager, *Canada 1922–1939: Decades of Discord* (Toronto, 1985), pp. 76–103, 330.

64. Edith Gaskell, 'Nurses Are Not Selfish or Overpaid', *CN* 18, 1 (Jan. 1922), p. 26.

65. Sibella Barrington, 'Report', *CN* 20, 9 (Sept. 1924), p. 560.

66. These figures are calculated from MARN Central Directory Committee, *Reports*, 1924–9, and the MARN registration cards. Not all nurses remained in the association pool. Many migrated elsewhere and others obtained work through means other than the local registry. The number of nurses on MARN's Winnipeg call list remained relatively stable, numbering 267 in both 1922 and 1932, in spite of the annual additions graduating from city training programs.

67. For example, WGH reduced the number of students accepted into its nursing program after 1933, with the graduating class of 1935 particularly affected. WGH, *Reports and Accounts*, 1933–40; Seeman interview.

68. P. Brownell, 'Report to Manitoba Hospital Association meeting with the MARN', 13 June 1939, p. 1, MARN, uncatalogued.

69. MARN Central Directory Committee, *Report*, 6 Jan. 1932, MARN, uncatalogued.

70. Helen Smith, tape-recorded interview by author, Winnipeg, 3 Aug. 1988; McMillan interview.

71. Asta Oddson, *Employment of Women in Manitoba* (Winnipeg, 1939), p. 99.

72. For a discussion of rural public health nursing in the prairie provinces, see Ina Bramadat and Marion Saydak, 'Nursing on the Canadian Prairies 1900–1930: Effects of Immigration', *Nursing History Review* 1 (1993), pp. 105–17; McPherson, '"The Country is a Stern Nurse"'.

73. VanGH, *Annual Report*, 1928.

74. This conflict is described in Irene Goldstone, 'The Origins and Development of Collective Bargaining by Nurses in British Columbia 1912–1976', M.Sc. thesis (Univ. of British Columbia, 1980), pp. 30–1.

75. See Robert Tyre, *Saddlebag Surgeon: The Story of Dr Murrough O'Brien* (Winnipeg, 1954), pp. 177–8, for a description of the hospital at Frontier, Saskatchewan, which during some months in the 1930s did not pay its nurses at all.

76. Lytle interview; Mann interview.

77. Catton, 'Special Nursing in the Hospital'.

78. Chapman interview.

79. K.B. McCallum, Reg.N., 'The Case of the Private Duty Nurse', *Manitoba Medical Association Review* (Feb. 1935), p. 12.

80. MARN, 'Schedule of Rates and Hours for the Members of Manitoba Nurses' Central Directory', 1928 (Mary Shepherd collection). 'A resident nurse on a case charges forty cents an hour for a fifteen-hour day, but if the patient's condition is critical and her services are required for a longer period, she gives that time gratuitously. This means that the nurse who is the only nurse on a private case in a home, and is entitled to have, out of every twenty-four hours, six hours undisturbed rest and three hours' recreation, far too frequently gets neither.' Gaskell, 'Nurses Are Not Selfish or Overpaid', p. 25.

81. Weir, *Survey of Nursing Education*, pp. 76–7.

82. Ibid., pp. 76, 103. Agnes Jamieson claimed in an Apr. 1928 article in *CN*: 'Over half of private duty nurses are supporting someone.' 'Problems of the Private Duty Nurse', *CN* 24, 4 (Apr. 1928), p. 197.

83. Weir, *Survey of Nursing Education*, p. 79.

84. Kathleen Snowdon, 'Why a Budget?' *CN* 23, 6 (June 1927), p. 312.

85. Edith Charlton Salisbury, 'Make Your Income Serve You', *CN* 22, 2 (Feb. 1926), p. 83. Salisbury admitted that budgeting alone would not ensure that incomes would be sufficient, but considered it important none the

less that a budget would 'help to determine what you need most, and it may, and undoubtedly will, give you a certain peace of mind because you will know you have done your best with the materials at your command.'

86. Flora Stewart, 'How Life Insurance Benefits Business and Professional Women', *CN* 22, 1 (Jan. 1926), p. 21.

87. Weir proposed a salary schedule for institutional nurses that would rectify the absence of any 'system of annual increments' in hospital work. Initial salaries in the Weir scheme started general-duty nurses at $85 and specialists, who had taken an additional year of training, at $100. Within 5 or 10 years these nurses were expected to reach the terminal salaries of $125 and $150 respectively. He offered his CNA benefactresses no suggestions as to further remuneration for more experienced nurses, such as the WGH's Margaret McGillvray who served as night superintendent for nearly 20 years. Weir, *Survey of Nursing Education*, pp. 107, 125.

88. Ibid., pp. 75, 102–3, 124–5.

89. Ibid., pp. 75–7, 102–3, 124–5, 150–1.

90. Edith Gaskell, 'Annuities', *CN* 18, 9 (Sept. 1922), p. 564. In a report of the CNA Private Duty Section, a committee charged with investigating insurance plans discovered that arranging for group insurance was impossible, 'as many companies refuse to consider insurance at all on female lives. Some companies that granted accident and health insurance to women, up to three months ago, now refuse to do so. Individual policies can, however, be secured in some good reliable companies . . . .' 'Private Duty Nursing Department', *CN* 18, 6 (June 1922), p. 352. See also Stewart, 'How Life Insurance Benefits Business and Professional Women'.

91. Weir, *Survey of Nursing Education*, p. 76.

92. M. Judson Eaton, 'A Vital Question', *CN* 22, 4 (Apr. 1926), p. 181.

93. Jamieson, 'Problems of the Private Duty Nurse'.

94. Riggs interview.

95. Ann M. Forrest, 'Increase of Tuberculosis Among Nurses', *CN* 27, 11 (Nov. 1931), p. 580.

96. Ibid.

97. Limited numerical evidence makes the assessment of changing health standards of nurses a difficult task. Hospital officials' concerns about student health were not new to the inter-war years, but during those decades health issues received substantially more attention. For example, in 1932 vanGH Superintendent Dr Haywood stressed that the question of tuberculosis among nurses 'is not a problem peculiar to this hospital, but has been receiving the attention of hospital authorities and

medical authorities the world over.' vanGH, *Annual Report*, 1932. Eaton, *Report of the Advisory Committee on Labour Conditions in Hospitals*, has several sections on the health of nurses in BC hospitals. Blanche Pfefferkorn, *A Study of the Incidence and Costs of Illness Among Nurses* (Joint Committee on the Costs of Nursing Service and Nursing Education of the American Hospital Association, National League of Nursing Education, American Nurses' Association, 1939), addressed the problem in the American context.

98. Weir, *Survey of Nursing Education*.
99. Ibid., pp. 69, 97, 118, 145.
100. Ibid., pp. 69, 100, 122, 123.
101. Ibid., p. 149.
102. For an analysis of their role in influencing the direction of Canadian nursing, see Margaret May Allemang, 'Nursing Education in the United States and Canada, 1873–1950: Leading Figures, Forces, Views in Education', Ph.D. diss. (Univ. of Washington, 1974).
103. Weir, *Survey of Nursing Education*, pp. 100–1, 123.
104. Ibid., pp. 68, 81.
105. A very small portion of this increase is attributed to the emergence of university schools of nursing. For example, in 1930 only 301 university-educated nurses graduated, whereas in 1931 over 11,000 student nurses were enrolled in all Canadian training programs, of whom approximately one-third or 3,300 graduated that year. By these calculations only one-tenth of all graduate nurses were products of university programs. F.H. Leacy, ed., 'Full-time university undergraduate enrolment, by field of specialization and sex, Canada, selected years, 1861–1975', Series W439–55, *Historical Statistics of Canada*, 2nd edn (Ottawa, 1983).

Year	# Grads. University Nursing Schools
1920	122
1925	188
1930	301
1935	372
1940	510

106. Riggs interview.
107. MARN, 'Registrar's Report', 1936, MARN Library, uncatalogued.
108. MARN, 'Registrar's report to MHA and MARN', 13 June 1939, pp. 2–3.
109. vanGH, Nurses Annual, 1926, p. 61.
110. Anne Glaz, 'We Accept the Challenge', wGHNAA, *Annual*, 1934, p. 19.
111. vanGH, *Nurses Annual*, 1937.
112. Veronica Strong-Boag, 'The Girl of the New Day: Canadian Working Women in the 1920s', *Labour/Le Travailleur* 4 (1979), pp. 131–64,

documents the continued difficulties faced by all working women in this decade.

113. See *cn* throughout the 1930s for examples of this. For an analysis of French-English relations that stresses the co-operation between the two groups of nurses in Quebec, see ARNPQ, *An Experiment in Mutual Understanding* (Montreal, 1946). La Garde-Malade canadienne-française was founded by Miss Charlotte Tassé, a 1917 graduate of Notre-Dame Hospital and, from 1919, director of nursing and nursing education at the Albert Prévost Sanitarium. Tassé was one of the new generation of lay nurses appointed to administrative positions in Quebec hospitals. Desjardins, Flanagan, and Giroux, *Heritage*, pp. 159, 160, 184.

114. On divisions within nursing organizations in the United States, see Barbara Melosh, *'The Physician's Hand': Work Culture and Conflict in American Nursing* (Philadelphia, 1982).

115. Even a brief reading of the CNA 'Official Directory', published monthly in *cn*, reveals this trend. In 1928, 1930, and 1932, for example, the members of the executive committee of the Canadian Nurses Association all listed hospitals or government offices as their mailing addresses. Provincial representatives from Manitoba tended to be split, with long-time nursing personalities such as Miss Jean Houston of the Manitoba Sanatorium in Ninette and Miss Mildred Reid of the WGH joining three other representatives from the province at the biennial convention. At the provincial and alumnae level, where geographic proximity might have facilitated more extensive private-duty participation, the presence of hospital personnel was even greater. In 1932, the Manitoba association listed Miss Houston, Miss Reid, Miss Christina Macleod of Brandon General, Miss Robertson of the Municipal Hospital, Miss Norah O'Shaughnessy and Miss A.E. Wells of the Provincial Health Department, and Miss LaPorte of the Misericordia Hospital as members of the executive. The remaining four positions were filled by women whose addresses did not suggest administrative postings. 'Official Directory', *cn* 28, 12 (Dec. 1932), p. 678.

116. MARN Board of Directors, *Minutes*, 6 Nov. 1931, 8 June 1933, 25 Apr. 1935, MARN Library, uncatalogued. By 1933 the Victoria General Hospital had decided that nurses in arrears of their fee had one month to clear their accounts or be stricken from the registry. VicGHNAA, *Minutes*, 6 Mar. 1933, VicGHNAAA, uncatalogued.

117. In 1935 the RNANS discussed the feasibility of asking local health officials to give Nova Scotia nurses preference when making appointments 'to various public positions in our Province'. VicGHNAA, *Minutes*, 2 Dec. 1935.

118. 'Application Form: Margaret Scott Nursing Mission', 20 July 1939, and letter to Miss M. Baird, RN, supt, MSNM, 30 Sept. 1939, PAM, MG 10 B 9.

119. 'As an Ex-Governor Sees It', CN 24, 4 (Apr. 1928), p. 178.

120. CNA, Minutes, 1938.

121. For a discussion of women's difficulties organizing within traditional union structures, see Ruth Frager, 'No Proper Deal: Women Workers and the Canadian Labour Movement, 1870–1940', in Linda Briskin and Lynda Yanz, eds, Union Sisters: Women in the Labour Movement (Toronto, 1983); Marie Campbell, 'Sexism in British Columbia Trade Unions, 1900–1920', in Barbara Latham and Cathy Kess, eds, In Her Own Right: Selected Essays on Women's History in BC (Victoria, 1980). Bryan Palmer has characterized the 1920s and 1930s as decades of 'Dissolution and Reconstitution'. See Palmer, Working-Class Experience: The Rise and Reconstitution of Canadian Labour, 1800–1980 (Toronto, 1983).

122. Glaz, 'We Accept the Challenge'; Ross interview.

123. 'Nurses walkout at Comox', Vancouver Sun, 13 Apr. 1939, cited in Goldstone, 'The Origins and Development of Collective Bargaining by Nurses in British Columbia 1912–1976'. Goldstone describes this conflict in some detail on pp. 35–7.

124. MARN, 'Registrars report to MHA and MARN', 13 June 1939, p. 5.

125. MARN Annual Meeting, Minutes, 1939.

126. Darlene Clark Hine commented on Johns's progressive attitudes in Black Women in White: Racial Conflict and Cooperation in the Nursing Profession, 1890–1950 (Bloomington, 1989).

127. CN 17, 3 (Mar. 1921), pp. 159–60.

128. CN 17, 4 (Apr. 1921), p. 226.

129. CN 17, 5 (May 1921), p. 295.

130. Randal adhered to her belief that anonymity was the 'only way to promote free discussion in the CN' and to her opinion that the anonymous letter was not a personal attack on Johns. Johns considered the letter an 'unprovoked attack'. The General Assembly passed by 66 votes a resolution in favour of continuing the editorial policy of permitting the publication of anonymous letters provided the editor possessed the author's name and address. 'Report of the CNATN Convention, Quebec, June 1921', CN 17, 7 (July 1921), pp. 416–17.

131. Ibid., pp. 416–17, 453–6.

132. Johns, 'The Biennial Meeting Canadian Nurses Association', CN 26 (1930), pp. 395–6.

133. Pearl Brownell, 'Changes in Private Duty', WGHNAA, Annual, 1937, p. 19.

134. CNA, 'Report of the Private Duty Section', *Minutes*, 1924, pp. 22–3.

135. CNA, *Minutes*, 1924, pp. 17–18. Gunn served as secretary of the CNA, 1914–17, and president, 1917–20, and was elected second vice-president of the International Congress of Nurses in 1925. A 1905 graduate of New York's Presbyterian Hospital, Gunn assumed the helm at TGH in 1913. 'International Congress of Nurses', *CN* Mar. 1929, p. 119. For a biography of Gunn, see Natalie Reigler, 'The Work and Networks of Jean I. Gunn, Superintendent of Nurses, Toronto General Hospital 1913–1941: A Presentation of Some Issues in Nursing During Her Lifetime', Ph.D. diss. (Univ. of Toronto, 1992).

136. CNA, *Minutes*, 1924, pp. 17–18.

137. CNA, 'Private Duty Section', *Minutes*, 1926, pp. 52, 63.

138. CNA, *Minutes*, 1928, p. 26.

139. Ibid., 1930, p. 14. A graduate of Swansea General Hospital in Wales, Fairley moved to Canada in 1912 and served as superintendent of nurses at Hamilton General Hospital, 1919–24, Victoria General Hospital, 1924–9, and Vancouver General Hospital, 1929–44. Barbara Tunis, *In Caps and Gowns: The Story of the School for Graduate Nurses, McGill University, 1920–1964* (Montreal, 1966), p. 3.

140. CNA, *Minutes*, 1938.

141. Jean Davidson, 'Are There Too Many Nurses?' *CN* 28, 7 (July 1932), p. 373.

142. Margaret L. Moag, 'Hourly Nursing', *CN* 27, 3 (Mar. 1929), pp. 138–41.

143. CNA, 'Private Duty Section', *Minutes*, 1928, p. 41.

144. Pearl Brownell, Convenor, 'Report', WGHAA, Journal, 1933, p. 41.

145. WGHAA, *Journal*, 1934, p. 25.

146. WGHAA, *Journal*, 1962, p. 49.

147. Doreene MacGuinness, 'Per Ardua Ad Astra', WGHAA, *Journal*, 1936, p. 18. MacGuinness was a 1935 grad of WGH.

148. Glaz, 'We Accept the Challenge', p. 19. A grad of 1934, Glaz wrote: 'As for alumnae assistance, it is only a relief measure which is temporary and cannot exist very long.'

149. RNANS, 'Survey Summary', 1935, PANS, MG 20, box 3.

150. CNA, *Minutes*, 1930, p. 16.

151. Ibid., 1932.

152 . Ibid., 1934, 1936, 1938, 1940.

153. RNANS, 'Survey Summary', 1935.

154. CNA, *Report to Dominion Council of Health*, 1947.

155. See Chapter 1 for a discussion of these historiographical positions.

156. VanGH, *Annual Report*, 1933.

157. RNANS, 'Survey Summary', 1935.

158. VanGH, *Annual Report*, 1937.

Chapter 5

1. Gary Kinsman, *The Regulation of Desire: Sexuality in Canada* (Montreal, 1987).
2. 'House Rules for Nurses approved by the board August 1920', WGH, House Committee, *Minutes*, 25 Aug. 1920, PAM, MG 10, B 2.
3. H.S. Stalker, MD, medical superintendent, Tranquille Sanatorium, to P. Walker, deputy provincial secretary, Victoria, BC, 25 Nov. 1940, and Walker to Stalker, 26 Nov. 1940, PABC, GR 496.
4. Unpublished history of the St Boniface School of Nursing, n.d. (*c.* 1976), pp. 14–15, St Boniface General Hospital School of Nursing Alumnae Room Archives.
5. Mariana Valverde, *The Age of Light, Soap, and Water: Moral Reform in English Canada, 1885–1925* (Toronto, 1991).
6. E.M. Knox, *The Girl of the New Day* (Toronto, 1919), p. 42.
7. Christina Simmons, 'Modern Sexuality and the Myth of Victorian Repression', in Kathy Peiss and Christina Simmons, eds, *Passion and Power: Sexuality in History* (Philadelphia, 1989), pp. 157–77. In the Canadian context, Veronica Strong-Boag's *The New Day Recalled: The Lives of Girls and Women in English Canada, 1919–1939* (Toronto, 1988) and Andrée Lévesque's *Making and Breaking the Rules: Women in Quebec, 1919–1939* (Toronto, 1994) focus on the continuing prescriptive emphasis on motherhood. Simmons acknowledges that 'Women's celebrated "new freedom" was most salient for single women since most white wives did not remain long in the labor force', but since most nurses were single the prescriptions for sexual 'liberation' continued to have resonance for them.
8. See Kathryn McPherson, 'Skilled Service and Women's Work: Canadian Nursing 1920–1939', Ph.D. diss. (Simon Fraser University, 1990), ch. 6.
9. Historians of fashion have analysed the relationship between costume and social role. For example, Jane Gaines has argued that in movies: 'Stepping into a costume, was like stepping into a role. Costumes, furthermore, were expected to express the same feelings . . . called for in the part.' She links this theatrical use of costume to the late nineteenth-century sense that, unlike earlier eras of dress: 'Clothes should thus be seen as the matter necessary to "body forth an idea." The problem of the public self which made immediate impressions and the true self which was within, was dealt with in the possibility of personality management and improvement which historians of modern society find emerging at the turn of the century.' If in motion pictures, then, costume is designed to support the narrative being presented on the screen, so, too, can uniforms like those worn by nurses be interpreted as supporting nursing's

occupational 'narrative' of femininity and respectability. See Jane Gaines, 'Costume and Narrative: How Dress Tells the Woman's Story', in Gaines and Charlotte Herzog, eds, *Fabrications: Costume and the Female Body* (New York, 1990), pp. 184–5, 194. See also Ann Hollander, *Seeing Through Clothes* (New York, 1975).

10. Martha Riggs, interview by author, Halifax, May 1982. The many references to bobbed hair in students' yearbooks suggests the degree of controversy over the new fashion in hair.

11. For a discussion of the influence of 'American' fashion on images of female sexuality in Quebec, see Lévesque, *Making and Breaking the Rules*, esp. pp. 55–7.

12. 'Miss Grant Addresses the Alumnae Association', WGHNAA, *Journal* 18, 73 (1927), pp. 13–14, WGHNAAA, uncatalogued.

13. Arthur Stringer, *The Prairie Mother* (Toronto, 1920), p. 1, 2–3.

14. Leslie Bell, 'Nurses and their Attitude Toward Sex', *CN* 24, 10 (Oct. 1928); H.B. Atlee, 'Uniforms and Stereotyped Minds', *CN* 29, 10 (Oct. 1933), pp. 515–18.

15. For example, there were no references to nurses in either the January 1920 or January 1930 issues of the *Vancouver Sun*.

16. See Philip A. Kalisch and Beatrice J. Kalisch, *The Changing Image of the Nurse* (Menlo Park, Calif., 1987).

17. CNA, *Minutes*, 1936, pp. 68–9.

18. 'Are Uniforms All Alike?' MGH, *Blue and Gold*, 1928, p. 57. See also 'New 1933 Styles in Crisp White Uniforms', *Blue and Gold*, 1933.

19. Donna Parker, 'Made to Fit a Woman: Riding Uniforms of the Frontier Nursing Service', *Dress* 20 (1993), pp. 53–64, argues that the distinctive uniforms of the American Frontier Nursing Service enhanced that organization's public image.

20. 'Want Ads', MGH, *Blue and Gold*, 1928, p. 36.

21. 'Don't!!!', MGH, *Blue and Gold*, 1927, p. 53.

22. VanGH, Nurses' Annual, 1939, p. 45.

23. 'The Nurse's Chance', WGH, *Blue and White*, 1928, p. 45.

24. 'Flattery and Frankness', VanGH, *Nurses' Annual*, 1926, p. 42.

25. VicGH, *Ward Nursing Register*, 1920–4, PANS, RG 25, B, X.10.

26. VanGH, *Minutes*, Special Meeting Training School Committee, 15 Sept. 1932, VCA, Add MSS 320.

27. 'The Ten Commandments', MGH, *Blue and Gold*, 1927, p. 42.

28. The theme of coming of age was common in nursing school yearbooks. See, for example, 'From Farm to Fame', WGH *Blue and White*, 1928, p. 44; 'The Devolution of a Nurse', Toronto General Hospital, *Annual*, 1928, p. 20.

29. Knox, *The Girl of the New Day*, p. 51.

30. Mr P. Walker, deputy provincial secretary, to [Florence Maitland], Salmon Arm Hospital, Salmon Arm, BC, 9 Oct. 1940, PABC, GR 496.
31. A.D. Lapp, superintendent of Tranquille Sanatorium, to Mr P. Walker, deputy provincial secretary, Victoria, BC, 9 Jan. 1936, PABC, GR 496.
32. VanGH, Special Committee Meeting, *Minutes*, 27 Sept. 1929.
33. WGH, 'Love', *Blue and White*, 1931, p. 61; VanGH, *Nurses' Annual*, 1928, p. 84.
34. MSNM, *Report*, Dec. 1935, PAM, MG 10, B 9.
35. Shepherd interview. Members of the American Frontier Nursing Service also celebrated the symbolic protection their uniform provided. FNS nurse Betty Lester recalled, 'It is one of our few rules that no nurse rides alone at night but . . . we nurses are safe. Our uniform allows us to go anywhere in the mountains, and it is only fear of accident which prevents our riding alone at night.' Cited in Parker, 'Made to Fit A Woman', p. 53.
36. See WGH, *Blue and White*, 1926, 1928, 1931, 1932, 1933, 1936. Torchy Adamson was the alumnae association archivist for the Vancouver General Hospital Alumnae Association until her death in 1992.
37. Cameron interview.
38. Letters to Kathleen Ellis, n.d., VCA, Add MSS 320, vol. 9, file 37.
39. Letter to Mrs Gordon, 29 Mar. 1937, PABC, Add MSS 2034, file 1.
40. 'Red Cross Workers From Outpost Here: Miss [Patrick] Nurse in Far-off, Lonely Cecil Lake' and 'Beloved Red Cross Nurse Dies in North', PABC, Add MSS 2034, file 1.
41. On interpreting women's same-sex relations in the past, see Carol Smith Rosenberg, 'The Female World of Love and Ritual', *Disorderly Conduct: Visions of Gender in Victorian America* (New York, 1985); Gerda Lerner, 'Where Biographers Fear to Tread', *Women's Review of Books* 4 (Sept. 1987), pp. 11–12; Blanche Wiesen Cook, *Eleanor Roosevelt*, vol. 1, 1884–1933 (New York, 1992).
42. Doris G. Daniels, *Always a Sister: The Feminism of Lillian D. Wald* (New York, 1989), p. 72.
43. One of the few sources describing an erotic, if not explicitly sexual, relationship that flourished in a nursing residence is Mary Renault's novel, *Purposes of Love* (London, 1939). Renault's biographer, David Sweetman, analyses the relationship sparked in their nursing residence between Renault and her life partner of 48 years. Sweetman, *Mary Renault: A Biography* (London, 1993).
44. For a discussion of the potential contribution nursing history can make to the historiography of sexuality, see Kathryn McPherson and Meryn Stuart, 'Writing Nursing History in Canada', CBMH 11, 1 (1994), pp. 10–11. On the question of female friendships within American nursing,

see Daniels, *Always a Sister*; Helen Lefkowitz Horowitz, *The Power and Passion of M. Cary Thomas* (New York, 1994).

45. Concerns about shortages of graduate nurses abounded throughout the post-war era. See, for example, VICGH, *Annual Report*, 1948, pp. 23–5; ibid., 1953, p. 30. See also John R. Smiley, Isabel Black, Andrew Kapos, and Boyde G. Gill, 'The Untapped Pool: A Survey of Ontario Nurses', unpublished report, Toronto, 1968, TGHA, sch. series IX i, box 2, F.F. #2; RNABC, *Submission to the Royal Commission on Health Services* (1962), pp. 11–24.

46. Ruth Roach Pierson, *'They're Still Women After All': The Second World War and Canadian Womanhood* (Toronto, 1986).

47. *Hamilton General Hospital School of Nursing* (Hamilton, 1956) describes that school's efforts to modernize its uniform. See also 'Trends in Nursing', *CN* 49, 3 (Mar. 1953), p. 209, for a discussion of the Demonstration School at Windsor that eliminated the capping ceremony and allowed students to wear the full uniform from the first day of training. This strategy was taken to '[protect] our new students from that feeling of being different, without a cap and not yet a nurse, [in order to apply] some of that mental hygiene we discuss so much about.' The article also applauded other changes to the regulation dress. 'Can you remember when short sleeves were rather looked down upon as being unprofessional? Better to dabble our cuffs in bath water than to show our elbows!' For other discussions of changes to nurses' costume, see Ethel Johns, '... Off ... Duty ...', *CN* 38, 5 (May 1942), p. 350; 'Is the Cap a Symbol?' *CN* 37, 4 (Apr. 1941), pp. 262–3; L. Grace Giles, 'A Cap Is Part of a Uniform', *CN* 37, 3 (Mar. 1941), pp. 173–4.

48. Maureen Turim, 'Designing Women: The Emergence of the New Sweetheart Line', in Gaines and Herzog, eds, *Fabrications*, pp. 225–6. In her exploration of why this particular design connoted the feminine image it did, Turim concludes (p. 227): 'Just as these decorative dresses were often very uncomfortable and impractical to wear, so the decorative and passive function assigned to women by their metaphorical inscription in such clothing was the ugly underside of the charming appearance. In fact, the sweetheart line can also be seen as a form of gilded bondage. . . . This style, by enforcing symbolic femininity, allowed for a great restriction of the female role to be attached to the very notion of the feminine.'

49. 'Toronto General Hospital Student Nurses' Uniform', *The Quarterly* 7, 6 (Winter 1949), p. 1. Calgary General Hospital adopted a redesigned uniform in 1952. The new style was decided on by the senior class, which voted in favour of 'a straight pattern with two rows of buttons on the bib. On the skirt the buttons will be concealed. . . . The uniforms are

to be made of poplin, have no crests and the collars and cuffs are pointed.' 'New Uniforms', *In Cap and Uniform*, 1952, p. 44, Calgary General Hospital Nurses' Alumnae Association Archives, uncatalogued.

50. 'High School Girls Are Shown Hospital Works', *Vancouver Daily Province*, 11 May 1943; 'High School Students See Nurses at Work', *Vancouver News-Herald*, 11 May 1943.

51. CNA, 'What Nursing Holds For You', n.d. In addition to celebrating the many job options nursing offered, the pamphlet underscored the important social role played by nurses. 'Her place in the community is an important one. She takes part in the drama of life and is often called upon to play many roles.'

52. Marjorie McLeod, tape-recorded interview by author, 6 Sept. 1992, possession of author.

53. 'The Ten Commandments of Nursing', vanGH, *Nurses' Annual*, 1957.

54. vanGH, Nurses' Annual, 1958. In a 1963 biographical newspaper article about vanGH grad Mary E. Lewis, Lewis explained that the 'problems of women and nursing are the same the world over.' Margaret Steen, 'A look at today's nurse', *Press-Enterprise*, 12 May 1963, VCA, Add MSS 320, vol. 11, file 99.

55. 'Woman in Service', *Vancouver Daily Province*, 8 July 1944, p. 8.

56. See Gaines, 'Costume and Narrative'.

57. *Canadian Home Journal* (Oct. 1940), front cover. For an analysis of Norman Rockwell's 'Rosie the Riveter', which appeared on the cover of the *Saturday Evening Post* on 29 May 1943, see Melissa Dabakis, 'Gendered Labor: Norman Rockwell's Rosie the Riveter and the Discourses of Wartime Womanhood', in Barbara Melosh, ed., *Gender and American History Since 1890* (London, 1993).

58. A 1945 *Halifax Herald* advertisement depicted a group of citizens staring up at a large microphone descending from the sky. Among the uniformed civilians was a nurse, dressed in sensible shoes, cape, and nurse's cap.

59. *CN* 40, 3 (Mar. 1944), p. 225; *CN* 42, 12 (Dec. 1946), p. 1005.

60. *CN* 50, 10 (Oct. 1954), p. 773.

61. *CN* 40, 5 (May 1944), p. 367.

62. *CN* 54, 3 (Mar. 1958), p. 249.

63. *CN* 49, 4 (Apr. 1953), p. 258. A similar message was conveyed in a 1943 advertisement for SMA baby food. The head-and-shoulder sketch of a nurse was accompanied by the text: 'Some men are so clever! Take my boss for instance . . .' Her boss, a medical doctor, was advising another doctor about the advantages of SMA infant formula. *CN*, 39, 11 (Nov. 1943), p. 713.

64. Ethel Johns, '. . . Off . . . Duty . . .', *CN* 39, 1 (Jan. 1943), p. 74.

65. Margaret Ann Jensen, *Love's Sweet Return: The Harlequin Story* (Toronto, 1984), Ann Snitow, '"Mass Market Romance: Pornography for Women Is Different', in Snitow, Christine Stansell, and Sharon Thompson, eds, *Powers of Desire: The Politics of Sexuality* (New York, 1983).
66. Jill Christian, *Nurse of My Heart* (Winnipeg, 1963).
67. Elizabeth Hoy, *Nurse in Training* (Winnipeg, 1963).
68. Anne Vinton, *Nurse Wayne in the Tropics* (Winnipeg, 1960).
69. Jensen, *Love's Sweet Return*, p. 81.
70. Christian, *Nurse of My Heart*, p. 49.
71. Ibid., pp. 64–5.
72. Vinton, *Nurse Wayne in the Tropics*, pp. 21, 151.
73. 'Red Cross Seeking Students' Red Blood', *The Manitoban* 37, 14 (10 Nov. 1950), p. 1.
74. For analyses of the sexualized image of nurses in American popular culture, see Kalisch and Kalisch, *The Changing Image of the Nurse*; Melosh, 'Doctors, Patients, and "Big Nurse"'.
75. VanGH, *Minutes*, Meeting, 15 Jan. 1959, 16 Jan. 1959, VCA, Add MSS 320.
76. Jeannine Locke, 'Nurses Denied Romance by Prudish Profession', *Toronto Daily Star*, VCA, Add MSS 320. See also 'Kissing Case: Nurses Threaten to Strike', Vancouver Sun, 15 Jan. 1959, p. 2; 'Hospital to "Kiss, Make Up" With its Student Nurses', ibid., 16 Jan. 1959, p. 17; 'At Hospital: "Kissing Nurse" Case Put on Ice', ibid., 17 Jan. 1959, p. 9; 'New Rule for Nurses', ibid., 27 Jan. 1959. A letter to the editor entitled 'Good Night, Nurse,' apparently written by an ex-patient of VanGH, defended the students' right to a social life on the grounds that they received so little financial remuneration for their hard work that the least they deserved was some romance to maintain their femininity: 'More power and happiness to her and student nurses like her . . . these student nurses . . . don't get enough pin money to keep them in lipstick or a few other female necessities. . . .'
77. Kinsman, *The Regulation of Desire*. See also John d'Emilio and Estelle Freedman, *Intimate Matters: A History of Sexuality in America* (New York, 1988).
78. Donna Penn, 'The Sexualized Woman: The Lesbian, the Prostitute, and the Containment of Female Sexuality in Postwar America', in Joanne Meyerowitz, *Not June Cleaver: Women and Gender in Postwar America, 1945–1960* (Philadelphia, 1994), pp. 358–81.
79. See, for example, Janet Muff, 'Why doesn't a smart girl like you go to medical school? The women's movement takes a slap at nursing', in Muff, ed., *Socialization, Sexism, and Stereotyping: Women's Issues in Nursing* (St Louis, 1982).

80. See Chapter 2. On the relationships between nurses and suffragists in the United States, see Sandra Beth Lewenson, *Taking Charge: Nursing, Suffrage, and Feminism in America, 1873–1920* (New York, 1993).

Chapter 6

1. See, for example, Dorothy J. Kergin, 'Nursing as a Profession', in Mary Quayle Innis, *Nursing Education in a Changing Society* (Toronto, 1970), pp. 46–63; Linda B. McIntyre, 'Towards a Redefinition of Status: Professionalism in Canadian Nursing, 1939–45', MA thesis (Univ. of Western Ontario, 1984); Tony Cashman, *Heritage of Service: The History of Nursing in Alberta* (Edmonton, 1966). Cashman (p. 304) writes: 'The modern era of nursing in Alberta began on November thirteenth, 1945. On that date . . . there opened the first course for certified nursing aides.'
2. See, for example, David Coburn, 'The Development of Canadian Nursing: Professionalization and Proletarianization', *International Journal of Health Services* 18, 3 (1988), pp. 437–56; Sarah Jane Growe, *Who Cares: The Crisis in Canadian Nursing* (Toronto, 1991), pp. 58–62.
3. Captain W.D.M. Sage, ed., *Battlefield Nurse: Letters and Memories of a Canadian Army Overseas Nursing Sister in World War II* (Vancouver, 1994), pp. 5–7.
4. G.W.L. Nicholson, *Canada's Nursing Sisters* (Toronto, 1975), pp. 130–1, 174–5; Cashman, *Heritage of Service*, p. 229. Ingibjorg Cross also tried to join the forces in 1942, but her sister insisted that Cross remain in civilian duty. Instead, Cross got a job working for Fisher and Burpey, a hospital equipment company for whom she demonstrated and instructed in the use of their equipment to doctors across Canada. Ingibjorg Cross, tape-recorded interview by author, Vancouver, 20 July 1988.
5. Pierson, *'They're Still Women After All'*.
6. VanGH, *Annual Report*, 1942, p. 19, VCA, Add MSS 320, series A.
7. Ibid., 1944, p. 18; WGH, *Reports and Accounts*, 1944, p. 41, PAM, MG 10, B 2.
8. BGNA, Minutes, 1 Oct. 1946, BGHNAAA, box 82.
9. Dr E.P. Scarlett, 'Values Old and New', *CN* 44, 1 (Jan. 1948), p. 15.
10. WGH, *Reports and Accounts*, 1942–66.
11. 'Nursing Personnel Employed in Hospitals', *British Columbia's Nursing Resources: Supply and Demand Source and Utilization*, Apr. 1958.
12. RNAPQ, *Brief to the Royal Commission on Education, Province of Quebec* (Montreal, 1962), p. 9.
13. John R. Smiley, Isabel Black, Andrew Kapos, and Boyde G. Gill, 'The Untapped Pool: A Survey of Ontario Nurses' (unpublished report, 1968) TGHA, sch. series IXI, box 2, FF #2, p. 17.

14. David Gagan, 'A Necessity Among Us': The Owen Sound General and Marine Hospital, 1891–1985 (Toronto, 1990), p. 121.

15. Malcolm G. Taylor, Health Insurance and Canadian Public Policy: The Seven Decisions that Created the Canadian Health Insurance System (Montreal, 1978), p. 11; George M. Torrence, 'Hospitals as Health Factories', in D. Coburn et al., eds, Health and Canadian Society: Sociological Perspectives, 2nd edn (Richmond Hill, Ont., 1987), p. 482.

16. DBS, Census of Canada, 1951, 1961.

17. For figures pertaining to the growth of the nursing and women's workforces, see ibid., 1961. The Canadian population increased from 12 million in 1946 to 18 million in 1961. See Marvin McInnis, Warren Kalbach, and Donald Kerr, 'Population Changes', in Donald Kerr and Deryck W. Holdsworth, eds, Historical Atlas of Canada III: Addressing the Twentieth Century (Toronto, 1990), plate 59.

18. In 1951, 33,204 of 35,138 or 94.5% of graduate nurses in Canada worked in the 'community service' sector. That would include hospitals and public health organizations. A 1947 CNA report revealed that in 1930, 6,370 graduate nurses had worked in private practice, as compared to 4,160 in hospital and public health work. By 1943, the same number of practitioners were in private health care, but 13,950 now worked in hospitals and public health. See CNA, 'Presentation to the Dominion Council of Health' (1947), cited in MARN, 'Binoculars Lifed' (unpublished report, May 1948), MARN Library; RNABC, 'Report of Sub-Committee, Joint Planning Committee on Nursing: Disposal of 1946 Graduates' (unpublished report, 1947), PABC, GR 281.

19. RNAPQ, Brief to the Royal Commission, p. 8.

20. CNA, 'Special Resolution', Minutes, Biennial Meeting, Appendix A, 1946. In 1951, 15,623 students were enrolled in Canadian nursing training programs; by 1961 this number had grown nearly 50% to 22,993. DBS, Census of Canada, 1951, 1961.

21. Mary Macfarland, 'Miss Macfarland's Annual Report', TGHNAA, The Quarterly 6, 4 (July 1946), p. 11; see also W.G. Cosbie, The Toronto General Hospital, 1819–1965: A Chronicle (Toronto, 1975), p. 269.

22. 'A Proposed Plan for the Orderly Development of Nursing Education in British Columbia', n.d., VCA, Add MSS 320.

23. On the MARN radio series, see BGNA, Minutes, 8 Jan. 1946; on the use of radio campaigns to encourage French-speaking women in Quebec to enter nursing, see Juliette Trudel, 'Report of French-Speaking Advisor', CN 42, 9 (Sept. 1946), p. 763. For a description of two recruiting campaigns, one by Sister Anna of All Saints Hospital in Springhill, Nova Scotia, and one by the alumnae association of Montreal's Homeopathic Hospital, see Vera Graham, 'An Experiment in Recruiting',

CN 38, 10 (Oct. 1942), pp. 783–4. See also Gena E. Bamforth, 'Selling Nursing', *CN* 39, 9 (Sept. 1943), pp. 595–7; Electa MacLennan, 'What Local Associations Can Do to Step up Student Nurse Recruitment', *CN* 41, 4 (Apr. 1945), pp. 302–3.

24. 'Special Radio Broadcast', *CN* 43, 1 (Jan. 1947), p. 79.
25. Christina Macleod, letter to BGH president and board of directors, 9 Sept. 1943, BGHA, 'Medical Staff Minutes and Correspondence'.
26. Of the half-million dollars awarded in 1943–5, $310,000 or 62% was earmarked for recruitment and training of students. 'A Government Grant', *CN* 39, 9 (Sept. 1943), p. 593; 'Government Grant Committee', *CN* 42, 9 (Sept. 1946), pp. 782–3.
27. Calculated from VicGH, *Annual Reports*, 1944–6, 1949, 1951–3, 1955. Seven students travelled to VicGH from other Maritime provinces, and one was born in Ireland.
28. MGH, *Student Register*, 1948, 1953, MGHNAAA, uncatalogued.
29. Calculated from VanGH, *Nurses' Annual*, 1942, 1947, VanGHNAAA, uncatalogued. Of 161 graduates in those two years, 24 and 45 students, respectively, called Vancouver, New Westminster, Burnaby, or Victoria home, 3 and 7 listed urban centres in the prairies as their home towns, 16 and 27 women hailed from rural British Columbia, and a further 22 and 13 came from rural parts of the three prairie provinces.
30. Calculated from VicGH School of Nursing, Class Lists, 1941–55, VicGHNAAA, uncatalogued.
31. RNAPQ, *Brief to the Royal Commission*.
32. 'Men in Nursing', *CN* 50, 12 (Dec. 1954), p. 992.
33. Eileen De Witt, 'Random Comments', *CN* 60, 3 (Mar. 1964), p. 198; Albert W. Wedgery, 'Random Comments', *CN* 60, 6 (June 1964), pp. 536–8; Richard Palmer, 'Random Comments', ibid., p. 538. Palmer remained active in the occupation through the 1960s. In 1964 he attended an RNAO conference and, as the only male among 150 participants, engaged in the discussion around encouraging men to enter the profession. 'As the Staff Nurse Sees It . . .', *CN* 60, 2 (Feb. 1964), p. 149.
34. Margaret Duffield, 'Nursing Care for Racial Groups', *CN* 37, 5 (May 1941), pp. 337–8.
35. 'No Racial Discrimination', *CN* 43, 12 (Dec. 1947), p. 953.
36. Nancy H. Watson, acting registrar, RNANS, *Letter: Re Exit Permits*, to Jean S. Wilson, CNA, 9 July 1943, PANS, MG 20.
37. I would like to thank Marg Gorrie for sharing this research with me. Council of Nurse Education, *Minutes*, 1944, PAO, RG 10–107–0–448.
38. 'Notes from National Office', *CN* 43, 12 (Dec. 1947), p. 953.
39. Conversation with Pearline Oliver, Halifax, 1981. See also Agnes Calliste, 'Women of "Exceptional Merit": Immigration of Caribbean

Nurses to Canada', *Canadian Journal of Women and the Law* 6, 1 (1993), p. 92.

40. Ibid., pp. 92–3, 98–9.

41. Irene Desjarlais, in *Speaking Together: Canada's Native Women* (Toronto, 1975), p. 46, cited in Prentice et al., *Canadian Women: A History* (Toronto, 1989), p. 369.

42. Cited in Brian Walmark, 'The Changing Role of the Healer in a Traditional Ojibwa Family' (unpublished paper submitted to the Life Histories Project, Royal Commission on Aboriginal Peoples, 1994), pp. 15–16.

43. Terry Wotherspoon, 'Nursing Education: Professionalism and Control', in B. Singh Bolaria and Harley D. Dickinson, *Health, Illness and Health Care in Canada,* 2nd edn (Toronto, 1994), p. 583.

44. Calculated from DBS, *Census of Canada*, 1941, 1951, 1961.

45. 'Assessing Values', *CN* 45, 7 (July 1949), p. 528.

46. Donald Moore, *Don Moore: An Autobiography* (Toronto, 1985), pp. 139–50.

47. Calliste, 'Women of "Exceptional Merit"', pp. 94–5.

48. Ibid.

49. Whether native or foreign trained, women of colour remained in a clear minority. A 1958 BC report calculated that in the 1955–7 years, 89% of the new RNs had been trained in British Columbia or other Canadian provinces, whereas only nine RNs from 'other countries', including South Africa, India, Korea, Southern Rhodesia, and Jamaica, migrated to Canada's west coast. 'Nursing Personnel Employed in Hospitals', *British Columbia's Nursing Resources: Supply and Demand Source and Utilization*, Apr. 1958.

50. DBS, *Census of Canada*, 1961.

51. 'Married Nurses and Income Tax', *CN* 38, 10 (Oct. 1942), p. 789.

52. 'Executive Decisions', *CN* 43, 3 (Mar. 1947), p. 205.

53. Mrs A. Chisholm, 'A Married Nurse Returns to Duty', *CN* 40, 7 (July 1944), pp. 491–2.

54. Jo Mann, tape-recorded interview by author, Burnaby, 22 July 1988.

55. Violet McMill, tape-recorded interview by author, Winnipeg, 23 June 1987. Stories abound of women returning to nursing in the post-war years to support their families. See, for example, Mary Shepherd, ed., 'The 1928 Class: 28 Years Later, 1956'.

56. Barbara Burr, tape-recorded interview by author, 28 Nov. 1992, possession of author.

57. MARN, 'Minimum Monthly Salary for General Staff Nurses in Manitoba', 1942, MARN Library, uncatalogued.

58. Burr interview.

59. Smiley *et al.*, 'The Untapped Pool', p. 9. This evidence contradicts

assertions that in this era nursing was 'increasingly middle-class'. See, for example, Pat Armstrong, 'Women's Health-Care Work: Nursing in Context', in Armstrong, Choiniere, and Day, eds, *Vital Signs: Nursing in Transition*, p. 37.

60. Hospital annual reports listing graduate nurses' 'reasons for leaving' included in their tabulations 'home responsibilities' as distinct from marriage, which articulated for the institutions' reading public that conflict persisted. WGH, *Annual Reports*, 1959, p. 30, reported that 39% of the 'reasons for resignations' of nursing staff were 'home and/or family', of which 'responsibilities' constituted 18 resignations, marriage 21, and pregnancy 17. In 1960, this figure grew to 43%, then dropped in 1961 to 36%. It remained in the mid-30s until 1965 when it dipped to 23% and then 29% in 1966. WGH, *Reports and Accounts*, 1960–6.

61. Marjorie McLeod, tape-recorded interview by author, 6 Sept. 1992, possession of author. For a sensitive discussion of how working mothers in post-war Ontario interpreted conflicting attitudes about 'why mothers work', see Joan Sangster, 'Doing Two Jobs: The Wage-Earning Mother, 1945–70', in Joy Parr, ed., *A Diversity of Women: Ontario, 1945–80* (Toronto, 1995).

62. Vera O'Dacre, 'It Can be Done', *CN* 49, 5 (May 1953), pp. 362–3. See also Mary Kinnear, *In Subordination: Professional Women, 1870–1970*, (Montreal, 1995), pp. 115–16.

63. Susan Rimby Leighow, 'An "Obligation to Participate"': Married Nurses' Labor Force participation in the 1950s', in Joanne Meyerowitz, ed., *Not June Cleaver: Women and Gender in Postwar America, 1945–1960* (Philadelphia, 1994).

64. Veronica Strong-Boag, 'Home Dreams: Women and the Suburban Experience in Canada, 1945–50', *Canadian Historical Review* 72, 4 (Dec. 1991), pp. 471–504. For a discussion of American post-war domestic ideology, see Elaine Tyler May, *Homeward Bound: American Families in the Cold War Era* (New York, 1988).

65. M. Dorothy Mawdsley, 'The Position of Women in the Post-War World', *CN* 40, 8 (Aug. 1944), p. 549.

66. 'Men in Nursing', *CN* 50, 12 (Dec. 1954), p. 992.

67. O'Dacre, 'It Can be Done', pp. 362–3.

68. Leighow, 'An "Obligation to Participate"'.

69. For example, see Coburn, 'The Development of Canadian Nursing: Professionalization and Proletarianization'.

70. Mary E. Macfarland, 'Notice to Head Nurses', 28 May 1948, TGHA, 0005 sch. series IV, box #1, FF #8. See also Sister Francoise de Chantal, 'Some Newer Drugs', *CN* 38, 3 (Mar. 1942), pp. 177–9; K.J.R. Wightman, 'Chemotherapy with Sulphonamide Drugs', *CN* 38, 11 (Nov.

1942), pp. 835–6; 'Streptomycin Being Studied', *CN* 41, 10 (Oct. 1945), p. 808; Soeur A. Rose, 'Observation sur la Penicillinothérapie', *CN* 42, 6 (June 1946), pp. 488–90; Sister M. Décary, 'Hospital Penicillin Treatment Centre', *CN* 43, 11 (Nov. 1947), pp. 847–50; Roger R. Dufresne, 'Les Médicaments Nouveaux', *CN* 45, 2 (Feb. 1949), pp. 127–9.

71. WGH, Annual Report, 1948, p. 79. See also Rose Mindorff, 'Intravenous Infusion', *CN* 37, 1 (Jan. 1941), p. 46.

72. David P. Boyd, 'Blood Transfusion', *CN* 38, 6 (June 1942), pp. 388–92.

73. TGH School of Nursing, *Nursing Procedures*, 'Blood Pressures July 1949', p. 103, TGHA, 0005 sch. series IV, box #1, FF #8. WGH, *Reports and Accounts*, 1965, p. 29, stated that: 'The IV team took on more responsibility as they now start blood for transfusions, and have had additional drugs added to the list which they may give with intravenous solutions.'

74. WGH, *Reports and Accounts*, 1965, p. 136.

75. A 1945 *CN* article listed nine universities and 20 hospitals that offered postgraduate courses. A further 16 hospitals arranged for graduates to gain 'added experience' in various clinical specialties. See 'Post-Graduate Work Available in Canada', *CN* 41, 7 (July 1945), pp. 552–5.

76. For example, Miss McNally explained to the BGH medical staff that the BGNA had created a scholarship program: 'The graduate nurse chosen for the course would be expected to serve on the staff or in the district for at least one year following her post-graduate work.' BGH, General Hospital Medical Staff Meeting, *Minutes*, 1 Feb. 1943, BGHA, 'Medical Staff Minutes and Correspondence'. See also WGH, *Reports and Accounts*, 1944, p. 41, and 1947, p. 68, for descriptions of the growing number of staff nurses who had received bursaries for postgraduate courses and 'returned to strengthen' the hospital staff.

77. On Kathleen Russell's struggle to secure Rockefeller funding for (and therefore a degree program at) University of Toronto, see Rondalyn Kirkwood, 'Blending Vigorous Leadership and Womanly Virtues: Edith Kathleen Russell at the University of Toronto, 1920–52', *CBMH* 11, 1 (1994), pp. 175–206. For an historical overview of university nursing programs, see Janet Ross Kerr, 'A Historical Approach to the Evolution of University Nursing Education in Canada', in Kerr and MacPhail, *Canadian Nursing: Issues and Perspectives*.

78. Wotherspoon, 'Nursing Education: Professionalism and Control', p. 583.

79. M. Louisa Parker, 'Training Auxiliary Workers', *CN* 42, 7 (July 1946), pp. 563–6; Frances Waugh, 'L'Aide ou Auxiliare en Manitoba', *CN* 43, 5 (May 1947), pp. 373–5.

80. Kathleen A. Dier, 'Nursing Auxiliary Programs', CN 60, 10 (Oct. 1964), pp. 995–8.

81. British Columbia Council of Practical Nurses, 'Outline of Duties to be Used as a Guide in the Employment of the Licensed Practical Nurse in British Columbia', 1966, p. 5, VCA, Add MSS 320.

82. Jannetta MacPhail, 'Men in Nursing', in Kerr and MacPhail, Canadian Nursing: Issues and Perspectives, pp. 68–9.

83. Helen M. King, 'Auxiliary Workers in Hospitals', CN 46, 7 (July 1950), p. 560. See also RNABC, Report of Sub-Committee of Joint Planning Committee.

84. WGH, Reports and Accounts, 1942, pp. 23, 42.

85. Ibid., 1947, p. 67.

86. In 1953 at WGH, 163 graduate nurses on permanent appointment were joined by 33.7 graduate nurses hired on a daily basis, 28.5 practical nurses, 70 nurses' aides, 12 diet maids, and 37 ward maids as compared to 151.5 permanent graduate nurses, 23.5 daily graduate nurses, 20 practical nurses, 58 nurses' aides, 15 diet maids, and 26 ward maids the previous year. Ibid., 1953, p. 78.

87. Ibid., 1958, p. 25. Twenty-seven ward clerks 'were functioning in the nursing stations, doing much of the clerical work.' Twelve orderlies passed the training program, and nurses' aides increased from 112 to 148. Ibid., 1960, pp. 30–1, for lists of nursing personnel, 1956–60.

88. King, 'Auxiliary Workers in Hospitals', p. 558.

89. WGH, Reports and Accounts, 1966, p. 33.

90. For example, the Ontario Nurses' Act was revised in 1947 to provide for licensing certified nursing assistants. Marjorie G. Russell, 'The Emergence of the Nursing Assistant', in Innis, Nursing Education in a Changing Society, p. 142.

91. King, 'Auxiliary Workers in Hospitals', p. 559.

92. Frances Fisher, 'School for Nursing Aides', CN 49, 7 (1953), pp. 542–5, describes the Montreal School for Nursing Aides, which trained aides for three months in the classroom followed by three months on the ward. For full job descriptions of the various categories of workers, see Sub-Committee of Joint Planning Committee, Report, Sept. 1946.

93. In 1951, there were more than 7,000 male practical nurses and over 18,000 female practical nurses. By 1961, 13,177 men were listed as practical nurses, while 49,376 women were included in the nurses' aides and assistance category. DBS, Census of Canada, 1951, 1961.

94. Ibid., 1961.

95. TGH, 'List of Employees, September 30th, 1947', TGHA Series II, 2, box 19. Large hospitals like TGH employed significant numbers of skilled male workers, including engineers, chefs, bricklayers, plumbers,

bakers, butchers, printers, machinists, electricians, carpenters, and fire-
men, all of whom earned slightly more than the general-duty nurses on
staff. See WGH, *Reports and Accounts*, for discussions of union con-
tracts signed with hospital employee unions.

96. DBS, *Census of Canada*, 1961.

97. Charlotte Whitton, 'The Nurse and the Social Revolution', *CN* 46, 1
(Jan. 1950), p. 28.

98. WGH, *Reports and Accounts*, 1963, p. 27.

99. See, for example, B. Orlo MacInnes, 'The Eight-hour Day for Student
Nurses', *CN* 42, 7 (July 1946), pp. 569–71. At WGH, the 48-hour work
week of the 1940s was reduced in 1953 to a 44-hour week and then
again to 40 hours in the 1960s. WGH, *Reports and Accounts*, 1953,
1963.

100. Jessie Law, tape-recorded interview by author, 7 Oct. 1986, possession
of author.

101. Frances Waugh, 'Motion and Time Study', *CN* 38, 5 (May 1942), pp.
321–2. On job analysis, see Gertrude M. Hall, 'The Why's and Where-
fore's of Your Job', *CN* 44, 5 (May 1948), pp. 370–1. In 1951 WGH
engaged a University of Minnesota nursing instructor to assess the
organization and efficiency of WGH's operating room. WGH, *Reports and
Accounts*, 1951, p. 76.

102. WGH, Reports and Accounts, 1951, p. 76.

103. Ibid., 1958, pp. 23–4.

104. Ibid., 1952, p. 21.

105. Ibid., 1958, p. 30.

106. Sister Marie Irenaeus, 'A Central Dressing Room', *CN* 38, 8 (Aug.
1942), p. 550. See also WGH, *Reports and Accounts*, 1965, p. 29, for a
discussion of efforts to make the central supply service and the laundry
more effective.

107. For example, a team was created in 1948 to administer the 400 doses of
penicillin given daily, an amount that 'required so much time for
administration, that it became necessary to find a means of relieving the
nurses on the wards for their routine duties.' WGH, *Reports and
Accounts*, 1948, p. 79.

108. Ibid., 1959; Sister Clare Marie, 'The Nursing Team in Action', *CN* 49, 9
(Sept. 1953), pp. 706–8; Lucy D. Willis, 'Team Leadership as It
Appears to the Leader', *CN* 50, 1 (Jan. 1954), pp. 39–41.

109. WGH, *Reports and Accounts*, 1961, p. 35.

110. Law interview.

111. VANGH, *Annual Report*, 1946, p. 20; 1947, p. 21.

112. See, for example, Edith Pringle, inspector of hospitals, BC, letter to
Vera B. Eidt, RN, superintendent of the Trail-Tadanac Hospital,

25 Sept. 1950, in which Pringle applauded Eidt's efforts to reduce the patient stay: 'Slowly but surely you are getting rid of your long stay cases.' PABC, GR 142, box 1, file 14.
113. WGH, *Reports and Accounts*, 1943, p. 29; ibid., 1964, p. 25.
114. For a description of the work of the nursing committee at WGH, chaired by Dr K.R. Trueman, see WGH, *Reports and Accounts*, 1955, pp. 76–7, and WGH, 'Procedures Committee', *Reports and Accounts*, 1956, p. 95.
115. Marie L. Campbell, 'The Structure of Stress in Nurses' Work', in Bolaria and Dickinson, eds, *Health, Illness and Health Care in Canada*, p. 596; Campbell, 'Productivity in Canadian Nursing: Administering Cuts', in Coburn, et al., eds, *Health and Canadian Society*, pp. 463–75.
116. WGH, *Reports and Accounts*, 1958, p. 27.
117. V.V. Murray, *Nursing in Ontario* (Toronto, 1970), p. 29.
118. 'Nursing Personnel Employed in Hospitals', *British Columbia's Nursing Resources*, Apr. 1958.
119. WGH, *Accounts and Reports*, 1950, p. 74. The 1957 Annual Report stated that 89% of the staff had resigned and been replaced that year.
120. Law interview.
121. Esther Beith, 'Labor Relations Committee', *CN* 42, 9 (Sept. 1946), pp. 786–7.
122. Phyllis Marie Jensen, 'The Changing Role of Nurses' Unions', in Baumgart and Larsen, eds, *Canadian Nursing Faces the Future*, pp. 459–73.
123. Peter Dent, 'The Beginnings', unpublished paper, British Columbia Nurses Union, 1982, pp. 2–11. The HEU is now affiliated with the Canadian Union of Public Employees (CUPE).
124. Irene Goldstone, 'The Origins and Development of Collective Bargaining by Nurses in British Columbia', MA thesis (Univ. of British Columbia, 1980). There is no evidence, to date, that VanGH's decision to abandon the HEFU provoked any conflict or controversy among hospital employees. Further research into the process whereby nurses unionized might reveal such conflict.
125. Executive, VicGHNAA, *Minutes*, 30 Jan. 1942, VicGHNAAA, uncatalogued.
126. Dorothy M. Percy, 'Alumnae Association, TGH School for Nurses: Report of the President', TGHNAA, *The Quarterly* 6, 8 (Summer 1947), p. 8.
127. Beith, 'Report of the Labour Relations Committee', pp. 693–5.
128. Elaine Day, 'The Unionization of Nurses', in Armstrong, Choiniere, and Day, *Vital Signs*, pp. 89–112.
129. M.E.K., 'Should We?' *CN* 42, 11 (Nov. 1946), p. 935.

130. Ibid.
131. Goldstone, 'The Origins of Collective Bargaining', p. 81.
132. Ibid., p. 72.
133. Ibid.
134. Ina Broadfoot, 'Labor Relations Committee', *CN* 46, 5 (May 1950), pp. 374–6.
135. 'Labor Relations Institute', *CN* 60, 3 (Mar. 1964), p. 281.
136. Advertised wages varied according to regional economy. BC was often at the top of the wage scales, while Quebec was often at the bottom. See, for example, 'Positions Vacant', *CN* 43, 8 (Aug. 1947), pp. 653–5; 'Employment Opportunities', *CN* 60, 1 (Jan. 1960), pp. 79–90.
137. Calculated from DBS, *Census of Canada*, 1961, vol. 3, part 3, table 21. Teachers, in particular, included a large proportion (85%) of employees who worked over 40 weeks per year.
138. Judi Coburn, '"I See and Am Silent": A Short History of Nursing in Ontario, 1850–1930' in J. Acton et al., eds, *Women at Work: Ontario, 1850–1950* (Toronto, 1974), pp. 127–58, concludes that the 'feminine mystification of [nurses'] work and the illusion of professionalism' are forces nurses still need to overcome. On the development of white-collar unions, see Bryan Palmer, *Working-Class Experience*, 2nd edn (Toronto, 1992), pp. 320–5.
139. Sub-Committee of Joint Planning Committee, *Report*, Sept. 1946, p. 2.
140. WGH, *Reports and Accounts*, 1965, p. 29.
141. Burr interview.
142. Murray, *Nursing in Ontario*.
143. D.J.R. Wightman, MD, 'Chemotherapy with Sulphonamide Drugs', *CN* 38, 11 (Nov. 1942), pp. 835–6.
144. When Marjorie McLeod began her training at WGH in 1945, hers was the first class to enjoy the eight-hour work day. McLeod interview. WGH student nurses had their hours cut further, from 44 to 40 per week, in 1959. WGH, *Reports and Accounts*, 1959, p. 25. See also Wotherspoon, 'Nursing Education: Professionalism and Control'.
145. WGH, *Reports and Accounts*, 1948, p. 77.
146. Calculated from ibid., 1966, pp. 30–1, 34.
147. Ibid., 1954, p. 72.
148. Burr interview.
149. Leonard Stein, 'The Doctor-Nurse Game', *Archives of General Psychiatry* 16 (June 1967), pp. 699–703. For an insightful discussion of how this 'game' continues to inform relations on the ward, see Growe, *Who Cares*, pp. 21–3.
150. For example, Beryl Seeman described the ambivalence of her medical colleagues when nurses started taking blood pressures. Beryl Seeman,

tape-recorded interview by author, Winnipeg, 8 July 1987; also Myrtle Crawford, tape-recorded interview by author, Vancouver, 5 Aug. 1988.

151. McLeod interview.

152. WGH, *Reports and Accounts*, 1943, p. 23; 1947, p. 21; 1966, p. 22.

153. Ibid., 1957, p. 99.

154. For instance, when the WGH nursing superintendent discussed high rates of staff resignations, she referred to the highly mobile general-duty group as 'younger personnel'. WGH, *Reports and Accounts*, 1952, p. 74.

155. Christina Macleod, letter to president and board of directors, BGH, 12 Aug. 1942, BGHA, 'Medical Staff Minutes and Archives'.

156. McMillan interview.

157. Harriet Pentland, tape-recorded interview by author, Winnipeg, 13 June 1986, possession of author.

158. The one institution of female authority that did inform nursing relations was that of female religious orders. However, the role of nuns in Catholic health-care institutions was itself waning.

159. Ives emphasized the differential for head nurses and said very little about the low salary range for the general-duty nurses.

160. Mary Macfarland, letter to TGH nursing staff, 2 Nov. 1950, TGHA, Acc 0030, container 5, series D6.

161. TGH nursing staff, letters to superintendent, Nov. 1950, ibid.

162. Cosbie, *The Toronto General Hospital*, p. 269.

Chapter 7

1. June Callwood, 'Suspicion leaves its scars', *Globe and Mail*, 18 Jan. 1985. In the wake of the Grange Commission's investigation into deaths at Toronto's Hospital for Sick Children, Callwood assessed the inquiry's devastating effect on nurses. She wrote: 'Though the nurses are exhausted from more than three years of stress marked by long periods of fear and humiliation, they can already see that what happened to them was sitting in the medical system for a century, waiting to explode. . . . The price of generations of conditioning is a profession marked by timidity.'

2. 'A Day on the Ward', *Vancouver Sun*, 24 May 1989, pp. A1, A15; 'Nurses Strike 12 Hospitals', ibid., 14 June 1989, pp. A1–A2.

3. 'Hospitals Strike Escalates as Employees' Union Joins Nurses', ibid., 22 June 1989, pp. A1, A13.

4. *The Province*, 26 June 1989, pp. 2–3.

5. 'Quebec Nurses Cheer Deal', ibid., 23 June 1989, p. A12. For a brief history of British Columbia nurses' first strike, the 10-day walkout in

May 1980, see Peter Dent, 'Anatomy of a Strike', unpublished paper, British Columbia Nurses Union, 1981. For an overview of developments in each province, see Janet Ross Kerr, 'Emergence of Nursing Unions as a Social Force in Canada', in Kerr and MacPhail, *Canadian Nursing: Issues and Perspectives*.

6. 'Nurses' splinter group still pushing for "no" vote', *Vancouver Sun*, 11 July 1989, p. A6; 'Nurses Reject Contract', ibid., 13 July 1989, pp. A1–A2.

7. 'The nurses: money isn't main target', ibid., p. A9; 'Denny Boyd', ibid., 28 June 1989, p. B1.

8. 'Nurses' President Weathering Storm', ibid., 7 July 1989, p. B2.

9. 'More Hospitals Picketed as Nurses Expand Strike', ibid., 15 June 1989, pp. A1–A2.

10. 'Denny Boyd', ibid., 15 June 1989, p. B1.

11. For a critique of femininity and gender roles in nurses' work, see Janet Muff, ed., *Socialization, Sexism and Stereotyping: Women's Issues in Nursing* (St Louis, 1982).

12. For discussions of feminist unions, see The Bank Book Collective, *An Account to Settle: The Story of the United Bank Workers (SORWUC)* (Vancouver, 1979); Linda Briskin and Lynda Yanz, eds, *Union Sisters: Women in the Labour Movement* (Toronto, 1983).

13. Callwood, in 'Suspicion Leaves Its Scars', claimed that 'Nurses were among the most reluctant women to accept the feminist movement.' For a discussion of the emergence of the 'rudiments of a feminist consciousness' among British Columbia nurses, see T. Rennie Warburton and William K. Carroll, 'Class and Gender: A Study of Registered Nurses in Victoria', paper presented to the Fourth BC Studies Conference, Victoria, 1986.

14. 'Denny Boyd', *Vancouver Sun*, 6 July 1989, p. B1.

15. Ibid. For a recent publication in nurses' union history, see Trudy Richardson, *United Nurses of Alberta, History: 1994 Edition* (Edmonton, 1994).

16. Kerr, 'Emergence of Nursing Unions as a Social Force in Canada', p. 212. See also Phyllis Marie Jensen, 'The Changing Role of Nurses' Unions', in A. Baumgart and J. Larsen, eds, *Canadian Nursing Faces the Future: Development and Change* (St Louis, 1988).

17. See, for example, Canada Committee on the Cost of Health Services, *Task Force Reports on the Cost of Health Services in Canada* (Ottawa, 1970).

18. Marie L. Campbell, 'The Structure of Stress in Nurses' Work', in B. Singh Bolaria and Harley D. Dickinson, eds, *Health, Illness and Health Care in Canada*, 2nd edn (Toronto, 1994), p. 602; Marie L. Campbell, 'Productivity in Canadian Nursing: Administering Cuts', in D. Coburn

et al, eds, *Health and Canadian Society: Sociological Perspectives* (Richmond Hill, 1987). On nurses' resistence and consent to managerial control, see also Jerry White, 'Changing Labour Process and the Nursing Crisis in Canadian Hospitals', *Studies in Political Economy* 40 (Spring 1993), pp. 103–34.

19. Joan Stelling, 'Staff Nurses' Perceptions of Nursing: Issues in a Woman's Occupation', in Bolaria and Dickinson, eds, *Health, Illness and Health Care in Canada*, pp. 609–26.

20. Jannice E. Moore, 'Nursing Manpower: The Supply and Demand Pendulum', in Kerr and MacPhail, *Canadian Nursing: Issues and Perspectives*; Stelling, 'Staff Nurses' Perceptions', p. 610.

21. Moore, 'Nursing Manpower', pp. 150–1.

22. Kerr, 'Emergence of Nursing Unions', pp. 216, 218.

23. For an analysis of the CUPE strike in the Ontario hospital sector in 1981, see Jerry White, *Hospital Strike: Women, Unions, and Public Sector Conflict* (Toronto, 1990).

24. Carolyn Egan and Lynda Yanz, 'Building Links: Labour and the Women's Movement', in Briskin and Yanz, *Union Sisters*. Egan and Yanz (p. 363) write: 'More and more union activists see themselves as *women* unionists, acting for women in the fight against women's inequality and oppression.' For an overview of women's position in the labour movement, see Linda Briskin, 'Women and Unions in Canada: A Statistical Overview', ibid.; Julie White, *Women and Unions* (Ottawa, 1980).

25. Major contributions to what became known as the 'domestic labour debate' are reprinted in Roberta Hamilton and Michèle Barrett, *The Politics of Diversity: Feminism, Marxism and Nationalism* (London, 1986). On the relationship between feminists and nurses, see Janet Muff, 'Why doesn't a smart girl like you go to medical school?' in Muff, *Socialization, Sexism and Stereotyping*.

26. Ann Oakley, *Essays on Women, Medicine and Health* (Oxford, 1993), p. 39.

27. For a perceptive overview of this tension, which has not completed disappeared, see Susan Reverby, '"Even her nursing friends see her 'only as a feminist'" . . . and other tales of the nursing feminism connection', *Nursing and Health* (1993).

28. Quoted in White, *Hospital Strike*, pp. 47, 48.

29. See White, *Women and Unions*, pp. 103–9, for a full description of this conflict.

30. Pat Armstrong, 'Nursing as Women's Work', in Armstrong, Choiniere, and Day, eds, *Vital Signs: Nursing in Transition*; Pat Armstrong, *Pay Equity in Predominantly Female Establishments: Health Care Sector* (Ontario, 1988).

31. Bernard Blishen, *Doctors in Canada: The Changing World of Medical Practice* (Ottawa, 1991), , pp. 134–6.

32. William K. Carroll and Rennie Warburton, 'Feminism, Class Consciousness and Household-Work Linkages Among Registered Nurses in Victoria', *Labour/Le Travail* 24 (Fall 1989), p. 135. Survey respondents were more divided over paid maternity/paternity leave benefits, homemaker pensions, and universal day care.

33. Elaine Buckley Day, *A 20th Century Witch-Hunt: A Feminist Critique of the Grange Royal Commission at the Hospital for Sick Children*, SNID Occasional Paper No. 87–103, Queen's University (Kingston, Ont., 1987).

34. Growe, *Who Cares*, p. 34.

35. Jannetta MacPhail, 'Organizing for Nursing Care: Primary Nursing, Traditional Approaches or Both?' in Kerr and MacPhail, *Canadian Nursing: Issues and Perspectives*, pp. 179–80.

36. For an overview of the debate over nurse-practitioners at Queen's University School of Nursing, see E. Jean M. Hill and Rondalyn Kirkwood, *Breaking Down the Walls: Nursing Science at Queen's University* (Kingston, 1991), pp. 48–54. Hill and Kirkwood (p. 51) conclude that the initial enthusiasm for nurse practitioners 'in primary care or in independent practice came to a dead end' because the mechanism for funding such personnel was not in place and when the shortage of physicians ended the incentive to find such a mechanism dwindled.

37. See, for example, Gail Donner, Dyanne Semogas, and Jennifer Blythe, *Towards an Understanding of Nurses' Lives: Gender, Power, and Control* (Toronto, 1994).

38. Agnes Calliste, 'Women of "Exceptional Merit": Immigration of Caribbean Nurses to Canada', *Canadian Journal of Women and the Law* 6, 1 (1993), p. 86.

39. Jean Cuthand Goodwill, 'Organized Political Action: Indian and Inuit Nurses of Canada', in Baumgart and Larsen, eds, *Canadian Nursing Faces the Future*, pp. 501–10.

40. Calliste, 'Women of "Exceptional Merit"', p. 86.

41. Ibid.

Suggested Readings in

Nursing History

Canadian Scholarship

Adams, Annmarie. 1994. 'Rooms of Their Own: The Nurses' Residences at Montreal's Royal Victoria Hospital'. *Material History Review* 40 (Fall):29–41.

Armstrong, Pat, Jacqueline Choiniere, and Elaine Day. 1993. *Vital Signs: Nursing in Transition*. Toronto: Garamond.

Baillargeon, Denyse. 1994. 'Care of Mothers and Infants in Montreal between the Wars: The Visiting Nurses of Metropolitan Life, Les gouttes de lait, and assistance maternelle'. In *Caring and Curing: Historical Perspectives on Women and Healing in Canada*, edited by Dianne Dodd and Deborah Gorham. Ottawa: University of Ottawa Press.

Baumgart, Alice, and Jenniece Larsen. 1988. *Canadian Nursing Faces the Future: Development and Change*. St Louis: C.V. Mosby.

Bramadat, Ina J., and Marion I. Saydak. 1993. 'Nursing on the Canadian Prairies, 1900–1930: Effects of Immigration'. *Nursing History Review* 1:105–7.

Buckley, Suzann. 1979. 'Ladies or Midwives: Efforts to Reduce Infant and Maternal Mortality'. In *A Not Unreasonable Claim: Women and Reform in Canada 1880s to 1920s*, edited by Linda Kealey. Toronto: The Women's Press.

Calliste, Agnes. 1993. 'Women of "Exceptional Merit": Immigration of Caribbean Nurses to Canada'. *Canadian Journal of Women and the Law* 6, 1:85–103.

Campbell, Marie L. 1994. 'The Structure of Stress in Nurses' Work'. In *Health, Illness and Health Care in Canada*, 2nd edn, edited by D. Coburn et al. Markham, ON: Fitzhenry and Whiteside.

Carroll, William K., and Rennie Warburton. 1989. 'Feminism, Class Consciousness and Household-Work Linkages Among Registered Nurses in Victoria'. *Labour/Le Travail* 24 (Fall):131–45.

Coburn, David. 1988. 'The Development of Canadian Nursing: Professionalization and Proletarianization'. *International Journal of Health Services* 18, 3:437–56.

————. 1994. 'Professionalization and Proletarianization: Medicine, Nursing and Chiropractic in Historical Perspective'. *Labour/Le Travail* 24 (Fall):139–62.

Coburn, Judi. 1974. '"I See and Am Silent": A Short History of Nursing in Ontario'. In *Women at Work: Ontario, 1850–1950*, edited by Janice Acton et al. Toronto: The Women's Press.

Cohen, Yolande, and Louise Bienvenue. 1994. 'Émergence de l'identité québécoises, 1890–1927'. *Canadian Bulletin of Medical History* 11, 1:119–51.

————, and Michèle Dagenais. 'Le métier d'infirmière: Savoirs féminins et reconnaissance professionnelle'. *Revue d'histoire de l'Amérique française* 41, no. 2 (automne):155–77.

Daigle, Johanne. 1991. 'Devenir infirmière: les modalités d'expression d'une culture soignante au XXe siècle'. *Recherches féministes* 4, 1:67–86.

Delhi, Kari. 1990. 'Health Scouts for the State: School and Public Health Nurses in Early Twentieth-Century Toronto'. *Historical Studies in Education* 1, no. 2:247–64.

Desjardins, Edouard, Eileen Flanagan, and Suzanne Giroux. 1971. *Heritage: History of the Nursing Profession in Quebec from the Augustinians and Jeanne Mance to Medicare*. Quebec: The Association of Nurses of the Province of Quebec.

Gibbon, John Murray, and Mary S. Mathewson. 1947. *Three Centuries of Canadian Nursing*. Toronto: Macmillan.

Growe, Sarah Jane. 1991. *Who Cares: The Crisis in Canadian Nursing*. Toronto: McClelland and Stewart.

Innis, Mary Q., ed. 1970. *Nursing Education in a Changing Society*. Toronto: University of Toronto Press.

Jardine, Pauline. 1989. 'An Urban Middle-Class Calling: Women and the Emergence of Modern Nursing Education at the Toronto General Hospital 1881–1914'. *Urban History Review* 17 (February):179–90.

Keddy, Barbara. 1984. 'Private Duty Nursing Days in the 1920s and 1930s in Canada'. *Canadian Woman Studies* 7, 3:99–102.

————, et al. 1987. 'Nurses' Work World: Scientific or "Womanly Ministering"?' *Resources for Feminist Research* 16, 4:37–9.

————. 1984. 'The Nurse as Mother Surrogate: Oral Histories of Nova Scotia Nurses from the 1920s and 1930s'. *Health Care for Women International* 5, 4:181–93.

Kerr, Janet Ross, and Jannetta MacPhail. 1988. *Canadian Nursing: Issues and Perspectives.* Toronto: McGraw-Hill Ryerson.

Kinnear, Mary. 1995. *In Subordination: Professional Women, 1870–1970.* Montreal and Kingston: McGill-Queen's University Press.

Kirkwood, Rondalyn. 1994. 'Blending Vigorous Leadership and Womanly Virtues: Edith Kathleen Russell at the University of Toronto, 1920–52'. *Canadian Bulletin of Medical History* 11, 1:175–206.

Laurin, Nicole, Danielle Juteau, and Lorraine Duchesne. 1991. *A la recherche d'un monde oublié, les communautés religieuses de femmes au Québec de 1900 à 1970.* Montreal: Le Jour.

McPherson, Kathryn. 1994. 'Science and Technique: The Content of Nursing Work at a Canadian Hospital, 1920–1939'. In *Caring and Curing: Historical Perspectives on Women and Health Care in Canada,* edited by D. Dodd and D. Gorham. Ottawa: University of Ottawa Press.

———. 1995. '"The Country Is a Stern Nurse": Rural Women, Urban Hospitals and the Creation of a Western Canadian Workforce, 1920–1940'. *Prairie Forum* 20, 2 (Fall):175–206.

———, and Meryn Stuart. 1994. 'Writing Nursing History in Canada: Issues and Approaches'. *Canadian Bulletin of Medical History* 11, 1:3–22.

Nicholson, G.W.L. 1975. *Canada's Nursing Sisters.* Toronto: Samuel Stevens Hakkert.

Paul, Pauline. 1994. 'The Contribution of the Grey Nuns to the Development of Nursing in Canada: Historiographical Issues'. *Canadian Bulletin of Medical History* 11:207–17.

Petitat, André. 1989. *Les infirmières: de la vocation à la profession.* Montreal: Boréal.

Royce, Marin. 1983. *Eunice Dyke: Health Care Pioneer.* Toronto: Dundurn Press.

Street, Margaret. 1973. *Watchfires on the Mountains: The Life and Writings of Ethel Johns.* Toronto: University of Toronto Press.

Strong-Boag, Veronica. 1991. 'Making a Difference: The History of Canada's Nurses'. *Canadian Bulletin of Medical History* 8, 2:231–48.

Stuart, Meryn. 1988. 'Ideology and Experience: Public Health Nursing and the Ontario Rural Child Welfare Project, 1920–1925'. *Canadian Bulletin of Medical History* 6, 2 (Winter):111–31.

———. 1992. '"Half a Loaf Is Better Than No Bread": Public Health Nurses and Physicians in Ontario, 1920–1925'. *Nursing Research* 41, 1 (January/February):21–7.

———. 1994. 'Shifting Professional Boundaries: Gender Conflict in Public Health, 1920–1925'. In *Caring and Curing: Historical Perspectives on Women and Healing in Canada,* edited by D. Dodd and D. Gorham. Ottawa: University of Ottawa Press.

White, Linda. 1994. 'Who's In Charge Here? The General Hospital School of

Nursing, St John's, Newfoundland, 1903–30'. *Canadian Bulletin for Medical History* 11:91–118.

White, Jerry. 1990. *Hospital Strike: Women, Unions, and Public Sector Conflict.* Toronto: Thompson Educational Press.

Whittaker, Joanne. 1984. 'The Search for Legitimacy: Nurses' Registration in British Columbia, 1913–1935'. In *Not Just Pin Money: Selected Essays on the History of Women's Work in British Columbia*, edited by Barbara K. Latham and Roberta J. Pazdros. Victoria: Camosun College Publishers.

Wotherspoon, Terry. 1994. 'Nursing Education: Professionalism and Control'. In *Health, Illness and Health Care in Canada*, 2nd edn, edited by B. Singh Bolaria and Harley D. Dickinson. Toronto: Harcourt, Brace and Co.

International Scholarship

Abel-Smith, Brian. 1964. *The Hospitals 1800–1948: A Study in Social Administration in England and Wales.* Cambridge, Mass.: Harvard University Press.

Bellaby, Paul, and Patrick Oribabor. 1980. 'Determinants of the Occupational Strategies Adopted by British Hospital Nurses'. *International Journal of Health Services* 10, no. 2:291–309.

Daniels, Doris G. 1989. *Always a Sister: The Feminism of Lillian D. Wald.* New York: The Feminist Press.

Davies, Celia. 1989. *Rewriting Nursing History.* London: Croom Helm.

Dingwall, Robert, Anne Marie Rafferty, and Charles Webster. 1988. *An Introduction to the Social History of Nursing.* London: Routledge.

Gamarnikow, Eva. 1978. 'Sexual Division of Labour: The Case of Nursing'. In *Feminism and Materialism: Women and Modes of Production*, edited by Annette Kuhn and Anne Marie Wolpe. London: Routledge and Kegan Paul.

Glazer, Nona. 1991. 'Between a Rock and a Hard Place: Women's Professional Organizations in Nursing and Class, Racial, and Ethnic Inequalities'. *Gender and Society* 5, 3 (September):351–72.

Helmstadter, Carol. 1993. 'Old Nurses and New: Nursing in the London Teaching Hospitals Before and After the Mid-Nineteenth-Century Reforms'. *Nursing History Review* 1:43–70.

———. 1994. 'The Passing of the Night Watch: Night Nursing Reform in the London Teaching Hospitals, 1856–90'. *Canadian Bulletin of Medical History* 11, 1:23–69.

Hine, Darlene Clark. 1989. *Black Women in White: Racial Conflict and Cooperation in the Nursing Profession 1890–1950.* Bloomington: Indiana University Press.

Horowitz, Helen Lefkowitz. 1994. *The Power and Passion of M. Cary Thomas*. New York: Alfred A. Knopf.

Jones, Anne Hudson, ed. 1988. *Images of Nurses: Perspectives from History, Art, and Literature*. Philadelphia: University of Pennsylvania Press.

Kalisch, Philip A., and Beatrice J. Kalisch. 1987. *The Changing Image of the Nurse*. Menlo Park: Addison-Wesley Publishing Company.

Lagemann, Ellen Condliffe, ed. 1983. *Nursing History: New Perspectives, New Possibilities*. New York: Teachers College Press.

Leighow, Susan Rimby. 1994. 'An "Obligation to Participate"': Married Nurses' Labor Force Participation in the 1950s'. In *Not June Cleaver: Women and Gender in Postwar America, 1945–1960*, edited by Joanne Meyerowitz. Philadelphia: Temple University Press.

Lewenson, Sandra Beth. 1993. *Taking Charge: Nursing, Suffrage, and Feminism in America, 1873–1920*. New York: Garland.

Maggs, Christopher. 1986. *The Origins of General Nursing*. London: Croom-Helm.

————. 1993. 'Nursing History: State of the Art'. in *Nursing: Art and Science*, edited by A. Kitson. London: Chapman Hall.

Marks, Shula. 1994. *Divided Sisterhood: Race, Class and Gender in the South African Nursing Profession*. New York: St Martin's Press.

Melosh, Barbara. 1982. *'The Physician's Hand': Work Culture and Conflict in American Nursing*. Philadelphia: Temple University Press.

————. 1984. 'Doctors, Patients, and 'Big Nurse': Work and Gender in the Postwar Hospital'. In *Nursing History: New Perspectives, New Possibilities*, edited by E.C. Lagemann. New York: Teachers College Press.

Muff, Janet. 1982. *Socialization, Sexism, and Stereotyping: Women's Issues in Nursing*. St Louis: C.V. Mosby.

Olson, Thomas. 1993a. 'Apprenticeship and Exploitation: An Analysis of the Work Pattern of Nurses in Training, 1897–1937'. *Social Science History* 17, 4 (Winter):559–76.

————. 1993b. 'Laying Claim to Caring: Nursing and the Language of Training, 1915–1937'. *Nursing Outlook* 41, 2 (March/April):68–72.

Poovey, Mary. 1988. *Uneven Developments: The Ideological Work of Gender in Mid-Victorian England*. Chicago: University of Chicago Press.

Poplin, Irene. 1994. 'Nursing Uniforms: Romantic Idea, Functional Attire, or Instruments of Social Change?' *Nursing History Review* 2:153–67.

Rafferty, Anne-Marie. 1993. 'Decorous Didactics: Early Explorations in the Art and Science of Caring, circa 1860–90'. In *Nursing: Art and Science*, edited by A. Kitson. London: Chapman Hall.

Renault, Mary. 1939. *Purposes of Love*. London: Longmans.

Reverby, Susan. 1987. *Ordered to Care: The Dilemma of American Nursing 1850–1945*. New York: Cambridge University Press.

Rosenberg, Charles. 1979. 'Florence Nightingale on Contagion: The Hospital as Moral Universe'. In *Healing and History: Essays for George Rosen*, edited by Charles Rosenberg. New York: Science History Publications.

Sweetman, David. 1993. *Mary Renault: A Biography*. London: Chatto and Windus.

Vicinus, Martha. 1985. *Independent Women: Work and Community for Single Women, 1850–1920*. Chicago: University of Chicago Press.

Wagner, David. 1980. 'The Proletarianization of Nursing in the United States, 1932–1946'. *International Journal of Health Services* 10, 2:271–90.

Index

THE CANADIAN SOCIAL HISTORY SERIES

Terry Copp,
The Anatomy of Poverty:
The Condition of the Working Class
in Montreal, 1897–1929, 1974.
ISBN 0–7710–2252–2

Alison Prentice,
The School Promoters:
Education and Social Class in
Mid-Nineteenth Century
Upper Canada, 1977.
ISBN 0–7710–7181–7

John Herd Thompson,
The Harvests of War:
The Prairie West, 1914–1918, 1978.
ISBN 0–7710–8560–5

Joy Parr, Editor,
Childhood and Family in Canadian
History, 1982.
ISBN 0–7710–6938–3

Alison Prentice and
Susan Mann Trofimenkoff, Editors,
The Neglected Majority:
Essays in Canadian Women's History,
Volume 2, 1985.
ISBN 0–7710–8583–4

Ruth Roach Pierson,
"They're Still Women After All":
The Second World War and
Canadian Womanhood, 1986.
ISBN 0–7710–6958–8

Bryan D. Palmer,
The Character of Class Struggle:
Essays in Canadian Working Class
History, 1850–1985, 1986.
ISBN 0–7710–6946–4

Alan Metcalfe,
Canada Learns to Play:
The Emergence of Organized Sport,
1807–1914, 1987.
ISBN 0–7710–5870–5

Marta Danylewycz,
Taking the Veil:
An Alternative to Marriage,
Motherhood, and Spinsterhood in
Quebec, 1840–1920, 1987.
ISBN 0–7710–2550–5

Craig Heron,
Working in Steel: The Early Years in
Canada, 1883–1935, 1988.
ISBN 0–7710–4086–5

Wendy Mitchinson and
Janice Dickin McGinnis, Editors,
Essays in the History of
Canadian Medicine, 1988.
ISBN 0–7710–6063–7

Joan Sangster,
Dreams of Equality: Women on the
Canadian Left, 1920–1950, 1989.
ISBN 0–7710–7946–X

Angus McLaren,
Our Own Master Race: Eugenics in
Canada, 1885–1945, 1990.
ISBN 0–7710–5544–7

Bruno Ramirez,
On the Move:
French-Canadian and Italian Migrants
in the North Atlantic Economy,
1860–1914, 1991.
ISBN 0–7710–7283–X

Mariana Valverde,
"The Age of Light, Soap and Water":
Moral Reform in English Canada,
1885–1925, 1991.
ISBN 0–7710–8689–X

Bettina Bradbury,
Working Families:
Age, Gender, and Daily Survival in
Industrializing Montreal, 1993.
ISBN 0–19–541211–7

Andrée Lévesque,
Making and Breaking the Rules:
Women in Quebec, 1919–1939, 1994.
ISBN 0–7710–5283–9

Cecilia Danysk,
Hired Hands: Labour and the
Development of Prairie Agriculture,
1880–1930, 1995.
ISBN 0–7710–2552–1

Kathryn McPherson,
Bedside Matters: The Transformation
of Canadian Nursing, 1900–1990, 1996.
ISBN 0–8020-8679-9

Edith Burley,
Servants of the Honourable Company: Work, Discipline, and Conflict in the Hudson's Bay Company, 1770–1870, 1997.
ISBN 0–19–541296–6

Mercedes Steedman,
Angels of the Workplace: Women and the Construction of Gender Relations in the Canadian Clothing Industry, 1890–1940, 1997.
ISBN 0–19–54308–3

Angus McLaren and Arlene Tigar McLaren,
The Bedroom and the State: The Changing Practices and Politics of Contraception and Abortion in Canada, 1880–1997, 1997.
ISBN 0–19–541318–0

Kathryn McPherson, Cecilia Morgan, and Nancy M. Forestell, Editors,
Gendered Pasts: Historical Essays in Feminity and Masculinity in Canada, 1999.
ISBN 0–19–541449–7

Gillian Creese,
Contracting Masculinity: Gender, Class, and Race in a White-Collar Union, 1944–1994, 1999.
ISBN 0–19–541454–3

Geoffrey Reaume,
Remembrance of Patients Past: Patient Life at the Toronto Hospital for the Insane, 1870–1940, 2000.
ISBN 0–19–541538–8

Miriam Wright,
A Fishery for Modern Times: The State and the Industrialization of the Newfoundland Fishery. 1934–1968, 2001.
ISBN 0–19–541620–1

Judy Fudge and Eric Tucker,
Labour Before the Law: The Regulation of Workers' Collective Action in Canada, 1900–1948, 2001.
ISBN 0–19–541633–3

Mark Moss,
Manliness and Militarism: Educating Young Boys in Ontario for War, 2001.
ISBN 0–19–541594–9

Joan Sangster,
Regulating Girls and Women: Sexuality, Family, and the Law in Ontario 1920–1960, 2001.
ISBN 0–19–541663–5

Reinhold Kramer and Tom Mitchell,
Walk Towards the Gallows: The Tragedy of Hilda Blake, Hanged 1899, 2002.
ISBN 0–19–541686–4

Mark Kristmanson,
Plateaus of Freedom: Nationality, Culture, and State Security in Canada, 1940–1960, 2002.
ISBN 0–19–541866–2